Metabolism and Nutrition

First and second edition authors:

Sarah Benyon

Jason O'Neale Roach

Third edition author:

Ming Yeong Lim

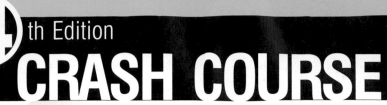

4th Edition
CRASH COURSE

SERIES EDITOR:
Dan Horton-Szar
BSc(Hons) MBBS(Hons) MRCGP
Northgate Medical Practice
Canterbury, Kent, UK

FACULTY ADVISOR:
Marek H. Dominiczak
dr hab med FRCPath FRCP(Glas)
Professor of Clinical Biochemistry and Medical Humanities
University of Glasgow; Consultant Biochemist
NHS Greater Glasgow and Clyde;
Docent in Laboratory Medicine
University of Turku, Finland

Metabolism and Nutrition

Amber Appleton
BSc(Hons) MBBS AKC
Academic Foundation Doctor (FY2), St George's Hospital,
London, UK

Olivia Vanbergen
MBBS MSc MA(Oxon) DIC
FY1 Doctor in Urology, Basingstoke and North Hampshire NHS
Foundation Trust, Basingstoke, UK

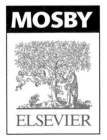

MOSBY

ELSEVIER

Edinburgh London New York Oxford Philadelphia St Louis Sydney Toronto 2013

MOSBY
ELSEVIER

Commissioning Editor: Jeremy Bowes
Development Editor: Sheila Black
Project Manager: Andrew Riley
Designer: Stewart Larking
Icon Illustrations: Geo Parkin
Illustration Manager: Jennifer Rose
Illustrator: Robert Britton and Marion Tasker

First edition 1998
Second edition 2003
Third edition 2007
Fourth edition 2013
  Reprinted 2013

ISBN: 978-0-7234-3626-3

British Library Cataloguing in Publication Data
A catalogue record for this book is available from the British Library

Library of Congress Cataloging in Publication Data
A catalog record for this book is available from the Library of Congress

Notices
Knowledge and best practice in this field are constantly changing. As new research and experience broaden our understanding, changes in research methods, professional practices, or medical treatment may become necessary.

Practitioners and researchers must always rely on their own experience and knowledge in evaluating and using any information, methods, compounds, or experiments described herein. In using such information or methods they should be mindful of their own safety and the safety of others, including parties for whom they have a professional responsibility.

With respect to any drug or pharmaceutical products identified, readers are advised to check the most current information provided (i) on procedures featured or (ii) by the manufacturer of each product to be administered, to verify the recommended dose or formula, the method and duration of administration, and contraindications. It is the responsibility of practitioners, relying on their own experience and knowledge of their patients, to make diagnoses, to determine dosages and the best treatment for each individual patient, and to take all appropriate safety precautions.

To the fullest extent of the law, neither the Publisher nor the authors, contributors, or editors, assume any liability for any injury and/or damage to persons or property as a matter of products liability, negligence or otherwise, or from any use or operation of any methods, products, instructions, or ideas contained in the material herein.

ELSEVIER your source for books, journals and multimedia in the health sciences
www.elsevierhealth.com

Printed in China

Series editor foreword

The *Crash Course* series was first published in 1997 and now, 15 years on, we are still going strong. Medicine never stands still, and the work of keeping this series relevant for today's students is an ongoing process. These fourth editions build on the success of the previous titles and incorporate new and revised material, to keep the series up-to-date with current guidelines for best practice, and recent developments in medical research and pharmacology.

We always listen to feedback from our readers, through focus groups and student reviews of the *Crash Course* titles. For the fourth editions we have completely re-written our self-assessment material to keep up with today's single-best answer and extended matching question formats. The artwork and layout of the titles has also been largely re-worked to make it easier on the eye during long sessions of revision.

Despite fully revising the books with each edition, we hold fast to the principles on which we first developed the series. *Crash Course* will always bring you all the information you need to revise in compact, manageable volumes that integrate basic medical science and clinical practice. The books still maintain the balance between clarity and conciseness, and provide sufficient depth for those aiming at distinction. The authors are medical students and junior doctors who have recent experience of the exams you are now facing, and the accuracy of the material is checked by a team of faculty advisors from across the UK.

I wish you all the best for your future careers!

Dr Dan Horton-Szar

Series Editor

Authors

Being a medical student is great but I know from experience the hard work involved; as a result, I advise using all tools you can find to make learning easier... including this book (as part of a vital survival strategy). This *Crash Course* aims to concisely bridge together core facts you need to know on nutrition and metabolism with relevant clinical scenarios.

The 4th edition of this book has been enhanced structurally and expanded clinically. The figures and text have been condensed, clarified and improved wherever possible. The aim has been to enhance your learning potential, while providing relevant, concisely presented, in-depth 'need to know' knowledge.

Finally, as I strongly believe that nutrition has an important role in life and medical practice, I hope you will find this book not only useful, user-friendly and informative for your exams, but also inspiring and applicable in your future clinical practice.

Amber Appleton
London, 2012

Rewriting the first half of the book completely for the 4th edition has been rewarding, although far more demanding than I had first anticipated. I truly hope the explanations and diagrams I have composed will make some of the more impenetrable aspects of metabolism comprehensible to both medical students and junior doctors.

I found metabolism the most challenging component of my undergraduate study. I hope this has ultimately contributed positively to the development of this book and that my own challenging experiences trying to identify the elements of (often complex) biochemistry topics relevant to medicine have helped to make the pertinent information accessible. My aim has been to enable readers to minimise the studying required to grasp the more esoteric concepts underlying biochemical theory.

Olivia Vanbergen
Basingstoke, 2012

Faculty Advisor

This book covers concisely aspects of biochemistry that are relevant to the medical course. Importantly, it also connects to the everyday clinical practice through the chapters on history taking, signs and symptoms, and laboratory investigations relevant to metabolic disease. Yet the most important thing about the *Crash Course* series is that these books are written by people with recent experience of examinations – on the side of the examined. Thus they are focused on helping the students to prepare for the exam. They also adopt a lighter tone than the conventional textbooks.

The *Crash Course in Biochemistry and Nutrition* is now in its 4th edition, and we have again updated the knowledge and carefully looked at the clarity of explanations. Many illustrations have been redrawn and large parts of the text completely rewritten. There are also changes to the structure of the book such as splitting chapters within the Nutrition section, to make them easier to read and assimilate.

Amber Appleton and Livvi Van Bergen did a superb job. I am sure the readers will benefit from it.

Marek Dominiczak
Glasgow, 2012

Acknowledgements

I would like to thank Dr. Dominiczak for all his patience, support and comments, also many thanks to Sheila Black for her fantastic organization and hard work.

A huge thank you to my parents, sister and brother for their enthusiasm and support.

Lastly, thank you to my wonderful friends for their ongoing encouragement.

Amber Appleton

Enormous thanks to Professor Dominiczak, Sheila Black and Dr Horton-Szar for their guidance and expertise. On a personal level, I wish to thank my family for their continual support and encouragement through the process of developing this book, and indeed my entire life. They are all individually, my inspirations.

Olivia Vanbergen

Figure acknowledgements

Figure 9.6 Reprinted by permission from Macmillan Publishers Ltd. Lowell, Spiegelman 2000 Towards a molecular understanding of adaptive thermogenesis. Nature Insight 404 (6 April).

Figure 12.7 Reproduced by kind permission of Dr R. Clarke (http://www.askdoctorclarke.com).

Figure 12.25 From Longmore, Murray et al. 2008 Oxford Handbook of Clinical Medicine, 7th edn. By permission of Oxford University Press (http://www.oup.com).

Contents

Contents

Introduction to metabolism

Objectives

After reading this chapter you should be able to:
- Define a reaction pathway
- Understand the definitions of catabolic and anabolic pathways
- Appreciate the vital role of enzymes in metabolism
- Understand the basic mechanisms of enzyme regulation
- Describe the different types of membrane transport, and appreciate the difference between active and passive transport
- Describe basic reaction bioenergetics, and understand redox reactions
- Become familiar with the pivotal molecules ATP, acetyl CoA, NAD^+, $NADP^+$ and FAD

INTRODUCTORY CONCEPTS

Metabolism

The term 'metabolism' describes the set of biochemical reactions occurring within a living organism. In humans these reactions allow energy extraction from food and synthesis of molecules required to sustain life. Key points to appreciate are:

- Reactions involve molecular conversion of substrates into products
- In living organisms, reactions never occur in isolation. The product of one reaction goes on to become a substrate in another subsequent reaction
- A set of consecutive reactions is described as a 'pathway'. Components of the pathway are known as 'intermediates' (Fig. 1.1).

In metabolism, pathways tend to be named for their overall role. A pathway with the suffix '-(o)lysis' is a reaction sequence devoted to degrading the molecule hinted at in the prefix. For example, 'glycogenolysis' pathway is a glycogen degradation pathway.

Since most molecules feature in more than one reaction pathway, different pathways tend to 'intersect' where they have a common participant. Therefore, metabolism is analogous to a route-map where the 'roads' representing reaction pathways criss-crossing one another.

Instead of traffic lights and speed humps, reaction pathway 'traffic' is regulated by various biological mechanisms. The rate at which molecules proceed through a pathway is governed by a number of regulatory mechanisms.

The key to understanding metabolism is to appreciate that the details are less important than the overall picture. It is more important that you understand the metabolic role, location and regulation of a pathway than memorize each individual reaction.

Enzymes

Enzymes are specialized, highly specific proteins. Each enzyme mediates a particular biochemical reaction by functioning as a biological catalyst. Without enzymes,

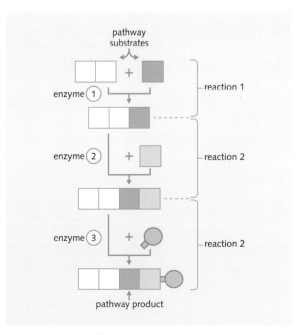

Fig. 1.1 Example of a short metabolic pathway. 1, 2 and 3 represent the enzymes catalysing each reaction.

biological reactions would occur too slowly for cellular viability.

Enzymes operate by temporarily binding to their substrate molecule, imposing molecular modification and finally releasing the altered molecule (the reaction product).

The efficiency of an enzyme at catalysing a reaction determines the rate the reaction proceeds at. In this way, enzyme function is comparable to a 'tuning dial' controlling the reaction's rate. Modulation of enzyme function ('activity') is therefore a major biological regulation strategy. A number of biochemistry terms are used in reference to enzymes, which you must understand the meaning of. These are shown in Fig. 1.2.

Enzyme nomenclature

Enzymes are named according to the reaction they catalyse, so their reaction can often be inferred from the name. Figure 1.3 provides common examples.

Fig. 1.2 Enzyme terms.

Term	Explanation
Active site	This is the region of the enzyme structure which physically binds to the substrate
Conformation	This term describes the 3D structure of a protein (enzyme). Changes in enzymatic conformation impose a change on enzymatic function. Any molecule binding an enzyme is likely to have an effect on the overall 3D structure, i.e. alter the conformation. Conformational changes may be subtle or dramatic and inevitably affect enzyme activity (either positively or negatively)
Activity	This is analogous to 'efficiency' in terms of enzyme performance. The rate of substrate → product conversions an enzyme performs is the enzyme's activity. Activity is affected by enzyme conformation, temperature, pH and the relative concentrations of enzyme and substrate. The presence of inhibitors or activators also influences enzyme activity
Affinity	Affinity describes the avidity of the association between an enzyme and its substrate. An enzyme with low affinity for its substrate binds only weakly, and vice-versa
Inhibitor	Inhibitors may compete with substrate for the active site of an enzyme (competitive inhibitors) or may bind to the enzyme away from the active site (non-competitive inhibitors). However, both types decrease the activity of an enzyme and therefore decrease the rate of a reaction
Activator	Enzyme activators increase the activity of an enzyme and therefore increase the rate of a reaction
Co-enzymes	Some enzymes require the presence of a co-enzyme to perform their catalytic function
Izoenzymes	Occasionally, different tissues of the body possess slightly different enzymes to catalyse the same reaction. These enzymes are referred to as 'isoenzymes', since they both catalyse the same reaction but are not the same enzyme

Fig. 1.3 Enzyme nomenclature.

Enzyme	Reaction catalysed
Kinase	Addition of a phosphate group ('phosphorylation')
Phosphatase	Removal of a phosphate group ('dephosphorylation')
Synthase	Synthesis of the molecule preceding the 'synthase'
Carboxylase	Incorporation of one carbon dioxide molecule into the substrate molecule
Decarboxylase	Removal of one carbon dioxide molecule from the substrate molecule
Dehydrogenase	Oxidation of the substrate via transfer of (one or more) hydride ions (H^-) to an electron acceptor, often NAD^+ or FAD
Isomerase	Rearrangement of existing atoms within the substrate molecule. The product has the same chemical formula as the substrate
Mutase	Transfer of a functional group within the substrate molecule to a new location within the same molecule

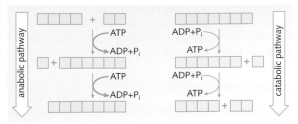

Fig. 1.4 Schematic of a catabolic (right) and anabolic (left) pathway. Enzymes are not shown for simplicity.

Anabolism and catabolism

Metabolic pathways are either anabolic or catabolic. Anabolic pathways generate complex molecules from smaller substrates, whilst catabolic pathways break down complex molecules into smaller products (Fig. 1.4). Metabolism itself is the integration of anabolic and catabolic processes. The balance between the two reflects the energy status of a cell or organism.

Anabolic pathways consume energy. They are synthetic, energy-demanding processes. The suffix of a synthetic pathway is '-genesis,' e.g. glycogenogenesis (glycogen synthesis). Anabolism is analogous to 'construction'; construction requires raw materials and energy.

Catabolic pathways release intrinsic chemical energy from biological molecules. They involve sequential molecular degradation. Catabolic pathways are suffixed with '-lysis', e.g. glycolysis (glucose degradation).

PATHWAY REGULATION

Different pathways have different maximum rates of activity. Since cellular metabolism is defined by the integration of intracellular pathways, every pathway cannot proceed at a rate independent of activity in co-existing pathways. Consider the scenario of synthetic pathways all operating at maximum capacity; products of high-rate pathways would be produced in excess at the expense of products synthesized by lower-rate pathways. Coordination and regulation of pathways are therefore vital aspects of metabolism.

There are three main control mechanisms exploited by cells to regulate metabolic pathways in an integrated and sensitive fashion. These include substrate availability, enzymatic modification and hormonal regulation.

Substrate availability

Pathway rate is limited by availability of the initial pathway substrate. An important mechanism cells use to regulate the quantity of substrate is the integrated control of membrane traffic of substrate molecules. Cells are not freely permeable to the majority of substrate molecules; so varying the supply of substrate by regulating cellular import/export adds an additional level of control.

Allosteric regulation

Cellular regulation of enzyme activity is a key pathway regulation tactic. Metabolic pathways inevitably contain at least one irreversible reaction, known as the rate-limiting reaction. The activity of the rate-limiting enzyme dictates the progression rate of the entire pathway, since an increase in the rate-limiting enzyme's turnover allows the entire pathway to proceed at the new increased rate.

When pondering the concept of 'rate-limiting', consider a study-class of varying ability. The class cannot move onto a new area until all students understand. Thus the least academic student sets the pace of learning for the entire class. This student is analogous to the rate-limiting enzyme in a metabolic pathway. The greatest impact on the class rate of learning can be made by modifications to the rate-limiting student, allowing the rest of the class to move on at a new increased rate.

> **HINTS AND TIPS**
>
> Recall that enzyme activity is analogous to a tuning dial controlling reaction rates. The rate-limiting enzyme may be thought of as a master dial controlling the pathway rate.

'Allosteric regulation' is the modification of an enzyme's activity by modifying the enzyme's structure. A structural modification may be positive (increasing enzyme activity) or negative (decreasing activity). Allosteric modulators are molecules that bind to enzymes, imposing the structural change. Enzyme inhibitors and activators are allosteric modulators. A very common example of allosteric modulation seen in metabolic pathways is 'negative feedback' (Fig. 1.5). This is where a downstream intermediate or final product of a pathway allosterically inhibits an upstream enzyme.

Phosphorylation

An extremely important allosteric modification to understand is 'phosphorylation'. Phosphorylation is the covalent addition of a phosphate moiety (PO_3^{2-}) to a molecule. This moiety is (relatively) large and strongly charged. It therefore has a major impact on the structure (and the activity) of the molecule (e.g. an enzyme) that it covalently binds to.

In the example of glucose, the presence of the phosphate moiety determines whether or not the glucose molecule can cross the cell membrane. When phosphorylated, glucose is rendered unrecognizable to the glucose-specific membrane transport apparatus that allow unphosphorylated glucose to pass across the membrane.

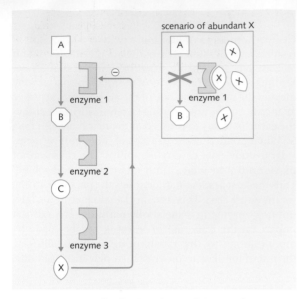

Fig. 1.5 Negative feedback. When pathway product X is abundant (inset), it inhibits the activity of upstream enzyme 1. If enzyme 1 is rate-limiting, this will slow the rate of the entire pathway. This is optimal, since abundant X implies that sustained pathway activity is superfluous to cellular requirements.

In enzymes, the phosphate moiety typically associates with amino acids serine and threonine. Depending on where exactly in the three-dimensional structure of the enzyme these amino acid 'residues' are situated, a phosphorylation can modulate enzyme activity positively or negatively (Fig. 1.6).

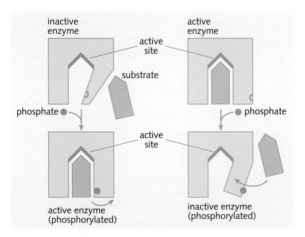

Fig. 1.6 In the scenario on the left, phosphorylation activates the enzyme by imposing a conformational change that exposes the active site (bold). On the right, the converse scenario is shown; phosphorylation inhibits the enzyme by imposing a conformational change that impedes substrate access to the active site.

This tricky concept of phosphorylation as both a positive and a negative allosteric regulator is vital to appreciate, since phosphorylation is the most ubiquitous allosteric modification that modulates enzyme activity.

Hormonal regulation

Hormones are molecular 'messengers', released from endocrine glands into the bloodstream. They may bind to external surface receptors (Fig. 1.7) or intracellular receptors, after diffusing passively across the cell membrane (Fig. 1.8).

Hormones ultimately exert their effect via alteration of the activity of various intracellular enzymes, allowing modulation of pathway activity. Altering the activity of

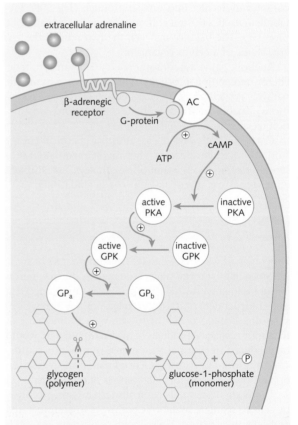

Fig. 1.7 Hormonal regulation: external cell-surface receptor binding. Extracellular adrenaline (epinephrine) binds to the receptor, activating the mobile Gγ subunit. This activates the membrane-embedded adenylate cyclase enzyme (AC), which synthesizes cyclic AMP (cAMP) from ATP. cAMP activates protein kinase A, which in turn activates (via phosphorylation) glycogen phosphorylase kinase. This activates glycogen phosphorylase, which releases glucose-1-phosphate from branched glycogen polymers. Via this intracellular cascade, extracellular adrenaline thus liberates glucose-1-phosphate from the intracellular storage polymer glycogen.

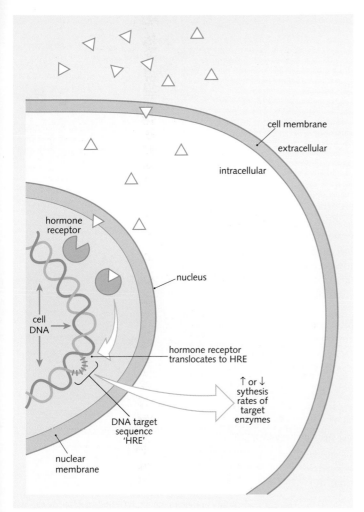

Fig. 1.8 Hormonal regulation: intracellular receptor binding. This example shows steroid hormone diffusing into a cell, accessing the nucleus and binding to its receptor. The activated receptor binds the relevant hormone-response element (HRE), leading to altered synthesis rates of target enzymes.

cell membrane

extracellular

intracellular

hormone receptor

nucleus

cell DNA

hormone receptor translocates to HRE

↑ or ↓ sythesis rates of target enzymes

DNA target sequence 'HRE'

nuclear membrane

either phosphorylation enzymes (kinases) or dephosphorylation enzymes (phosphatases) is a common strategic mechanism.

Some hormones (e.g. steroid hormones) bind to DNA within the cell nucleus at target DNA sequence ('hormone-response elements', HRE), directly influencing the rate of synthesis of enzymes. Increased enzyme availability ('enzyme induction') positively influences the pathway in which the enzyme participates, and vice-versa.

In human metabolism, hormonal control is a mechanism by which intracellular events are appropriately controlled according to the current energy needs of the body. Insulin and glucagon are two important examples.

Insulin is produced by the pancreas in response to a rise in blood [glucose], such as which occurs following absorption of a meal; the 'fed' state. Travelling in the bloodstream, insulin binds to cell membrane receptors. Acting through its receptor, it promotes intracellular anabolic pathway activity (such as lipid synthesis) when the body is in the fed state. Glucagon, conversely, is released into the bloodstream in response to a fall in blood [glucose], which may occur in the 'fasting' state. It promotes various intracellular pathways, for example one which responds to correct low blood [glucose]; gluconeogenesis (de novo glucose synthesis).

Membrane traffic

Cell membranes are composed of a phospholipid bilayer, studded with membrane proteins and cholesterol. They are impermeable to most molecules, necessitating specialized transport structures which function as focal access points. These transport proteins, along with ion channels and membrane receptors, account for the majority of the membrane proteins.

Intracellular metabolism relies on substrates gaining access to the cellular interior. This includes both complex molecules, which can be catabolized to generate

ATP, and simple molecules required for synthesis of complex molecules via anabolic pathways.

Symports ('co-transports') and antiports

Often, transport proteins allow passage of two different ions or molecules. If both travel in the same direction across the membrane, the structure is a symport, or co-transport. If however the direction of travel is opposite for both species, the structure is an antiport (Fig. 1.9).

Active and passive transport

When the direction of travel is from a high concentration to a low concentration, molecules will 'flow' passively in the direction of the gradient. If the membrane is freely permeable to the particular molecule (e.g. steroid hormones), diffusion is passive. If however the membrane is impermeable to a molecule, it must passively flow through a transport protein. This is known as 'facilitated diffusion' (Fig. 1.10).

If the direction of movement is against a concentration gradient, transport is described as 'active'. ATP hydrolysis powers active transport. This may be coupled directly to the transport protein ('primary active transport'), or may occur indirectly ('secondary active transport').

Primary active transport

Primary active transport is where the movement of a molecule or ion against its concentration gradient is coupled directly to ATP hydrolysis. Often the suffix '-ATPase' is used to indicate the primary active nature of transport (Fig. 1.11).

The most ubiquitous example of this is the sodium/potassium ATPase. This antiport imports two K^+ ions into the cell and exports three Na^+ ions out of the cell

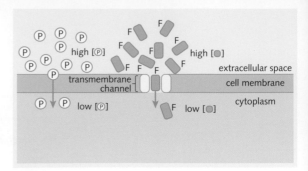

Fig. 1.10 Molecule 'P' is hydrophobic, allowing it to freely diffuse across the membrane (passive diffusion). Molecule 'F' requires a specialized channel to traverse the membrane (facilitated diffusion). Both can only travel down their electrochemical gradients.

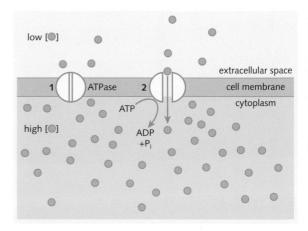

Fig. 1.11 Primary active transport. ATP hydrolysis provides the energy to elicit conformational changes necessary in the ATPase to transport X against concentration gradient.

per cycle (both against their concentration gradients). For every 'cycle' of transport, an ATP is hydrolyzed.

Secondary active transport

Instead of directly coupling with ATP hydrolysis, some transport systems exploit the intrinsic chemical potential energy of a previously accumulated ion gradient to drive the energy-demanding movement of an ion or molecule against its concentration gradient. The 'active' energy-consuming action (the build-up of the driving gradient) has already occurred previously. For example, the high transmembrane $[Na^+]$ gradient (high $[Na^+]$ extracellularly, low intracellularly) is maintained by primary active transport by the Na^+/K^+ ATPase, coupled to ATP hydrolysis (Fig. 1.12). The $[Na^+]$ gradient is allowed to 'run down' across the sodium–glucose symport; Na^+ ions flood into the cell down their concentration gradient, through the sodium–glucose symport.

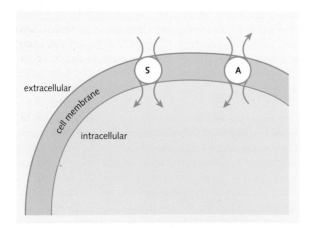

Fig. 1.9 Schematic illustration of a symport (S) and an antiport (A).

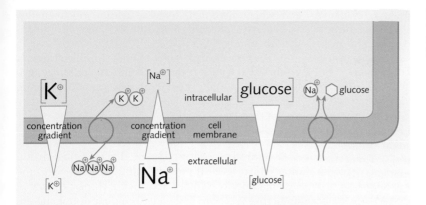

Fig. 1.12 Secondary active transport; the sodium–glucose symport. The Na/K ATPase maintains low intracellular [Na$^+$].

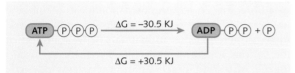

Fig. 1.13 ATP hydrolysis. This reaction permits energetically unfavourable (endergonic) reactions to occur simultaneously, giving an overall exergonic (favourable) reaction which may occur spontaneously. In this way, ATP 'powers' endergonic reactions.

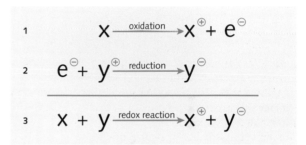

Fig. 1.14 Example redox reaction. X loses an electron, i.e. is oxidized; X is the 'reductant' (1). Y gains an electron, i.e. is reduced; Y is the 'oxidant' (2). These reactions are each 'half-reactions' since together they comprise a complete redox reaction (3).

Bioenergetics

Reactions are described as exergonic (energy-releasing) or endergonic (energy-requiring). Reactions will occur only if they are energetically favourable. Energetic favourability is quantified by the 'Gibbs free energy' (ΔG) of a reaction. Exergonic reactions have negative ΔG values, whilst endergonic reactions have positive ΔG values. A positive ΔG value has the consequence that the reaction cannot occur spontaneously unless coupled to another energy-releasing reaction, such as ATP hydrolysis. An illustrative example is shown in Fig. 1.13.

REDOX REACTIONS

Reduction and oxidation

In biochemistry, **oxidation** of a molecule (Fig. 1.14) means that it has lost an electron(s).

This is usually associated with:

- *Losing* a hydrogen atom or
- *Gaining* an oxygen atom.

The molecule undergoing oxidation is termed the 'reductant'.

Reduction of a molecule (Fig. 1.14) means that it has gained an electron(s).

This is usually associated with:

- *Gaining* a hydrogen atom or
- *Losing* an oxygen atom.

The molecule undergoing reduction is termed the 'oxidant'.

The word 'redox' is a combination of 'reduction' and 'oxidation'. It highlights that neither process can occur without the other. Whenever a reduction occurs, an oxidation must also occur. X and Y in Fig. 1.14 are redox partners. This is always the case; an oxidation reaction must accompany a reduction reaction and vice-versa. Note in Fig. 1.14 that the division into 'half-reactions' is to aid comprehension – electrons never 'float' around freely on their own in reality.

Free radicals

Free radicals are molecules or atoms containing an unpaired electron. Due to this unpaired electron, they are extremely reactive and indiscriminately enter undesirable redox reactions with other biological molecules such as DNA or proteins. This is known as 'oxidative damage', as the free radicals are reduced during the process (acting as oxidants). Free radical damage is thought to contribute to cell damage associated with ageing, inflammation and the complications of diabetes.

Numerous exogenous factors such as radiation, smoking and various chemicals all promote free radical formation. Surprisingly, free radicals are also produced in normal cellular metabolism. However, excessive oxidative damage is prevented by 'antioxidant' compounds such as glutathione and vitamins C and E. These 'scavenge' (mop-up) free radicals, limiting potential damage. Enzymes also exist to inactivate free radicals, e.g. catalase.

HINTS AND TIPS

When referring to oxygen atoms/molecules with an unpaired electron, one uses the term 'reactive oxygen species' (ROS). These include the superoxide anion O_2^-, peroxide (H_2O_2) and hydroxyl, OH^-. All are highly reactive.

KEY PLAYERS

Adenosine triphosphate (ATP): Cellular 'energy currency'

ATP is a molecule composed of an adenine ring attached to C1 of a ribose sugar. A 'tail' of three phosphate groups is attached to the C5 of the ribose (Fig. 1.15). The two phospho anhydride bonds illustrated in Fig. 1.15 are responsible for the high chemical energy content of the molecule. These bonds require much energy to form,

and when disrupted, likewise release much energy. The energy is released on hydrolysis of the phosphoanhydride bonds.

ATP is never stored; it is continuously utilized and resynthesized. It thus cycles between ATP and the hydrolyzed product ADP. The hydrolysis reaction is shown in Fig. 1.13.

Roles of ATP

ATP is critical for nearly all known life forms to function at a cellular level. It powers (indirectly or directly) the vast majority of cellular activities. ATP participates in numerous reactions as a vital phosphate donor and energy source. It also has important roles in intracellular signalling. It is required for synthesis of adenine nucleotides necessary for RNA and DNA synthesis. ATP is responsible for an enormous amount of membrane traffic; all ATP-ase transport systems require uninterrupted supply in order to maintain active transport of the various ions and molecules necessary to sustain the cell. All secondary active transport systems indirectly rely on concentration gradients maintained by primary transport as described earlier.

Sources of ATP

ATP is generated by two principal mechanisms; substrate-level phosphorylation and oxidative phosphorylation. The 'phosphorylation' refers to the phosphorylation of ADP. 'Oxidative' refers to ATP synthesis coupled to oxidation of the reduced intermediates $FADH_2$ and $NADH + H^+$ in the electron transport chain (Chapter 3). 'Substrate-level' refers to all phosphorylation of ATP occurring outside the electron transport chain, for example during glycolysis and the tricarboxylic acid (TCA) cycle.

Fig. 1.15   Molecular structure of ATP.

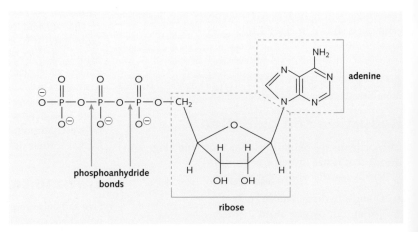

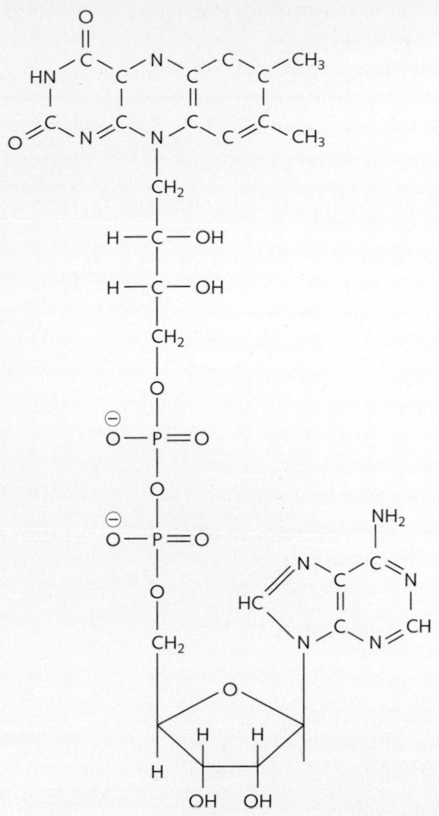

NAD$^+$ and FAD

NAD$^+$ (nicotinamide adenine dinucleotide) and FAD (flavin adenine dinucleotide) are two crucial team players in cellular metabolism. Their structures are given in Fig. 1.16. They usually function as redox partners in substrate oxidation reactions and act as cofactors for the enzymes mediating these reactions.

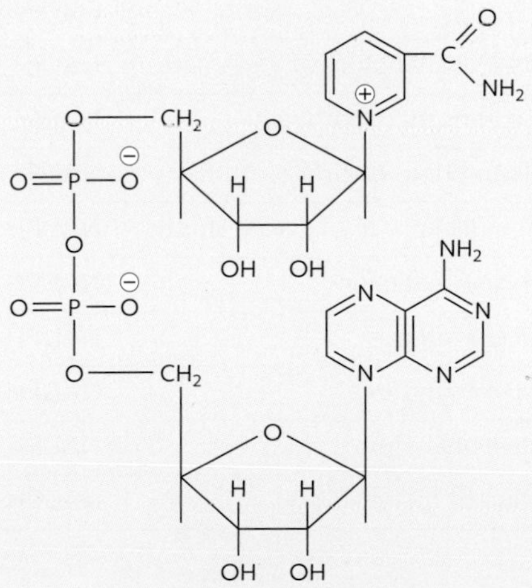

Both NAD$^+$ and FAD function as 'electron carriers', since they readily accept and donate electrons (associated with H atoms) during interaction with other molecules. They participate in catabolic oxidation reactions (as the oxidant, where they are reduced). Once reduced (as 're-duced intermediates'), they each transfer an electron pair (in association with H atoms) to electron transport chain complexes within the mitochondria. This fuels oxidative phosphorylation, in which they act as reductants and are re-oxidized, reforming NAD$^+$ and FAD. Their redox behavior is illustrated in Fig. 1.17, where 'X' represents a substrate molecule undergoing oxidation in any catabolic pathway (such as glycolysis).

Some scientists prefer to write 'NADH$_2$' rather than 'NADH$+$H$^{+'}$ for simplicity. This can cause confusion as it implies that the second hydrogen atom is covalently associated with NADH. The second 'atom' is in fact a hydrogen ion, and since it 'disappears' into solution in cellular media some scientists prefer to completely omit the H$^+$ ion from equations. This also causes confusion as the equation then appears unbalanced. Understand that

flavin adenine
dinucleotide

nicotinamide adenine
dinucleotide

Fig. 1.16 Structures of NAD$^+$ and FAD.

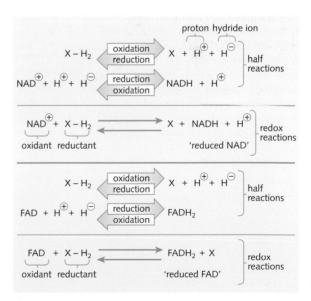

Fig. 1.17 Redox reactions of NAD$^+$ and FAD. Note in both reactions that X is oxidized, whilst NAD$^+$ or FAD are reduced, as seen in the half-equations. The two H atoms are removed from X-H$_2$ in the form of a hydride ion (H$^-$) and a proton (H$^+$ ion).

whenever you see 'NADH' written alone, the writer has assumed you appreciate that a free H^+ ion was also produced. Also, when you see 'NADH$_2$', mentally recognize that this is being used interchangeably with 'NADH+H$^+$'.

Role of NAD$^+$ and FAD in ATP generation

NAD$^+$ and FAD integrate catabolism of all the major energy substrates (carbohydrates, lipids and proteins). Energy released from oxidation of these molecules is used to reduce NAD$^+$ and FAD (by addition of a hydrogen ion (H^+) and a hydride ion (H^-)). This forms the reduced intermediates NADH+H$^+$ and FADH$_2$. NADH+H$^+$ and FADH$_2$ are then re-oxidized when they later transfer their two hydrogen atoms (and associated electrons) to the complexes of the electron transport chain.

NADP$^+$

NADP$^+$ (nicotinamide adenine dinucleotide phosphate) shares a structure with NAD$^+$ but has an additional phosphate group at C2 of the ribose moiety. The structure is shown in Fig. 1.18. The reduced form of NADP$^+$ is NADPH+H$^+$, and this is produced from NADP$^+$ in the pentose phosphate pathway (Chapter 4). NADPH+H$^+$ functions as a redox partner in a number of reductive biosynthesis reactions, including nucleotide, fatty acid and cholesterol synthesis (Fig.1.19). The redox behaviour of NADP+ is shown in Fig. 1.20.

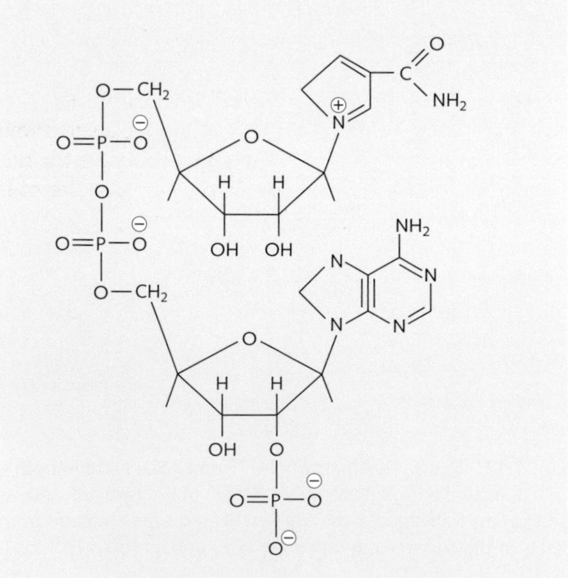

Fig. 1.18 Structure of NADP$^+$.

Fig. 1.19 Metabolic pathways requiring NAD$^+$/NADH+H$^+$ and FAD$^+$/FADH$_2$.

Pathway required	Cofactor
Glycolysis	NAD$^+$
Synthesis of serine and glycine	NAD$^+$
Oxidative deamination of glutamate	NAD$^+$
Catabolism of ethanol	NAD$^+$
Mitochondrial phase of citrate shuttle	NAD$^+$
Mitochondrial phase of malate-aspartate shuttle	NAD$^+$
Ketone oxidation	NAD+
TCA cycle	NAD$^+$, FAD
β-oxidation of fatty acids	NAD$^+$, FAD
Mitochondrial component of the carnitine shuttle	NAD$^+$, FAD
Mitochondrial component of the glycerol-3-phosphate shuttle	FAD
Cytoplasmic component of citrate shuttle	NADH+H$^+$
Cytoplasmic phase of the glycerol-3-phosphate shuttle	NADH+H$^+$
Glycerol synthesis	NADH+H$^+$
Acetoacetate→3-hydroxybutyrate conversion (ketone synthesis)	NADH+H$^+$
Oxidative phosphorylation	NADH+H$^+$, FADH$_2$
Oxidative deamination of glutamate	NADP$^+$
Pentose phosphate pathway	NADP$^+$
Cytoplasm phase of citrate shuttle	NADP$^+$
Mitochondrial phase of citrate shuttle	NADPH+H$^+$
Glutathione reduction	NADPH+H$^+$
Fatty acid synthesis	NADPH+H$^+$
Cholesterol synthesis	NADPH+H$^+$
Reductive animation	NADPH+H$^+$
Reduction of folate	NADPH+H$^+$

Acetyl CoA

The structure of **acetyl CoA** consists of an acetyl group (CH$_3$COO$^-$) covalently linked to coenzyme A (CoA). The functional group of CoA is a thiol group ($-$SH), and to highlight this CoA is sometimes written as CoA-SH. The structure is shown in Fig. 1.21.

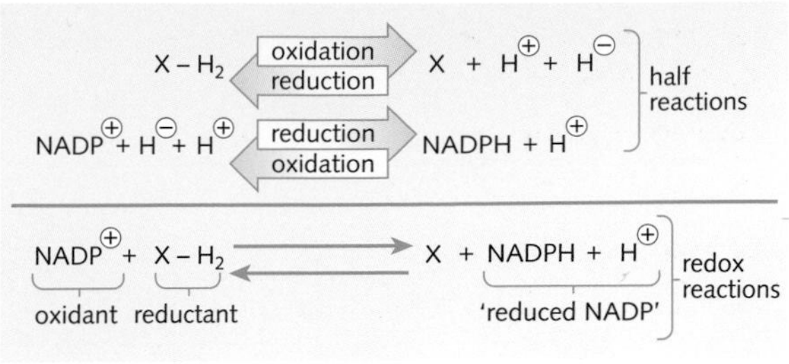

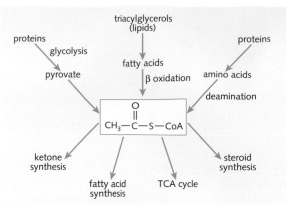

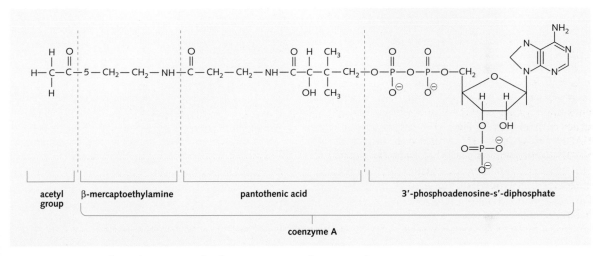

Fig. 1.20 Redox reaction of NADP$^+$. Note in this reaction that X is oxidized, and NADP+reduced. The two H atoms are removed from X-H$_2$ in the form of a hydride ion (H$^-$) and a proton (H$^+$ ion).

Fig. 1.22 Central role in metabolism of acetyl CoA. Dotted lines indicate anabolic pathways.

Fig. 1.21 Structure of acetyl CoA. Note the three components of coenzyme A.

This molecule is central to metabolism (Fig. 1.22). Most cellular catabolic pathways (including carbohydrate, fat and protein) eventually lead to acetyl CoA. Oxidation of the acetyl residue of acetyl CoA in the TCA cycle (Chapter 2) generates ATP directly (substrate-level phosphorylation) and indirectly (via oxidative phosphorylation of TCA cycle-generated FADH$_2$ and NADH+H$^+$). It is also a substrate for numerous synthetic pathways, including fats, steroids and ketones.

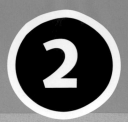
After reading this chapter you should be able to:

- Recognize the TCA cycle reactions
- Describe the energy-generation role of the cycle
- Recognize the biosynthetic significance of the cycle
- Appreciate how intermediates from different pathways enter the cycle
- Understand how the TCA cycle is regulated
- Describe the concept of an anaplerotic reaction/pathway

THE TRICARBOXYLIC ACID (TCA) CYCLE

The TCA cycle (aka the 'Krebs cycle' or the 'citric acid' cycle) is a cyclical reaction sequence (Fig. 2.1). Sequential oxidation reactions generate metabolic energy.

Key points to note are:

- The cycle occurs in the **mitochondrial matrix** of all mitochondria-containing cells

- It requires the presence of oxygen, i.e. is **aerobic**
- There are **eight** reactions in the cycle
- The cycle 'kicks off' by accepting an **acetyl CoA** molecule; this combines with an **oxaloacetate** (generated by a previous 'turn' of the cycle) to form **citrate**
- The TCA cycle generates a molecule of **GTP** directly by substrate-level phosphorylation during reaction 5. This is turn generates further ATP
- The TCA cycle generates **ATP** indirectly via production of the high energy intermediates **FADH₂** and $NADH + H^+$ in reactions 3, 4, 6 and 8.

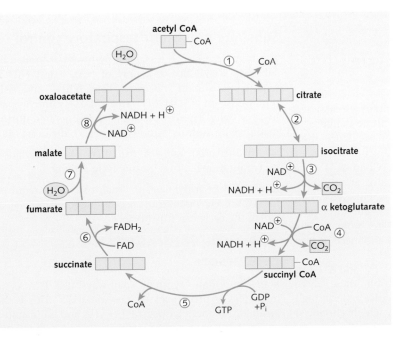

Fig. 2.1 The TCA cycle. 1=citrate synthase, 2=aconitase, 3=isocitrate dehydrogenase, 4=α-ketoglutarate dehydrogenase, 5=succinyl CoA synthetase, 6=succinate dehydrogenase, 7=fumarase, 8=malate dehydrogenase. Note each square represents a carbon atom.

Reactions 1, 3 and 4 are irreversible, rate-limiting reactions. They form the main regulation points for the cycle.

Role in metabolism

Since acetyl CoA is produced from catabolism of carbohydrates, fatty acids and amino acids (the three main dietary sources of energy), the TCA cycle is pivotal in metabolism. It functions as a common pathway for energy generation. Cycle intermediates also function as 'raw materials' for numerous anabolic (synthetic) pathways. As the TCA cycle possesses both catabolic (breakdown of energy-rich molecules to release energy) and anabolic (synthetic) elements, it is known as an 'amphibolic' pathway.

Energy yield of the TCA cycle

GTP is directly generated by substrate-level phosphorylation (reaction 5). ATP, however, is generated indirectly, via production of the reducing equivalents $FADH_2$ and $NADH + H^+$.

One 'turn' of the TCA cycle generates one molecule of $FADH_2$ and three $NADH + H^+$. $FADH_2$ and $NADH + H^+$ equate to approximately 1.5 and 2.5 ATP respectively (Chapter 3). The single GTP generated in reaction 5 equates to 1 ATP. Thus, 10 ATP are generated (per acetyl CoA molecule) by one complete 'turn' of the cycle:

$$Acetyl\ CoA + 2\ H_2O + 3\ NAD^+ + FAD + GDP + P_i$$
$$\rightarrow 2\ CO_2 + 3\ (NADH + H^+) + FADH_2 + GTP + CoA$$

Regulation of the TCA cycle

Allosteric regulation

The three irreversible reactions (1, 3 and 4) are catalysed by the enzymes citrate synthase, isocitrate dehydrogenase and α-ketoglutarate dehydrogenase. Since their reactions are rate-limiting, modulating the activity of these enzymes controls cycle activity (Chapter 1).

These enzymes are all allosterically activated by calcium ions. Intracellular $[Ca^{2+}]$ is elevated when energy-demanding processes are active. The three rate-limiting enzymes of the cycle operate more rapidly when $[Ca^{2+}]$ is high. Cycle activity is enhanced, generating more metabolic energy (Fig. 2.2).

Conversely, cycle products $NADH + H^+$ and ATP (an indirect product) allosterically inhibit these three enzymes. Abundance of these molecules reflects high cellular energy level, i.e. contexts in which enhanced TCA cycle activity is not required.

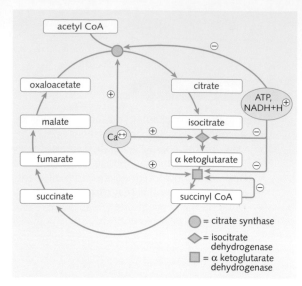

Fig. 2.2 TCA cycle regulation. Note that the figure only illustrates the key regulatory enzymes.

HINTS AND TIPS

High intracellular $[Ca^{2+}]$ correlates with ATP-demanding cellular activities. This is because Ca^{2+} ions are chemical 'signals' initiating a vast number of key biochemical processes. Examples include muscle contraction, cell division and neurotransmitter release (exocytosis). This explains why Ca^{2+} has such a powerful influence on cellular energy homeostasis.

Substrate provision/'respiratory control'

The TCA cycle, like all metabolic pathways, is limited by substrate availability. A supply of NAD^+ and FAD is required to sustain the cycle. Thus NAD^+ and FAD renewal (from $NADH + H^+$ and $FADH_2$) controls pathway activity. These molecules are regenerated during oxidative phosphorylation (Chapter 3), meaning that:

- An increased rate of oxidative phosphorylation (respiration) allows greater cycle activity.

Availability of acetyl CoA, the major substrate required for TCA cycle operation, also influences the rate at which the cycle can function.

TCA cycle intermediates as precursors

Many important synthetic pathways use TCA cycle molecules as precursors, or 'raw materials'. This is the synthetic (anabolic) aspect of the cycle, and is illustrated in Fig. 2.3. Key examples include:

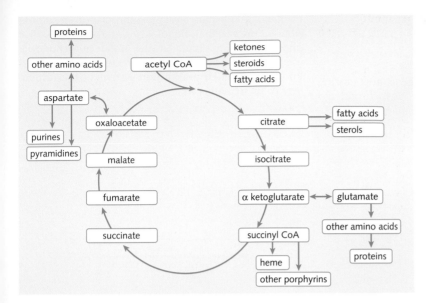

Fig. 2.3 Biosynthetic utility of TCA cycle intermediates.

- Gluconeogenesis (glucose production) utilizes oxaloacetate (Chapter 4)
- Fatty acids and cholesterol are synthesized using acetyl CoA, which may be derived from citrate (Chapter 5)
- Amino acid synthesis uses both oxaloacetate and α-ketoglutarate (Chapter 6)
- Porphyrin synthesis requires succinyl CoA (Chapter 7).

Anaplerotic reactions

When TCA cycle molecules are recruited for use in synthetic pathways, they must be replenished so the cycle can continue to operate (Fig. 2.4). Pathways and reactions that replenish pathway molecules are known as 'anaplerotic'. For example, carboxylation of pyruvate forming oxaloacetate replenishes oxaloacetate withdrawn from the cycle to participate in nucleotide synthesis or gluconeogenesis.

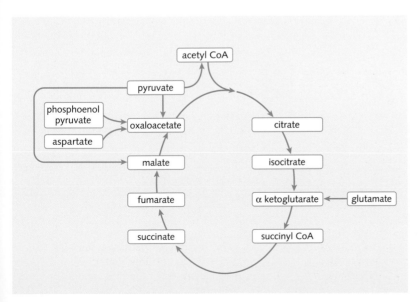

Fig. 2.4 Anaplerotic reactions of the TCA cycle.

TCA-generated reducing equivalents enter the electron transport system

The key role of the TCA cycle is that it generates reducing equivalents ($FADH_2$ and $NADH + H^+$) which undergo oxidative phosphorylation. Oxidative phosphorylation (rather than substrate-level phosphorylation) is responsible for the vast majority of ATP generation. Oxidative phosphorylation occurs at the inner mitochondrial membrane, which is studded with an array of proteins known as the electron transport system, or the 'respiratory chain' (Chapter 3).

Energy metabolism II: ATP generation

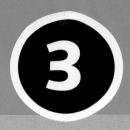

3

Objectives

After reading this chapter you should be able to:
- Describe the process of oxidative phosphorylation
- Identify the components of the electron transport chain
- Appreciate the role of NADH+H$^+$ and FADH$_2$
- Understand how electron transfer provides energy for generating the proton gradient
- Understand how discharge of the proton gradient provides energy for ATP synthesis
- Describe the glycerate-3-phosphate and the malate-aspartate shuttles
- Define the significance of uncoupling
- Understand substrate-level phosphorylation

ATP GENERATION

ATP molecules are all created by phosphorylation of ADP. This occurs by either 'substrate-level' phosphorylation or 'oxidative' phosphorylation.

SUBSTRATE-LEVEL PHOSPHORYLATION

This describes the reaction where ATP (or GTP) is synthesized from ADP (or GDP) by transfer of a phosphoryl group (PO_3^{2-}). The phosphoryl group is derived from a substrate and is transferred to ADP or GDP (Fig. 3.1). Substrate-level phosphorylation is an endergonic reaction, and is therefore always accompanied by an exergonic reaction, which provides the energy required to drive the reaction forward.

Substrate-level phosphorylation does not require oxygen, and thus is vital for energy generation in anaerobic environments, such as rapidly contracting skeletal muscle. This form of ATP generation is seen during glycolysis (reactions 7 and 10), the TCA cycle (reaction 5) and creatine kinase-mediated hydrolysis of phosphocreatine in muscle cells.

OXIDATIVE PHOSPHORYLATION

This type of ATP production does require oxygen, and occurs only at the **inner mitochondrial membrane** (IMM). The energy required to perform the phosphorylation reaction is derived from the electron pairs associated with NADH+H$^+$ and FADH$_2$, which are in turn generated during catabolism of high-energy molecules such as carbohydrates, fatty acids and amino acids. The electron pairs are transferred from NADH+H$^+$ and FADH$_2$, along with pairs of H$^+$ ions, to the acceptor 'complexes' of the **electron transport chain** (ETC). The electrons then transfer between the ETC complexes.

Every electron pair transfer between ETC complexes results in both:

- The protein complex that donates the electrons being oxidized
- The protein complex that receives the electrons being reduced.

Electron movement in an electronegative direction releases energy. This is used to generate a chemical gradient of hydrogen ions (protons) across the IMM, with higher [H$^+$] in the intermembrane space than the mitochondrial matrix. This sequential oxidation of ETC complexes is the 'oxidative' component of 'oxidative phosphorylation'.

The exergonic (energy-releasing) discharge of protons back into the mitochondrial matrix through the ATP synthase pore (also located in the IMM) provides the energy required for formation of the phosphoanhydride bond between P$_i$ and ADP, forming ATP. This is the 'phosphorylation' part of the 'oxidative phosphorylation'.

The electron transport chain (ETC)

The ETC consists of four protein structures embedded in the IMM. Each contains structural features that allow complexes to readily accept and release electrons. Each

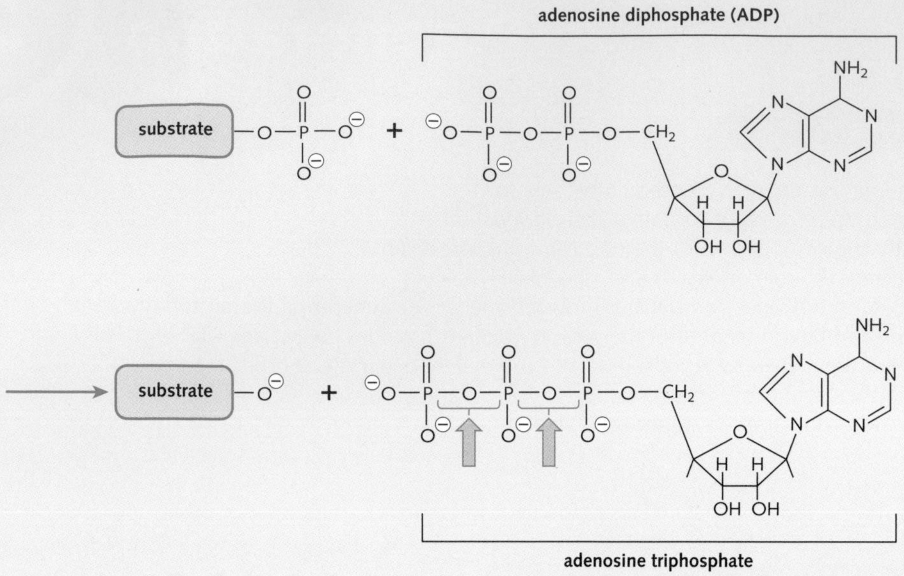

Fig. 3.1 Substrate-level phosphorylation. No oxygen is involved in this reaction. Note the two high-energy phosphoanhydride bonds in ATP are illustrated with arrows.

structure or 'complex' is numbered in order of increasing electron affinity and redox potential.

Two mobile transfer proteins also participate in oxidative phosphorylation. Coenzyme Q (aka ubiquinone) ferries two e^- and two H^+ between complexes I and III and between complexes II and III. Cytochrome c transfers the electron and proton pair from complex III to complex IV (Fig. 3.2).

Electron pairs: where do they come from?

Electron pairs arrive at the ETC incorporated within NADH+H^+ and FADH$_2$. NADH+H^+ transfers two e^- (and two H^+) to complex I and FADH$_2$ transfers an e^- pair (and a H^+ pair) to complex II. NADH+H^+ and FADH$_2$ are thus converted back to NAD$^+$ and FAD. In receiving the e^- and H^+ ion pairs, each complex is itself reduced.

Electron pair transfer between ETC complexes

Having accepted an e^- pair (and a H^+ pair), complexes then switch function, acting as e^- donors to the following unit of the ETC. Complex III receives electron and proton pairs from either complex I or II via coenzyme Q, and complex IV receives electron and proton pairs from complex III via cytochrome c. The final

transfer occurs when complex IV transfers both the electron pair and the proton pair to molecular oxygen (O_2). This requirement for oxygen as the terminal electron pair acceptor explains why the process of oxidative phosphorylation requires oxygen (Fig. 3.3).

Generation of the proton gradient

The significance of electron transfer between complexes of the ETC is that it is highly exergonic. Electron transfer releases energy. This energy is harnessed by complexes I, III and IV and utilized to transfer ('pump') protons from the mitochondrial matrix into the intermembrane space (across the IMM). This transfer is endergonic (requires energy), as this direction is against a H^+ (proton) concentration gradient. In this way, receipt of the e^- pairs is like an 'energy delivery', providing complexes with the energy needed to transport protons across the IMM against their concentration gradient.

Different ATP generation capacity of NADH+H^+ and FADH$_2$

Note that electron pairs originating from FADH$_2$ arrive at complex II, bypassing complex I. Oxidation of FADH$_2$ leads to proton pumping at complexes III and IV, compared to NADH+H^+ oxidation, which leads to proton pumping at complexes I, III and IV. This

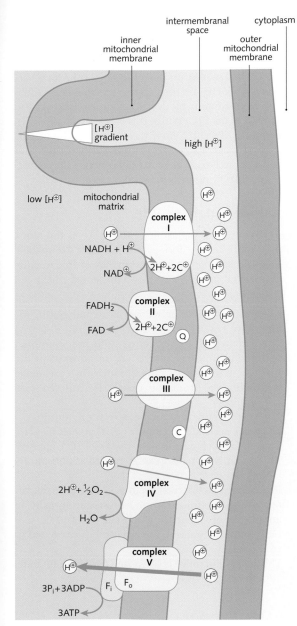

Fig. 3.2 Schematic of oxidative phosphorylation. Note the direction of the proton concentration gradient. C = cytochrome C, Q = coenzyme Q.

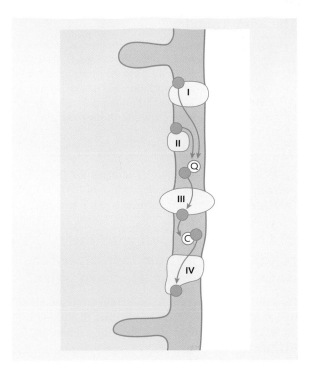

Fig. 3.3 Pathway of electron and hydrogen ion transfer. Note that the dark circle represents the transferred electron and proton pair. C = cytochrome C, Q = coenzyme Q.

a proton gradient is formed by the action of complexes I, III and IV, the intrinsic chemical energy contained within the gradient (the 'proton-motive force') can be utilized by ATP synthase.

> **HINTS AND TIPS**
>
> Exploiting a chemical gradient as a source of chemical energy to power an energy-demanding biological process, is conceptually similar to secondary active transport (Chapter 1).

ATP synthase (complex V)

ATP synthase, also located at the IMM, binds ADP and P_i and catalyses the bond formation between the two species, generating ATP. The enzyme contains an intrinsic pore, connecting the mitochondrial matrix with the intermembrane space. Protons travel down their concentration gradient; however in doing so they impose a transient structural alteration in the enzyme protein. This results in the ADP and P_i substrates being forced into close contact by ATP synthase, so that the formation of the phosphoanhydride bond becomes energetically favourable.

accounts for why 1 $FADH_2$ leads to generation of less ATP per molecule than 1 $NADH+H^+$ (~ 1.5 ATP and ~ 2.5 ATP respectively).

ATP synthesis

Formation of the second phosphoanhydride bond of ATP (from ADP and P_i) is highly endergonic. Once

The term 'coupling'

ATP synthesis occurring in this manner is intimately associated with discharge of the proton gradient. Generation of which is powered by electron transfer between ETC complexes. This association is termed 'coupling'; ATP synthesis is coupled with proton gradient discharge. This is often referred to as 'chemiosmotic coupling'.

Sources of NADH+H$^+$ and FADH$_2$

Catabolism of carbohydrates, fatty acids and the carbon skeletons of amino acids, all produce NADH+H$^+$ and FADH$_2$ from their redox partners NAD + and FAD.

ETC complexes: why do they readily accept and then transfer onward incoming electron pairs?

For a protein to function as an electron acceptor and donor, it must contain structural features that allow it to do so. Specific features present in the proteins of the ETC are shown in Fig. 3.4.

Transfer of NADH+H$^+$: from cytoplasm to the mitochondria

Both β-oxidation of fatty acids and the TCA cycle occur in the mitochondrial matrix. NADH+H$^+$ produced by these pathways is therefore already in the appropriate location for accessing the ETC and participate in oxidative phosphorylation. However, NADH+H$^+$ is also generated in cell cytoplasm by glycolysis. The mitochondria are impermeable to NADH+H$^+$. So how does NADH+H$^+$ gain access to the mitochondrial interior? There are two ways, described below.

Glycerol-3-phosphate shuttle

This mechanism recruits cytoplasmic NADH+H$^+$ into a redox reaction with dihydroxyacetone-phosphate (DHAP). NADH+H$^+$ is oxidized to NAD$^+$ whilst DHAP is reduced to glycerol-3-phosphate (G3P). G3P can diffuse across the outer mitochondrial membrane (OMM) and into the intermembrane space. Here, G3P is re-oxidized

back to DHAP. This is mediated by glycerol-3-phosphate dehydrogenase, an enzyme spanning the IMM. The relevance of this second redox reaction is that the redox partner for the second oxidation is FAD, located in the mitochondrial matrix, on the other side of the IMM. Reduced FAD (FADH$_2$) is then able to participate in oxidative phosphorylation by donating the electron pair to complex II of the ETC. Whilst this is not a scenario identical to an NADH+H$^+$ itself travelling into the matrix, there is no longer an NADH+H$^+$ in the cytoplasm and there is a reduced equivalent in a site where it may participate in oxidative phosphorylation.

Malate-aspartate shuttle

This system uses cytoplasmic NADH+H$^+$ as the redox partner in the reduction of oxaloacetate to malate. This shuttle exploits the fact that malate is able to cross mitochondrial membranes. It is represented in Fig. 3.5 and described here:

* Cytoplasmic malate dehydrogenase catalyses the oxidation of NADH+H$^+$ to NAD$^+$
* The malate then travels across both mitochondrial membranes into the matrix via an antiport in the inner mitochondrial membrane; in exchange, α-ketoglutarate from the matrix is extruded into the cytoplasm
* Once in the matrix, the reaction reverses, re-forming oxaloacetate and reducing matrix NAD$^+$ to NADH+H$^+$. Thus the reducing equivalent (NADH+H$^+$) 'appears' in the matrix to participate in oxidative phosphorylation
* Regenerated oxaloacetate is then converted to aspartate, which is extruded from the mitochondria by an antiport in exchange for glutamate
* Once in the cytoplasm, the aspartate is converted to oxaloacetate
* The matrix glutamate is converted to α-ketoglutarate, completing the cycle.

NAD$^+$ regeneration

Activity of malate-aspartate or glycerol-3-phosphate shuttles ensures that cytoplasmic NAD$^+$ is continuously available. Shuttle activity is driven by oxidative

Fig. 3.4	Structural features of proteins of the electron transport chain.
Feature	**Description**
Iron–sulphur centres	Iron ions are complexed with cysteine residue, sulphur atoms or inorganic sulphide groups. Iron in this configuration can undergo oxidation and reduction by cycling between the ferric and ferrous states
Haem groups	These also contain an iron ion associated with four nitrogen atoms. The iron ion likewise can undergo oxidation and reduction by cycling between the ferric and ferrous states

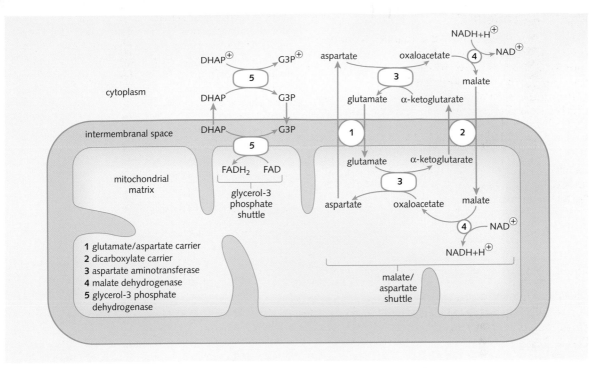

Fig. 3.5 The glycerol-3-phosphate and malate-aspartate shuttles. DHAP = dihydroxyacetone phosphate, G3P = glycerol phosphate. Note that there are both mitochondrial and cytoplasmic isoforms of the enzymes aspartate aminotransferase (3) and glycerol-3-phosphate dehydrogenase (5).

phosphorylation, since this is the process that consumes the reducing equivalents in the mitochondrial matrix. Thus sustained oxidative phosphorylation ensures the maintenance of an available pool of NAD^+ in the cytoplasm.

Under anaerobic conditions, when oxidative phosphorylation cannot occur, NAD + is regenerated from $NADH+H^+$ by a different mechanism. It acts as a redox partner in the reduction reaction pyruvate → lactate.

Uncoupling

Recall that 'coupling' describes the simultaneous discharging of the H^+ gradient with ATP synthesis. 'Uncoupling' describes the scenario where the permeability of the IMM to H^+ ions is increased. H^+ ions are then able to discharge back into the matrix without travelling through the ATP synthase pore. This route of return cannot generate ATP; instead, the energy is dissipated as heat.

This uncouples ATP synthesis from discharge of the H^+ gradient. Any molecule that increases permeability of the IMM to H^+ ions is capable of uncoupling. 2,4-Ninitrophenol (2,4-DNP) and FCCP (carbonyl cyanide p-(trifluoromethoxy)-phenyl hydrazone) uncouple mitochondria, short-circuiting the H + gradient accumulated by the ETC and blockading the main source of ATP production.

Uncoupling is only physiologically advantageous if heat is required, for example, in hairless newborn mammals. Newborn babies possess specialized heat-generating cells, termed 'brown fat' cells. These contain large numbers of uncoupled mitochondria, which are devoted to heat production. The mitochondria are uncoupled by the presence of proteins in the IMM that contain a proton pore, allowing the accumulated H^+ gradient to discharge. These proteins are known as 'uncoupling proteins' or UCPs.

Carbohydrate metabolism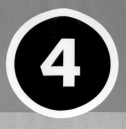

CARBOHYDRATES: A DEFINITION

A carbohydrate (aka 'saccharide') is a molecule containing only carbon, hydrogen and oxygen. The ratio of these atoms is always C:H:O = 1:2:1. The basic example of a carbohydrate 'unit' is the 6-carbon 'monosaccharide' such as glucose, fructose (Fig. 4.1) or galactose. Disaccharides comprise two linked monosaccharides. Sucrose (glucose + fructose) and lactose (glucose + galactose) are shown in Fig. 4.1. The more complex 'polysaccharides' consist of numerous monosaccharide units linked by glycosidic bonds. A physiological example is glycogen (Fig. 4.2).

In biochemistry, metabolism of carbohydrates includes glycolysis, glycogen synthesis and degradation,

Fig. 4.1 Monosaccharides; formula $C_x(H_2O)_y$. Glucose and fructose are shown. The disaccharides lactose and sucrose are also shown.

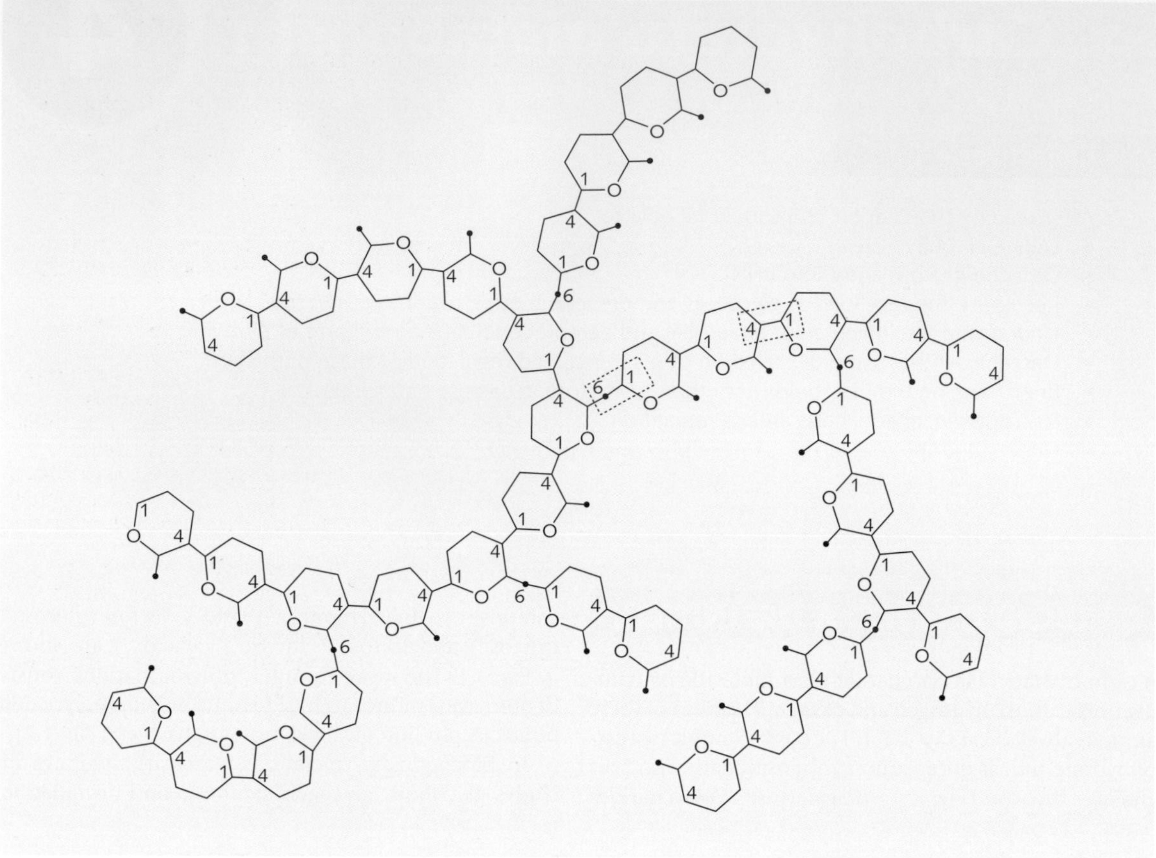

Fig. 4.2 Macroscopic structure of glycogen. Hexagons represent glucose monomers. Note that both (1–4) and (1–6) carbon-to-carbon bonds are present (examples shown within the dotted boxes). These bonds are detailed in Fig. 4.12.

gluconeogenesis and the pentose phosphate pathway. These will be discussed in turn.

HINTS AND TIPS

Six-carbon carbohydrates are also known as 'hexose' sugars. 'Pentose' sugars are five-carbon carbohydrates. 'Triose' sugars are three-carbon carbohydrates.

Glucose entry into cells

Glucose (or its derivatives, such as glucose-6-phosphate) participates in all the carbohydrate pathways of metabolism. As phospholipid bilayers are impermeable to polar molecules, glucose cannot directly diffuse across plasma cell membranes. To allow glucose to move into and out of cells, specialized transporter structures span the membranes. Regulating transporter function therefore allows integrated regulation of glucose traffic across the cell membrane.

Facilitated diffusion

In certain environments, glucose is a greater extracellularly than intracellularly. The concentration gradient is thus favourable for glucose to passively enter the cell. However, a route is required to traverse the phospholipid bilayer. This is provided by the GLUT facilitated diffusion transporters. The different characteristics of the most important subtypes are shown in Fig. 4.3.

Secondary active transport

When the extracellular glucose is lower than the intracellular glucose, glucose entry is coupled to sodium transport, via the sodium–glucose symport (Chapter 1). This allows the Na^+ gradient to 'power' the energy-demanding import of glucose against its concentration gradient. Such a system operates, for instance, in the gastrointestinal tract, allowing the absorption of glucose.

Subtype	Transports	Expression	Insulin dependence	Affinity	Role
GLUT 1	Glucose	Erythrocytes (adult) Blood–brain barrier endothelia (adult) Astrocyte glia (adult) Widespread (fetus)	Independent	High	Responsible for the basal uptake of glucose that is necessary to sustain cellular viability Delivers glucose from the circulation into the brain
GLUT 2	Glucose, fructose, galactose	Renal tubular cells Pancreatic beta cells Hepatocytes Enterocytes	Independent	Low	Allows absorption of digested saccharides from gut lumen to intestinal cells The low-affinity high-capacity characteristics allow the intracellular glucose of pancreatic beta 'sensor' cells to closely resemble plasma glucose, allowing for regulation of pancreatic glucose-stimulated insulin secretion This is also the main transporter for hepatic glucose absorption
GLUT 3	Glucose	Neurons Placental cells	Independent	High	Allows glucose entry into neuronal and placental tissue
GLUT 4	Glucose	Cardiac and skeletal muscle Adipose tissue	Expression of GLUT 4 is proportional to insulin levels. This accounts for increased uptake of glucose from plasma in the presence of insulin	High	Mediates blood glucose regulation by allowing insulin to control the extent of glucose uptake from the circulation
GLUT 5	Fructose	Skeletal muscle Enterocytes Spermatozoa Testis Kidney	Independent	High	Imports fructose

Fig. 4.3 Glucose transporters. Note that 'high-affinity' transporters allow more rapid glucose traffic across membranes

GLYCOLYSIS

Overview

Glycolysis is catabolism of glucose and the equation is as follows ($CH_3COCOOH$ is the formula of pyruvate):

$$C_6H_{12}O_6 + 2NAD^+ + 2ADP + HPO_4{}^{2-}$$
$$\rightarrow CH_3COCOOH + 2\ NADH+H^+ + 2\ ATP$$

Glycolysis occurs in the cytoplasm of all cells. It can occur in both aerobic and anaerobic environments. In ten reactions, one glucose molecule is sequentially oxidized, ultimately forming two molecules of pyruvate (Fig. 4.4A).

During glycolysis, two ATP are generated via substrate-level phosphorylation (in fact, four are generated, but two are consumed). Two $NADH+H^+$ are also generated, each representing $\sim$2.5 ATP. Thus the ATP yield of glycolysis is 7 ATP per glucose molecule oxidized:

$$2\ ATP + 2\ (\sim 2.5\ ATP)\ =\ 7\ ATP$$

Much of the pyruvate generated in glycolysis is decarboxylated, forming acetyl CoA. Recall that acetyl CoA may enter the TCA cycle for further oxidation (Chapter 2), generating further ATP and $NADH+H^+$. Alternatively it may participate in a number of synthetic pathways.

Glycolysis: the reaction pathway

'Energy investment' phase

- Reaction 1: Glucose is phosphorylated, forming glucose-6-phosphate (Glc-6-P). ATP donates the phosphoryl group

Fig. 4.4A Glycolysis. Enzymes shown in bold represent the regulation points of the pathway

Reaction	Enzyme	Type of reaction	Reaction equation	ΔG_O
1	**Hexokinase** (HK) (or **Glucokinase** in pancreatic islet cells and liver cells)	Phosphorylation	Glucose + ATP → Glucose-6-phosphate + ADP + H$^+$	− 16.7 kJ/mol
2	Phospho glucoisomerase	Isomerization	Glucose-6-phosphate → Fructose-6-phosphate	+ 1.7 kJ/mol
3	**Phosphofructokinase**	Phosphorylation	Fructose-6-phosphate + ATP → Fructose-1,6-bisphosphate + ADP + H$^+$	− 18.5 kJ/mol
4	Aldolase	Cleavage	Fructose-1,6-bisphosphate → dihydroxyacetone phosphate + glyceraldehyde-3-phosphate	+ 28 kJ/mol
5	Triose phosphate isomerase	Isomerisation (ketose→aldose)	Dihydroxyacetone phosphate → glyceraldehyde-3-phosphate	+ 7.6 kJ/mol
6	Glyceraldehyde-3-phosphate dehydrogenase	Oxidation and phosphorylation	Glyceraldehyde-3-phosphate + NAD$^+$ + HPO$_4^{2-}$ → 1,3-bisphosphoglycerate + NADH + H$^+$	+ 6.3 kJ/mol
7	Phosphoglycerate kinase	Substrate-level phosphorylation	1,3-bisphosphoglycerate + ADP → ATP + 3-phosphoglycerate	− 18.8 kJ/mol
8	Phosphoglycerate mutase	Isomerization	3-phosphoglycerate → 2-phosphoglycerate	+ 4.4 kJ/mol
9	Enolase	Dehydration	2-phosphoglycerate → phosphoenolpyruvate + H$_2$O	+ 1.7 kJ/mol
10	**Pyruvate kinase**	Substrate-level phosphorylation	Phosphoenolpyruvate + ADP → Pyruvate + ATP	− 31.4 kJ/mol

- Reaction 2: Glc-6-P isomerizes, forming fructose-6-phosphate (Fru-6-P)
- Reaction 3: Fru-6-P is phosphorylated, generating fructose-1,6-bisphosphate (Fru-1,6-BP). Again, ATP is the phosphoryl donor
- Reaction 4: Fru-1,6-BP is split into two three-carbon molecules, glyceraldehyde-3-phosphate (GAP) and dihydroxyacetone phosphate (DHAP)
- Reaction 5: DHAP isomerizes, producing GAP.

'Energy generation' phase

HINTS AND TIPS

It is important to understand that the following glycolysis reactions occur in duplicate, since the original six-carbon glucose molecule is split into two three-carbon molecules, each of which progresses through reactions 6–10.

- Reaction 6: The two three-carbon GAP molecules undergo dehydrogenation and phosphorylation to form 1,3-bisphosphoglycerate (1,3-BPG). NAD$^+$ is reduced to NADH + H$^+$. Note that two NADH + H$^+$ are actually produced, one per GAP molecule
- Reaction 7: 1,3-BPG donates a phosphate group to ADP, forming 3-phosphoglycerate (3-PG) and ATP. This is a substrate-level phosphorylation
- Reaction 8: 3-PG is isomerized; the phosphate group is transferred from the 3rd to the 2nd carbon atom, forming 2-phosphoglycerate (2-PG)
- Reaction 9: 2-PG is dehydrated, forming phospho-enolpyruvate (PEP)
- Reaction 10: The final step of glycolysis is transfer of the phosphoryl group from PEP to ADP. This generates pyruvate and ATP (the second substrate-level phosphorylation) (Fig. 4.4B).

Glycolytic intermediates as biosynthetic precursors

The pathway also acts as an essential source of intermediates for other pathways, which therefore rely on glycolysis for substrate provision. These include:

- The TCA cycle (Chapter 2)
- The pentose phosphate pathway (PPP)

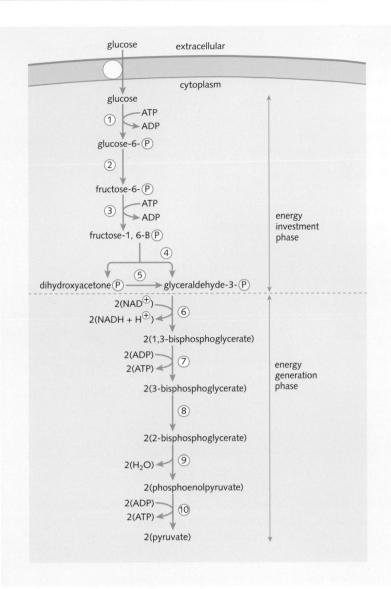

Fig. 4.4B The glycolysis pathway. Numbers refer to Fig. 4.4A.

- Gluconeogenesis (glucose synthesis from non-carbohydrate precursors)
- Lipid synthesis (Chapter 5)
- Synthesis of several non-aromatic amino acids (Chapter 6)
- Synthesis of aromatic amino acids (Chapter 6) (Fig. 4.5).

Regulation of glycolysis

The enzymes catalysing reactions 1, 3 and 10 of the pathway function as glycolysis regulation points, since these reactions are all highly exergonic and as such are essentially irreversible.

Reaction 1: Glucose phosphorylation

Reaction 1 of glycolysis is catalysed by hexokinase (HK). This enzyme is allosterically inhibited by the reaction product Glc-6-P. Insulin up-regulates HK transcription, whilst glucagon down-regulates HK transcription. Insulin and glucagon thus comprise the main hormonal regulation of this reaction.

Note that glucokinase (GK; the isoform of HK present in liver, pancreatic beta cells and hypothalamic cells) is insensitive to product-mediated inhibition by Glc-6-P. Glucose phosphorylation will persist in these locations even when the remainder of the pathway is less active and Glc-6-P accumulates. This isoform also differs from HK by affinity; GK requires 100 times

Fig. 4.5 Glycolytic intermediates in biosynthetic pathways. PPP = pentose phosphate pathway, Glc-1-P = glucose-1-phosphate, G3P = glycerol-3-phosphate, 2,3-BPG = 2,3-bisphosphoglycerate.

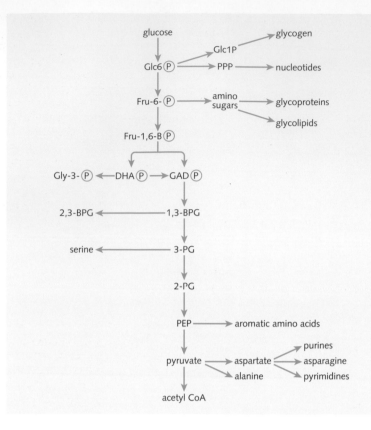

greater concentration of glucose than HK to function. This means that GK will only catalyse glucose phosphorylation at high intracellular glucose, unlike HK, which will operate at low concentrations.

Reaction 3: Fructose-6-phosphate phosphorylation

The enzyme catalysing this reaction (phosphofructokinase) is an important site of glycolysis regulation, since reaction 3 is the rate-limiting step of the pathway. Accelerating this pathway accelerates glycolysis. Various factors influence (PFK-1) activity, including:

* ATP. ATP allosterically inhibits PFK-1. When ATP is abundant, reflecting high cellular energy status, PFK-1 operates at a lower rate
* Citrate. This is not a direct product of reaction 3; the final product, pyruvate, is decarboxylated to acetyl CoA which combines with oxaloacetate to form citrate. Citrate allosterically inhibits PFK-1. When glycolysis is highly active, citrate is abundant and has an inhibitory effect on the pathway
* AMP and ADP. These allosterically activate PFK-1. They are abundant in cells when energy status is low, reflecting the need for more ATP to be generated
* Fructose-6-phosphate. Fru-6-P (a reaction 3 substrate) allosterically activates PFK-1; accumulation

of substrate feeds-forward positively on PFK-1 activity, increasing glycolysis
* Fructose-2,6-bisphosphate (Fru-2,6-BP). This allosterically activates PFK-1. Note that Fru-2,6-BP is synthesized by phosphofructokinase-2 (PFK-2), not PFK-1. When [Fru-2,6-BP] is high, glycolysis predominates over gluconeogenesis (see 'Gluconeogenesis' section later in this chapter)
* Insulin. Insulin regulates glycolysis by increasing synthesis of PFK-1. More enzyme means that glycolysis can function at a greater rate under the influence of insulin
* Glucagon. Glucagon regulates glycolysis, by decreasing synthesis of PFK-1. This means that glycolysis operates at a lower rate under the influence of glucagon.

Reaction 10: Phosphoenolpyruvate → pyruvate

Pyruvate kinase (PK) catalyses reaction 10 of glycolysis. It is influenced by:

* ATP. This allosterically inhibits PK by decreasing the affinity of the enzyme for its substrate PEP. When cellular energy status is high and ATP is abundant, PK is less active

- Acetyl CoA allosterically inhibits PK. Acetyl CoA reflects high cellular energy status; in this context PK is less active
- Fructose-1-6-bisphosphate. This allosterically activates PK in a feed-forward manner, reducing the probability of disadvantageous accumulation of substrate
- Insulin. Insulin brings about intracellular dephosphorylation of PK. Dephosphorylation activates PK
- Glucagon. Glucagon exposure results in intracellular PK phosphorylation. Phosphorylation inactivates PK.

Clinical Note

Phosphofructokinase-1 is an enzyme of the glycolysis pathway. In contrast, phosphofructokinase-2 does not participate directly in glycolysis, but produces fructose-2,6,-bisphosphate (Fru-2,6-BP), which powerfully influences glycolysis via its effect on PFK-1. Importantly, however, Fru-2,6-BP also inhibits one of the enzymes of the gluconeogenesis pathway. This ensures that glucose is not degraded and synthesized simultaneously. Figure 4.6 elaborates this concept.

The insulin:glucagon ratio influence on glycolysis

Insulin is secreted when plasma glucose is high, i.e. in the 'fed' state. When glucose is abundant, glucose oxidation to provide ATP (via glycolysis) is advantageous. Insulin promotes glycolysis by various effects on key regulatory enzymes. Glucagon, on the other hand, is released in the bloodstream when plasma glucose is low,

i.e. in the 'fasting' state. It has the converse effect on the regulatory enzymes of glycolysis; it dampens down (rather than promotes) pathway activity.

Physiologically, insulin and glucagon are usually released by the pancreas reciprocally. This means that if one is high, the other should be low. The relationship between the two is reflected in the insulin:glucagon ratio. If insulin is high and glucagon low, this ratio is high, and likewise vice-versa. In health, the response of the pancreas to changes in blood glucose is swift. Thus the insulin:glucagon ratio both reflects the nutritional state of the organism in terms of carbohydrate intake and determines the metabolic fate of glucose.

Regarding glycolysis, when the insulin:glucagon ratio is high ('fed' state), pathway activity is also high. When the ratio is low ('fasting' state), glycolysis activity is low.

Aerobic glycolysis vs. anaerobic glycolysis

Glycolysis occurs whether or not oxygen is present. It is the only pathway that produces ATP in the absence of oxygen, and therefore is of paramount importance in cells lacking mitochondria, such as erythrocytes, and in hypoxic (low-oxygen) environments such as ischaemic tissue or rapidly contracting skeletal muscle.

The key difference between aerobic and anaerobic glycolysis is that $NADH + H^+$ generated during glycolysis undergoes oxidative phosphorylation in the presence of oxygen (Chapter 3), producing ~ 2.5 ATP per $NADH + H^+$ molecule. However, when oxygen is not present to act as a terminal electron acceptor, oxidative phosphorylation cannot occur. Instead, $NADH + H^+$ is oxidized to NAD^+ as a redox partner for the reaction pyruvate→lactate, catalysed by lactate dehydrogenase. This reaction yields no ATP. This lowers the ATP yield of glycolysis in anaerobic conditions to 2 ATP per glucose molecule. To compound the situation, since pyruvate is converted to lactate it cannot enter the TCA cycle. This would yield 10 further ATP per pyruvate molecule, but does not happen in anaerobic conditions.

Hyperlactataemia

Cells and tissues cannot perform oxidative phosphorylation if they are not supplied with oxygen. Pathophysiologically, the state of insufficient oxygen is known as 'hypoxia', and is seen in many disease states, for example, ischaemia (restriction in blood supply). In this anaerobic environment, pyruvate is converted to lactate. When lactate rises above approximately 2.5 mmol (hyperlactataemia), it is suggestive of tissue hypoxia,

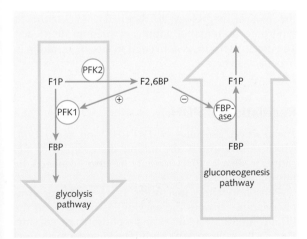

Fig. 4.6 Dual role of fructose-2,6-bisphosphate (F2,6BP) as a regulator of both glycolysis and gluconeogenesis. PFK = phosphofructokinase.

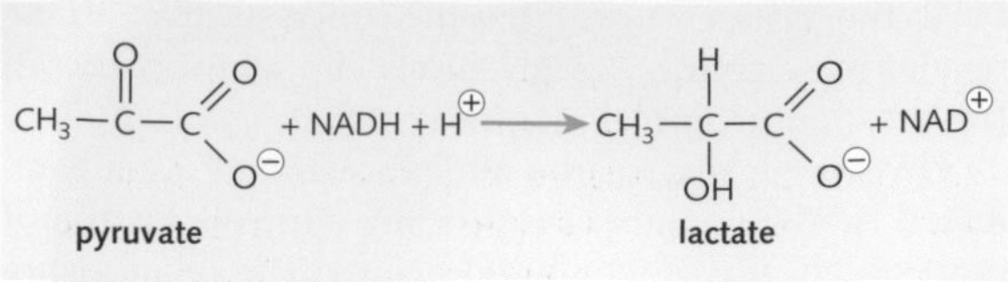

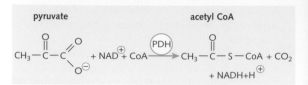

Fig. 4.7 Lactate production.

Fig. 4.8 Formation of acetyl CoA from pyruvate.

and is pathological unless appearing transiently during intense exercise.

If the patient is at rest and has elevated lactate levels and blood pH < 7.35, i.e. is also 'acidotic', this is pathological, and the condition is misleadingly termed 'lactic acidosis'. It is important to appreciate that lactate does not cause the acidosis that often accompanies elevated lactate (although it serves as its clinical marker) (Fig. 4.7).

Clinical Note

Any scenario imposing anaerobic conditions will cause lactate elevation, as pyruvate is oxidized to lactate in order to regenerate NAD^+. For example; compromised oxygen delivery to respiring tissues resulting from haemorrhage, insufficient perfusion pressure, insufficient oxygen levels in the blood ('hypox**aemia**') or excessive tissue demand. All of these scenarios will generate H^+ ions and can cause acidosis, but this acidosis is not due to lactate production.

Hereditary red cell enzymopathies

Mutations in the gene coding for one of the glycolysis enzymes are known as inherited red cell enzymopathies. These conditions are extremely rare; however, amongst these glycolytic enzyme deficiencies, pyruvate kinase deficiency is the most common. Inheritance is autosomal recessive for all but enolase (autosomal dominant) and phosphoglycerate kinase (X-linked recessive) deficiencies.

Deficiencies in glycolytic pathway enzymes damage red blood cells, which, lacking mitochondria, rely solely on glycolysis for ATP generation. Unable to produce sufficient ATP to maintain viability, their lifespan is dramatically shortened. This manifests clinically as chronic haemolytic anaemia.

THE PYRUVATE → ACETYL COA REACTION

Acetyl CoA is formed from pyruvate. This reaction is shown in Fig. 4.8. It is an irreversible oxidative decarboxylation, catalysed by pyruvate dehydrogenase

(PDH). This reaction is important, since it allows the final common product of carbohydrate catabolism (pyruvate) access to the TCA cycle. Note that this reaction also reduces NAD^+ to $NADH + H^+$, which can generate further ATP via oxidative phosphorylation in the presence of oxygen (Chapter 3).

Pyruvate dehydrogenase

PDH is in fact a trio of enzymes (E1, E2 and E3) that are all physically and spatially associated. It is located in the **mitochondrial matrix**; thus the reaction occurs in this location. There are in fact five steps in the pyruvate → acetyl CoA reaction, which are not essential to learn for medicine (however it does explain why so many coenzymes are necessary!). These coenzymes are:

- Thiamine pyrophosphate (TPP)
- Lipoic acid
- CoA
- FAD
- NAD^+.

TPP is deficient in thiamine-deficient states, resulting in failure of the pyruvate → acetyl CoA reaction and thus accumulation of pyruvate. This in part contributes to the clinical pathology of beriberi and Wernicke's syndrome, both manifestations of thiamine deficiency. The excess pyruvate is converted to lactate, resulting in hyperlactataemia.

Regulation of PDH

The reaction generates $NADH + H^+$ and acetyl CoA, which both allosterically inhibit the complex by negative feedback. PDH activity is also regulated by phosphorylation.

Phosphorylation inactivates PDH, whilst dephosphorylation activates the enzyme. Associated with the PDH complex are a kinase and a phosphatase enzyme. These act on the enzyme itself. The kinase (inactivator) is itself allosterically activated by PDH reaction products ($NADH + H^+$ and acetyl CoA). The phosphatase (activator) is activated by insulin (Fig. 4.9).

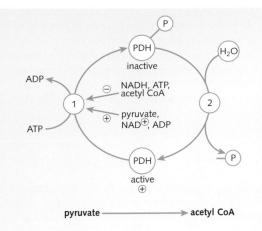

Fig. 4.9 Regulation of pyruvate dehydrogenase (PDH) activity. 1 = PDH kinase, 2 = PDH phosphatase.

GLUCONEOGENESIS

Gluconeogenesis is the production of glucose from non-carbohydrate molecules. It mainly occurs in **hepatocytes**. Most gluconeogenesis reactions occur in the **cytoplasm**, but two reactions occur in **mitochondria**. The substrate molecules are derived from breakdown of lipids, carbohydrates and protein.

Recall that glycolysis includes a number of highly exergonic reactions that are essentially irreversible. Different enzymes take over at these steps, so the actual reaction is not simple reversal of glycolysis. Gluconeogenesis is an energy-consuming pathway: 6 ATP are consumed per molecule of glucose produced. This energetic 'expense' is justified by the physiological importance of glucose (Chapter 8).

Necessity of a synthetic pathway for glucose

Even when fasting, blood glucose levels must be maintained within the range 3–6 mmol. This is achieved through ingestion of exogenous glucose (eating), endogenous release of stored glucose (glycogenolysis) or endogenous synthesis of glucose (gluconeogenesis).

Clinical Note

Straying outside the range 3–6 mmol may have serious consequences; both severe hypoglycaemia and hyperglycaemia are dangerous (Chapter 8).

Timescale of glycogenolysis vs. gluconeogenesis

Glycogen breakdown (glycogenolysis) is the 'first-line' mechanism preventing glucose levels falling below normal. However, glycogen reserves are quickly exhausted during fasting or prolonged exercise. Metabolism must therefore be able to compensate by producing glucose from other sources.

Gluconeogenesis substrates

Various types of molecules may be degraded in order to provide substrates for gluconeogenesis. These include:

- Proteins. Muscle protein is degraded to form amino acids, some of which ('glucogenic' amino acids) participate in gluconeogenesis
- Lipids. Mobilized fat stores or ingested fats ('triacylglycerols') are hydrolyzed, releasing glycerol and fatty acids (Chapter 5). Glycerol enters gluconeogenesis. **Propionyl CoA** (a product of β-oxidation of odd-numbered fatty acids) also enters gluconeogenesis. However, fatty acids themselves do not give rise to glucose
- Carbohydrates. Glycolysis under anaerobic conditions ultimately generates lactate, which can be converted back to pyruvate by lactate dehydrogenase. Pyruvate in turn is a gluconeogenic substrate.

Sequence of reactions

This is best illustrated as a diagram (Fig. 4.10).

Key differences between gluconeogenesis and glycolysis

- The conversion of pyruvate to PEP in gluconeogenesis is a two-step reaction, rather than the single PEP → pyruvate reaction (glycolysis reaction 10). Also, it requires both ATP and GTP. The responsible enzymes are mitochondrial pyruvate carboxylase and cytoplasmic phosphoenolpyruvate carboxykinase
- Between these first two reactions, oxaloacetate 'leaves' the mitochondria and 'enters' the cytoplasm via the malate–aspartate shuttle (Chapter 3)
- Fru-1,6-BP is converted to Fru-6-P via a hydrolytic reaction, with no involvement of ADP or ATP (compare with glycolysis reaction 3)
- The final reaction of gluconeogenesis is dephosphorylation of Glc-6-P, catalysed by glucose-6-phosphatase in a hydrolytic reaction, with no involvement of ADP or ATP (compare with glycolysis reaction 1)

- Gluconeogenesis occurs only in cells possessing the appropriate enzymes, i.e. in hepatocytes and to a certain extent in cells of the renal cortex
- Gluconeogenesis occurs in both the cytoplasm and the mitochondria, as opposed to purely cytoplasmic glycolysis
- Gluconeogenesis activity tends to be reciprocal with glycolysis.

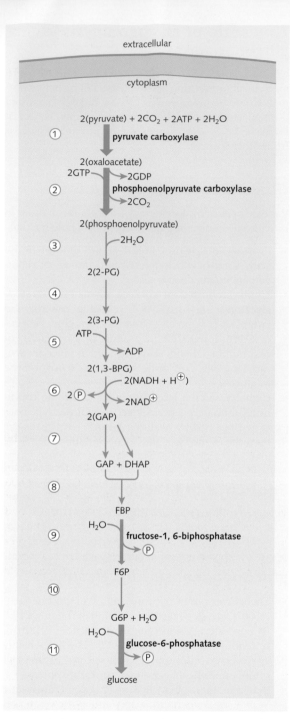

Fig. 4.10   Gluconeogenesis. The reactions that are not simply a reversal of glycolysis are shown in bold, annotated with the responsible enzyme. Glycolysis enzymes not shown. Please note that two 3-carbon pyruvate molecules enter the pathway to form one 6-carbon molecule of glucose.

Regulation of gluconeogenesis

This pathway is appropriately active in contexts which require endogenous glucose production, e.g. fasting, starvation, prolonged exercise and low-carbohydrate diets. It is also inappropriately active in insulin deficiency.

Bearing in mind the reciprocity between glycolysis and gluconeogenesis, it follows that intracellular conditions that inhibit one pathway would activate the other.

The reactions of gluconeogenesis (reactions 1, 2, 9 and 11) that differ from glycolysis are also highly exergonic and essentially irreversible. The enzymes catalysing these reactions function as points of regulation for gluconeogenesis.

Reaction 1: Pyruvate $\longrightarrow$ oxaloacetate (carboxylation)

Pyruvate carboxylase is allosterically activated by acetyl CoA. Remember that acetyl CoA inhibits pyruvate kinase (glycolysis reaction 10). High [acetyl CoA] promotes gluconeogenesis but inhibits glycolysis. Acetyl CoA is generated by β-oxidation of fatty acids (Chapter 5), which is maximal during fasting, and therefore is an appropriate activator of gluconeogenesis.

Reaction 2: Oxaloacetate $\longrightarrow$ phosphenolpyruvate (decarboxylation)

Phosphoenolpyruvate carboxykinase expression is enhanced by glucagon and inhibited by insulin. A low insulin:glucagon ratio, therefore inhibits glycolysis but promotes gluconeogenesis.

Reaction 9: Fructose-1,6-bisphosphate $\longrightarrow$ fructose-6-phosphate (hydrolysis)

AMP promotes glycolysis (AMP activates PFK) but inhibits gluconeogenesis, by virtue of allosterically inhibiting Fru-1,6-BP. Similarly, Fru-2,6-BP promotes glycolysis (Fru-2,6-BP activates PFK) but is inhibitory to gluconeogenesis, since it functions as an allosteric inhibitor of fructose-1,6-bisphosphatase.

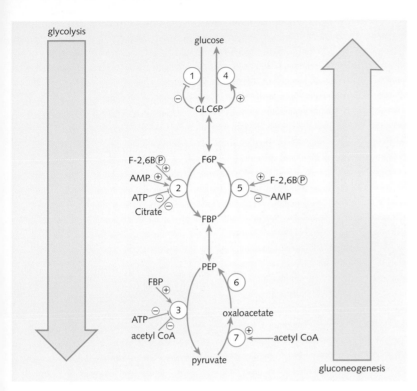

Fig. 4.11 Regulation mechanisms of gluconeogenesis and glycolysis. 1 = hexokinase, 2 = phosphofructokinase, 3 = pyruvate kinase, 4 = glucose-6-phosphatase, 5 = fructose-1,6-bisphosphatase, 6 = phosphoenolpyruvate carboxykinase, 7 = pyruvate carboxylase.

Reaction 11: Glc-6-P → glucose (hydrolysis)

Glucose-6-phosphatase is allosterically activated in a feed-forward fashion by the reaction substrate Glc-6-P. Remember that Glc-6-P conversely inhibits hexokinase. High Glc-6-P promotes gluconeogenesis and inhibits glycolysis (Fig. 4.11).

GLYCOGEN METABOLISM

Glycogen is a polysaccharide: a polymer of glucose molecules (monomers). It is stored as intracellular granules in liver and muscle cell cytoplasm. Glycogen is synthesized from excess dietary glucose. Glycogen breakdown ('glycogenolysis') allows rapid mobilization of glucose. This can stave off acute hypoglycaemia until gluconeogenesis can pick up its pace (or until the next meal takes place), or provide intracellular fuel for muscle contraction. Adrenaline (epinephrine) and glucagon stimulate glycogenolysis and insulin stimulates glycogen synthesis (glycogenesis).

Glycogen stores

Liver glycogen accounts for 10% of the liver's mass. It functions as a systemic reserve for maintenance of blood glucose levels during fasting. Once released into the blood, glucose liberated from hepatic glycogen can be utilized by any tissue of the body.

Muscle, however, lacks the necessary enzyme (glucose-6-phosphatase) to convert Glc-6-P (generated by glycogenolysis) to free glucose. Since Glc-6-P cannot cross cell membranes, it remains intracellularly and is exclusively used by the cell it originates from. The role of muscle glycogen is to provide glucose for oxidation in glycolysis when glucose demand exceeds the maximum that can be absorbed from the circulation, for example during rapid muscle contraction.

Glycogen structure

Glycogen consists of chains of glucose molecules, linked by glycosidic bonds between the C1 of one glucose and the C4 of the next. The polymer is branched; a branch point occurs every 8–12 glucose units (residues). Branch bonds are between the C6 of the residue on the main strand and the C1 of the terminal glucose of the incoming branch (Fig. 4.12).

The branched structure allows for a large number of 'ends' or termini. Enzymes that degrade glycogen can only operate on these termini; thus the more termini available, the more rapidly glycogen can be degraded. This allows for rapid mobilization of glucose, e.g. the adrenaline-fuelled 'fight-or-flight' response.

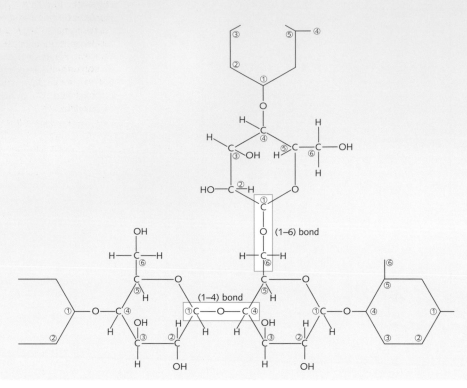

Fig. 4.12 Glycogen structure. The (1–4) and (1–6) linkages are highlighted. Ringed numbers illustrate the numbering of carbon atoms within each glucose monomer.

Glycogen synthesis (glycogenesis)

This occurs in the cytoplasm. The process requires:

- **UDP-glucose**, the glucose donor. UDP is uridine diphosphate (a nucleotide). It is required to 'activate' glucose molecules so they are recognizable by the glycogenetic enzymes.
- Four enzymes: **phosphoglucomutase**, **glycogen synthase**, **branching enzyme** (amylo $(1,4{\rightarrow}1,6)$ transglycosylase) and **uridyl transferase**.
- ATP.
- A pre-existing glycogen chain to link additional glucose molecules to; in absence of this **glycogenin** (a molecular 'primer') is required.

Stage I: Formation of glucose-1-phosphate (Glc-1-P)

Glucose-6-phosphate (Glc-6-P) is converted to glucose-1-phosphate (Glc-1-P) by phosphoglucomutase.

Stage II: Formation of 'activated' glucose (UDP-glucose)

UDP-glucose is synthesized from Glc-1-P and UTP by uridyl transferase (aka 'UDP-glucose pyrophosphorylase').

Glucose in this form is now 'eligible' to join the growing glycogen chain.

Stage III: Elongation

Glycogen synthase now transfers the glucose from UDP-glucose to the C4 of the terminal glucose in an existing glycogen strand (Fig. 4.13). It is linked via a (1–4) glycosidic bond. Elongation requires a strand of at least four glucose residues to exist before it can occur; either an existing 4-plus residue strand or the protein glycogenin ('primers') must be present.

Stage IV: Branch formation

Glycogen synthase can only lengthen strands: it cannot create branches. For this, branching enzyme is required. This enzyme cleaves off a length from a separately growing glycogen strand, usually around seven residues long, and transfers this to another strand (Fig. 4.14). This generates a branch point. A (1–4) bond is broken, but a (1–6) bond is formed (between the C1 of the incoming fragment and the C6 of the 'branch' residue on the main strand).

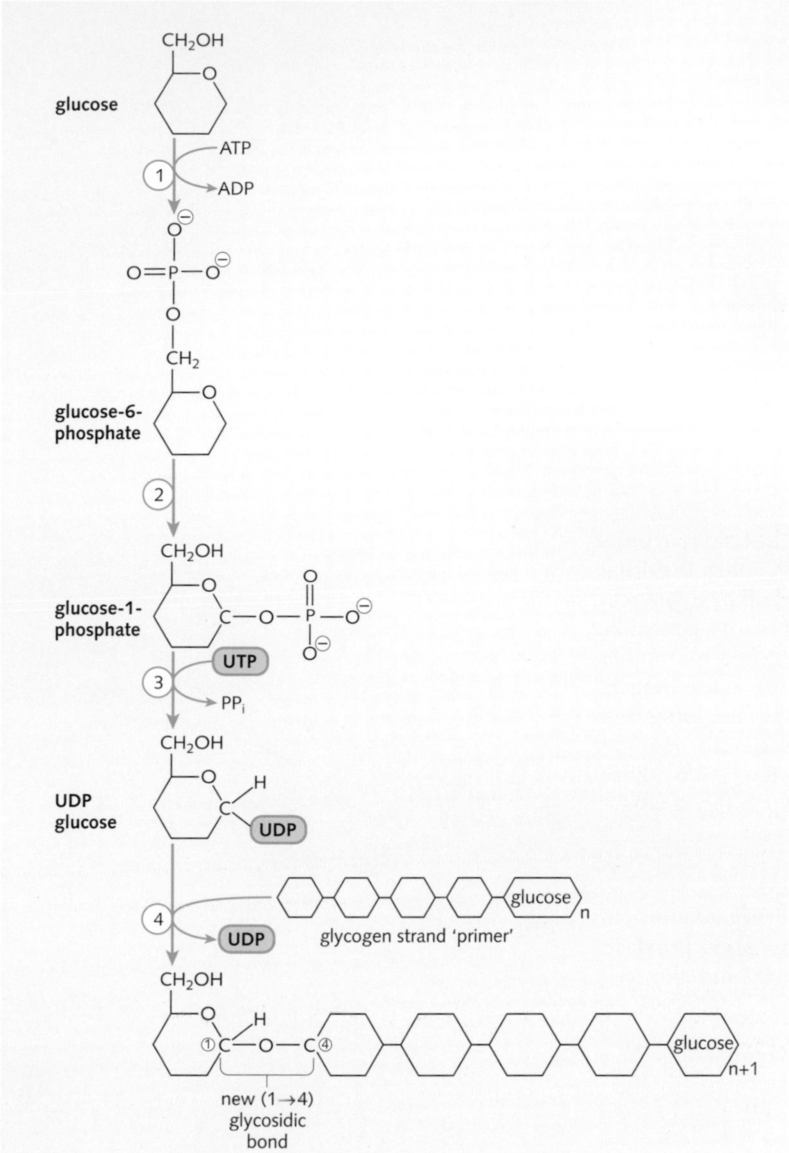

Fig. 4.13 Glycogen polymer synthesis: chain elongation. For simplification, only the main carbon skeleton structure is shown for glucose. Please refer to Fig. 4.1 for the precise structure. UTP=uridine triphosphate, UDP=uridine diphosphate, PP_i=pyrophosphate. 1=hexokinase, 2=phosphoglucomutase, 3=UDP glycogen pyrophosphorylase, 4=glycogen synthase. Note that glycogenin can replace an existing strand of residues as the primer.

Glycogen breakdown ('glycogenolysis')

This occurs in the cytoplasm. It is stimulated by glucagon and adrenaline. There are two elements to glycogenolysis; strand-shortening and branch removal. The enzymes involved are glycogen phosphorylase (which requires pyridoxal phosphate (PLP) as a cofactor), debranching enzyme (aka $(1,4) \to (1,4)$ glucan transferase) and amylo-α-1,6-glucosidase.

Strand shortening

Glucose units are cleaved off strand termini, one by one. The cleavage of the $(1 \to 4)$ glycosidic bond linking terminal and penultimate units is performed by glycogen phosphorylase; 'phosphorolysis', and within intracellular organelles called lysosomes by lysosomal α-1,4-glucosidase. Glucose-1-phosphate (Glc-1-P) is released.

Unhelpfully, glycogen phosphorylase will only remove units if the chain is four residues or longer. It also cannot process branch-point residues. Thus the enzyme stops short when the strand/branch diminishes to four residues in length (not including the 'branch' unit). This leaves a number of branch-remnant 'stubs' (Fig. 4.15).

Glc-1-P released by glycogenolysis may be converted by phosphoglucomutase to Glc-6-P, which can enter glycolysis. In hepatocytes, Glc-6-P may be converted to glucose itself by hepatocyte glucose-6-phosphatase.

Fig. 4.14 Glycogen polymer synthesis: branch formation. Each hexagon represents a glucose residue. Stage 1 = excision of terminal six residues of a strand via hydrolysis of a (1→4) bond, stage 2 = transfer to a proximal residue and formation of a (1→6) glycosidic bond. To facilitate understanding, the transferred segment residues are shaded.

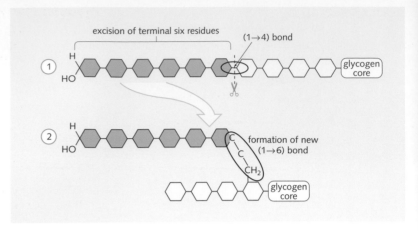

Branch removal

Once a branch has been shortened to the final four units of a branch (stemming from a 'branch' unit), the distal three units of this branch are trimmed off by debranching enzyme, which hydrolyzes the (1→ 4) glycosidic bond. These three units are then attached to another strand elsewhere in the polymer. This leaves the 'branch' unit of the main strand with just one remaining unit (step 1, Fig. 4.16). This protruding unit requires amylo-α-1,6-glucosidase to hydrolyse the (1→ 6) glycosidic bond, releasing free glucose (step 2, Fig. 4.16).

Regulation of glycogen metabolism

The activity of the key synthesis and degradation enzymes (glycogen synthase and glycogen phosphorylase, respectively) is modulated via hormonal and allosteric mechanisms.

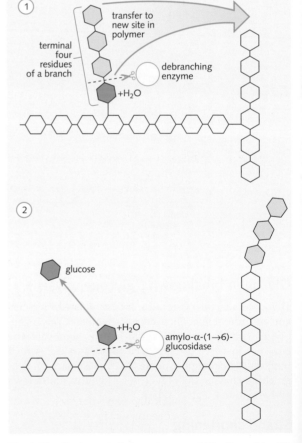

Fig. 4.15 Glycogenolysis. Strand /branch shortening via sequential phosphorylysis. Ringed numbers indicate carbon numbers within each glucose monomer.

Fig. 4.16 Glycogenolysis: branch removal. The 'branch' unit is shaded heavily, whilst the terminal three residues on the 'stub' are shaded lightly to facilitate visualization.

Hormonal control

Hormones regulate these enzymes via phosphorylation. Glycogen phosphorylase is activated by phosphorylation. Glycogen synthase is deactivated by phosphorylation. Refer to Fig 1.7.

- The same kinase enzyme (protein kinase A; PKA) phosphorylates both enzymes
- PKA itself is activated by cyclic AMP (cAMP)
- Intracellular cAMP is elevated by binding of adrenaline or glucagon to membrane receptors associated with adenylate cyclase (AC). This enzyme synthesizes cAMP from AMP
- Glucagon and adrenaline therefore elevate intracellular cAMP, activating PKA, which phosphorylates (deactivates) glycogen synthase and (activates) glycogen phosphorylase
- This promotes glycogenolysis and inhibits glycogen synthesis
- Insulin has the opposite effect, since insulin binding to its intracellular receptors results in up-regulation of intracellular protein phosphatase-1 (PP-1). This dephosphorylates the two enzymes, with the opposing outcome: glycogen synthesis is promoted and glycogenolysis is inhibited.

Allosteric regulation

The scenario differs according to the location of glycogen: hepatocytes or muscle cells.

Hepatic glycogen

Glucose allosterically inhibits glycogen phosphorylase, inhibiting glycogenolysis. Glucose binds to glycogen phosphorylase, causing a conformational change that exposes its phosphate group. This phosphate group is the target for hydrolytic cleavage by PP-1. Thus, glucose binding increases the probability of dephosphorylation and consequent deactivation of glycogen phosphorylase, and inhibition of glycogenolysis. Conversely, glucose allosterically activates glycogen synthase, promoting glycogen synthesis. Glc-6-P too, allosterically inactivates phosphorylase and activates synthase.

Muscle glycogen

Ca^{2+} ions, intracellularly elevated during skeletal muscle contraction, allosterically activate glycogen phosphorylase. Thus glycogenolysis is promoted in a context where glucose mobilization is desirable. Similarly, AMP, plentiful in active cells undergoing high levels of ATP hydrolysis, allosterically activates glycogen phosphorylase.

Glycogen storage diseases

This term describes genetic diseases arising from deficiencies of one of the enzymes of either glycogen synthesis or degradation. They result in clinical manifestations reflecting the resulting abnormalities of glycogen synthesis or degradation (Fig. 4.17).

THE PENTOSE PHOSPHATE PATHWAY (PPP)

The PPP, aka the 'hexose monophosphate shunt', is a primarily anabolic pathway that uses glucose-6-phosphate (Glc-6-P) as an initial substrate. The PPP generates $NADPH + H^+$, pentose sugars and other intermediates. $NADPH + H^+$ is both vital for fatty acid and cholesterol synthesis (Chapter 5) and also regeneration of glutathione. Pentose sugars are required for nucleotide and nucleic acid synthesis. Other pathway intermediates are important raw materials for numerous synthetic reactions.

Processing of dietary pentose sugars

Whilst not the pathway's primary role, the PPP allows conversion of dietary pentose sugars into hexose and triose intermediates that are then able to enter glycolysis, conserving energy substrates.

Reactions of the PPP

The pathway (Fig. 4.18) has two stages:

- An initial oxidative phase. Three exergonic reactions ultimately generate ribulose-5-phosphate, CO_2 and two molecules of $NADPH + H^+$ per Glc-6-P oxidized
- A reversible non-oxidative phase, consisting of a series of reactions converting ribulose-5-phosphate into intermediates with varying carbon numbers.

Regulation of the PPP

The main regulatory influence is exerted at the glucose-6-phosphate $\rightarrow$ 6-phosphogluconolactone reaction. The substrate:product ratio drives the reaction forward; the higher the $[NADP^+]$ (substrate) relative to the $[NADPH + H^+]$ (product), the greater the pathway activity. Higher activity results in more Glc-6-P entering the PPP (and less participating in glycolysis).

Demand for intermediates (generated during the second, non-oxidative phase) determines which products are predominantly generated. For example, if ribose-5-phosphate is withdrawn from the PPP to enter nucleic acid synthesis, it will not be able to combine with xylulose-5-phosphate and progress along the PPP to produce downstream intermediates (Fig. 4.18).

Fig. 4.17 Glycogen storage diseases

Type	Name	Defective enzyme	Pathology	Clinical consequences
I	Von Gierke's disease	Glucose-6-phosphatase *or* debranching enzyme	Glucose-6-phosphate from gluconeogenesis or glycogenolysis cannot be converted to glucose and thus released from liver cells. Glycogen accumulates within liver and renal cells (gluconeogenesis sites)	Hepatomegaly (enlarged liver) and enlarged kidneys; both due to accumulated unmobilized glycogen. Fasting hypoglycaemia from inability to release glucose from glycogen or gluconeogenesis (glucose-6-phosphatase deficiency) or from glycogenoloysis (debranching enzyme)
II	Pompe's disease	Lysosomal α-(1,4)-glucosidase (aka maltase)	Glycogen strands cannot be shortened lysosomally. Glycogen accumulates intralysosomally within heart muscle, skeletal muscles, liver and CNS	Hepatomegaly, cardiomegaly (enlarged heart), muscular and neurological symptoms. Restrictive cardiomyopathy can develop from glycogen accumulation in the myocardium. Inheritance is autosomal recessive
III	Cori's disease	Debranching enzyme	The final four residues of shortened branches cannot be removed. Glycogen has abnormal structure, with large numbers of short 'branchlets'	Hepatomegaly, hypoglycaemia, late-onset muscle weakness and cardiomyopathy. Inheritance is autosomal recessive
IV	Andersen's disease	Branching enzyme	Glycogen synthesis is abnormal; long unbranched strands accumulate. This abnormal structure is less soluble than normal glycogen	Accumulation is most pronounced in the heart muscle and the liver. Progressive causes death, usually before the age of 5. A number of genes can cause this syndrome; inheritance varies according to the particular gene
V	McArdle's disease	Muscle isoform of glycogen phosphorylase	Muscles cannot perform glycogenolysis, therefore must rely on glucose absorbed from the bloodstream	Decreased exercise tolerance, (increased fatigue and muscle cramps) on sustained exercise since local glycogen mobilisation is impossible. No hypoglycaemia, since hepatic glycogenolysis is unimpaired
VI	Hers disease	Glycogen phosphorylase	Impaired glycogenolysis results in normal-structured glycogen accumulation in liver and muscle	Hepatomegaly. Hypoglycaemia on fasting. 75% cases are X-linked recessive, remaining cases are autosomal recessive
VII	Tarui's disease	Phospho fructokinase (muscle isoform)	Complex. Essentially, glycogen synthase is abnormally activated, resulting in glycogen accumulation in muscles	Muscle cramps, exercise intolerance, myoglobinuria, haemolytic anaemia

Glutathione

Glutathione is a 'tripeptide'; a trio of amino acids (glutathione, cysteine and glycine). Glutathione is the primary intracellular antioxidant, neutralizing harmful intracellular reactive oxygen species (ROS) (Chapter 1) and limiting oxidative damage. This function is particularly important in immune cells. Glutathione also plays fundamental roles in many vital metabolic processes, including enzyme activation, protein synthesis, DNA synthesis and DNA repair.

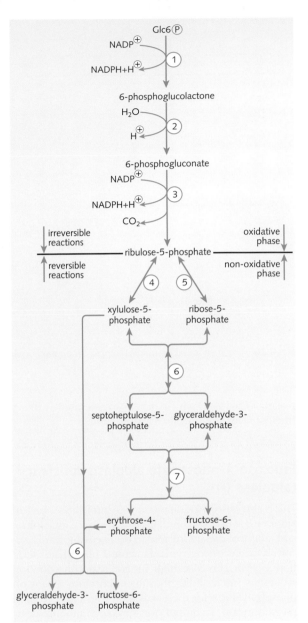

Fig. 4.18 Pentose phosphate pathway. 1 = glucose-6-phosphate dehydrogenase, 2 = gluconolactonase, 3 = 6-phosphogluconate dehydrogenase, 4 = ribulose-5-phosphate-3-epimerase, 5 = ribulose-5-phosphate isomerase, 6 = transketolase, 7 = transaldolase.

Mechanism of action of glutathione

Glutathione operates to neutralize ROS by donating H^+ and e^- (from the thiol group of the cysteine residue) to the unstable ROS. In donating reducing equivalents, glutathione is itself oxidized, and becomes unstable. It then rapidly reacts with another (unoxidized) glutathione molecule, forming glutathione disulphide (GSSG). GSSG is inactive in

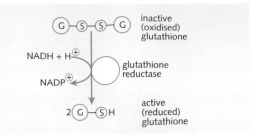

Fig. 4.19 Glutathione regeneration.

terms of its antioxidant role. To return glutathione to its active, unoxidized form, $NADPH + H^+$ is required (Fig. 4.19).

Role of glutathione in drug metabolism

Glutathione is of key importance in hepatocytes. They require a constant supply of active (unoxidized) glutathione for participation in conjugation (excretion) of numerous foreign compounds – including dietary molecules, drugs and toxins. If active glutathione becomes unavailable, these substances accumulate to toxic levels. As a constant supply of $NADPH + H^+$ is required in order to maintain a constant supply of active glutathione, the PPP assumes partial responsibility for maintaining the liver's excretion role.

Glutathione in erythrocytes

When high levels of ROS are present in a context of cellular oxidative stress, the cytochrome b_5 reductase system (which normally maintains haemoglobin in the reduced state (Fe^{2+})) becomes overwhelmed. Active glutathione protects against oxidation of haemoglobin (to a nonfunctional methaemoglobin (Fe^{3+})) and allows erythrocytes to continue performing their oxygen-carrying role. In this way, the PPP is also very important in the context of oxidative stress in erythrocytes, since PPP mediated $NADPH + H^+$ production ensures that sufficient glutathione is available to sustain Hb function.

Glutathione: the γ-glutamyl cycle

The γ-glutamyl cycle is a mechanism for importing various amino acids into cells (Chapter 6). Glutathione is required for this import process to operate.

Glucose-6-phosphate dehydrogenase deficiency; the failure of the PPP

Glucose-6-phosphate dehydrogenase deficiency is an X-linked recessive condition, affecting over 400 million persons worldwide, making it the most common enzymopathy. Since inheritance is X-linked and recessive, females are rarely seriously affected.

Absence of functioning glucose-6-phosphate dehydrogenase results in failure of the PPP. The mitochondrial citrate shuttle (Chapter 5) is the only other mechanism generating $NADPH + H^+$. Erythrocytes, however, lack mitochondria, and so cannot counteract the $NADPH + H^+$ deficit. Absence of active glutathione leaves erythrocytes unable to survive oxidative assaults, dramatically shortening their lifespans. This manifests clinically as haemolysis in situations of oxidative stress.

Precipitating factors

There are a number of factors that enhance cellular oxidative stress. For example:

- Broad beans (fava beans) contain high levels of vicine compounds, which are potent cellular oxidants
- Various drugs, in particular sulphonamides, certain antibiotics, aspirin and antimalarials
- Infection.

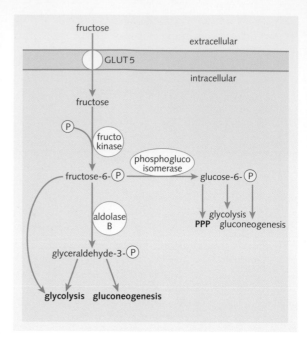

Fig. 4.20 Fructose metabolism in a liver cell. In a muscle cell, hexokinase would perform the first phosphorylation.

FRUCTOSE, GALACTOSE, SORBITOL AND ETHANOL

Fructose metabolism

Fructose is a hexose ($C_6H_{12}O_6$). This formula is the same as glucose; however fructose is altered in structure. Its main dietary source is the disaccharide sucrose. Gut sucrase hydrolyzes sucrose to component monosaccharides glucose and fructose. Absorption of fructose into intestinal cells (enterocytes) is via the GLUT-5 transporter. Fructose then leaves the enterocytes into the bloodstream (this time via GLUT-2) (Fig. 4.20).

Fructose is phosphorylated by hepatocyte fructokinase, forming fructose-1-phosphate. This is further metabolized to glyceraldehyde-3-phosphate (GAP) by aldolase B, which enters glycolysis or gluconeogenesis according to cellular energy status (Fig. 4.11). In muscle cells, fructose is phosphorylated to Fru-6-P by HK (like glucose) and enters glycolysis.

Genetic deficiencies of fructose metabolism

The two main enzymopathies of fructose metabolism are fructokinase deficiency and fructose-1-phosphate aldolase deficiency. Both are autosomal recessive conditions.

Fructokinase deficiency

Deficiency of fructokinase results in failure of hepatic fructose catabolism. Fructose therefore can only be degraded by muscle hexokinase. This leads to increased plasma fructose, which leads to elevated urinary fructose. This is clinically asymptomatic.

Fructose-1-phosphate aldolase deficiency (aldolase B)

This is also called 'hereditary fructose intolerance'. Lack of aldolase B leads to accumulation of fructose-1-phosphate and failure of dietary fructose to be diverted towards glycolysis or gluconeogenesis. Fructose-1-phosphate elevation is toxic, because high intracellular concentration sequesters intracellular phosphate. Enzymes reliant on phosphorylation for their activation thus fail. Glycogen phosphorylase (required for glycogen mobilization) and aldolase A (required for gluconeogenesis) are inactivated. Therefore the two mechanisms for maintaining plasma glucose on fasting fail, and fasting hypoglycaemia soon occurs following fructose exposure in deficient individuals. Treatment is by complete dietary exclusion of anything containing fructose, including sucrose.

Fructose-6-phosphate

Recall that Fru-6-P participates in glycolysis, when PFK-1 mediates addition of a second phosphate, generating Fru-1,6-BP. In the liver, Fru-6-P can also participate in gluconeogenesis or the PPP, after conversion to Glc-6-P by phosphoglucoisomerase.

In erythrocytes, fructose-derived Glc-6-P enters the PPP or glycolysis (gluconeogenesis does not occur in erythrocytes), allowing $NADPH + H^+$ production.

Galactose metabolism

Galactose is also a hexose, and shares the formula $C_6H_{12}O_6$ with fructose and glucose. The main dietary source is the disaccharide lactose, found in milk products. Gut lactase hydrolyzes lactose to its components glucose and galactose. Absorption into enterocytes is via the sodium/glucose symport. Like glucose, diffusion into the bloodstream from the enterocytes is via the GLUT-2 transporter. Galactose is converted into Glc-6-P, which can then enter gluconeogenesis (in the liver), glycolysis or the PPP (Fig. 4.21).

Galactose $\longrightarrow$ Glucose-6-phosphate

This occurs in several stages:

- Galactose is converted to galactose-1-phosphate by galactokinase
- Galactose-1-phosphate then reacts with UDP-glucose, forming glucose-1-phosphate and UDP-galactose. This is catalysed by galactose-1-phosphate uridyl transferase
- Glucose-1-phosphate is then converted to glucose-6-phosphate by phosphoglucomutase
- The UDP-galactose is re-converted to UDP-glucose by galactose-6-phosphate epimerase.

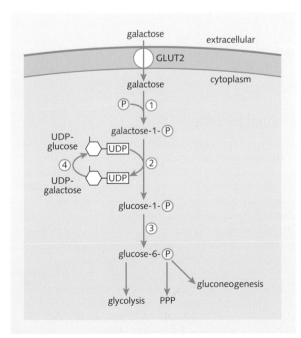

Fig. 4.21 Galactose metabolism. 1 = galactokinase, 2 = galactose-1-phosphate uridyltransferase, 3 = phosphoglucomutase, 4 −galactose-6-phosphate epimerase.

Galactosaemia

This is a rare, autosomal recessive condition, arising from deficiency of either galactose-1-phosphate uridyl transferase, galactokinase or galactose-6-phosphate epimerase. Failure of galactose catabolism results in toxic accumulation of galactose or galactose-1-phosphate in various tissues, particularly the liver, kidney, lens and CNS. These serious and irreversible events occur soon after feeding commences postpartum; even breastfeeding galactosaemic infants exposes them to galactose. Treatment is complete exclusion of all galactose-containing foods from the diet.

Sorbitol metabolism

Sorbitol (aka glucitol) is a sugar-alcohol, produced endogenously from excess glucose via the polyol pathway. It can also be obtained from the diet. Tissues containing sorbitol dehydrogenase (such as the liver or sperm cells) oxidize sorbitol to fructose. This reaction uses NAD^+ as a redox partner, thus generating $NADH + H^+$. This can then undergo oxidative phosphorylation. The fructose may ultimately feed into glycolysis or the PPP (or gluconeogenesis in the liver) (Fig. 4.22).

At high plasma glucose, such as is seen in uncontrolled diabetes for example, aldose reductase upregulates. As this enzyme is part of the sorbitol synthesis (polyol) pathway, this results in enhanced sorbitol production. This is significant for two reasons:

- The polyol pathway utilizes $NADPH + H^+$ as a redox partner in the glucose $\rightarrow$ sorbitol reduction, resulting in lower availability of $NADPH + H^+$ for regeneration of glutathione. This renders cells less able to survive oxidative assaults
- Certain tissues lack sorbitol dehydrogenase and cannot divert sorbitol into glycolysis via fructose. Sorbitol accumulates and exerts a pathological osmotic effect, leading to structural damage and impaired function. This is seen in Schwann cells and retinal cells in particular.

Ethanol metabolism

Ethanol (C_2H_5OH) is a component of alcoholic beverages. It binds to many CNS receptors, including acetylcholine, serotonin, GABA and glutamate, with an overall depressant effect on neuronal activity.

Enzyme systems

Ethanol detoxification occurs in liver cells via two sequential oxidations, culminating in the less toxic **ethanoic acid** (aka 'acetic acid'). There are three different systems that mediate the first oxidation, which

Fig. 4.22 Polyol pathway. 1 = aldose reductase, 2 = sorbitol dehydrogenase.

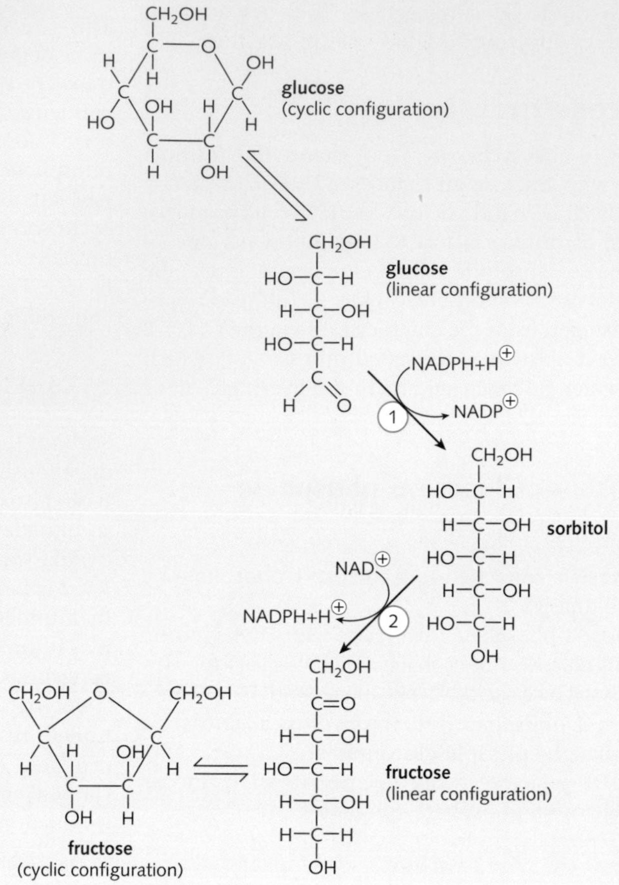

produces the even more toxic aldehyde ethanal (aka 'acetaldehyde'):

- Cytoplasmic oxidation by alcohol dehydrogenase
- Microsomal ethanol oxidizing system, which uses the P450 enzyme system
- Peroxisomal metabolism, which uses peroxisomal oxidative enzymes.

Mitochondrial processing

Ethanal (produced by one of the mechanisms above) enters the mitochondria, where it is further oxidized to **ethanoate** (acetate) by mitochondrial aldehyde dehydrogenase. A cytoplasmic isoform of this enzyme also exists. The acetate produced can then be coupled with coenzyme A by the enzyme acetyl CoA synthetase, forming acetyl CoA.

Ethanal toxicity

Aldehydes are highly reactive and react promiscuously with numerous biological molecules. The ethanal arising from biological ethanol processing is responsible for the unpleasant effects of ethanol consumption. These are usually seen when individuals consume excessively and exceed their own personal capacity for maintaining ethanal at an asymptomatic concentration. Nausea, vomiting, flushing, dizziness, elevated heart rate, headache and shortness of breath are seen.

These symptoms are exploited by Disulfiram (Antabuse), a drug used to deter recovering alcoholics from consuming alcohol. Disulfiram inhibits aldehyde dehydrogenase (mitochondrial and cytoplasmic), resulting in rapid ethanal accumulation following ethanol consumption. The unpleasant symptoms of ethanal toxicity act as a deterrent against repeated consumption.

Approximately 50% of Oriental individuals lack the mitochondrial isoform of aldehyde dehydrogenase. With only the cytoplasmic isoform to deal with an ethanal load following ethanol consumption, degradation is retarded, leading to accumulation of ethanal. These individuals manifest early signs of ethanal toxicity such as flushing, nausea and vomiting.

Impact of ethanol catabolism

Both reactions of ethanol catabolism consume NAD^+ (Fig. 4.23). This depletes the NAD^+ available to act as a redox partner in numerous metabolic reactions, including:

- Glycolysis. Less carbohydrate catabolism occurs, with the consequence of less ATP production
- Pyruvate→acetyl CoA reaction. Pyruvate must instead convert to lactate
- The TCA cycle. Less oxidation of TCA cycle substrates occurs, with the consequence of less ATP generation
- Gluconeogenesis. Inhibition of this pathway causes hypoglycaemia once glycogen reserves are exhausted.

Clinical Note

Lactate and urate compete for the same cellular excretion apparatus in the renal tubules. Thus excess lactate results in proportional retention of urate. This may crystallize in connective tissue, leading to an inflammatory reaction. This causes the substantial pain of gout, and explains its association with excessive ethanol intake (Chapter 7).

Ethanol influence on drug metabolism

Ethanol consumption causes an up-regulation in synthesis of alcohol-detoxifying enzymes. This includes the cytochrome P450 system. However, these enzymes

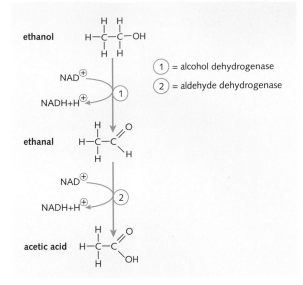

Fig. 4.23 Ethanol catabolism.

are also solely responsible for metabolism and clearance of many individual therapeutic drugs. An alcohol-induced increase in enzyme presence results in increased clearance of such drugs. This can result in drug levels falling to sub-therapeutic, i.e. ineffective levels.

Clinical Note

Warfarin, for example, is metabolized and cleared from the body via the cytochrome P450 system. Alcohol-induced up-regulation of the P450 system means that the usual dose of warfarin will be degraded too rapidly reach a sufficient level to exert therapeutic anticoagulative effects. This can be catastrophic for those relying on warfarin anticoagulation to prevent thrombotic events such as stroke, pulmonary embolism and myocardial infarction.

Lipid transport and metabolism (5)

Objectives

After reading this chapter you should be able to:
- Define lipid structure and understand the nomenclature
- Appreciate the mechanism of the citrate shuttle in fatty acid transport
- Describe fatty acid synthesis and degradation
- Describe mobilization of fatty acids from triacylglycerols, and conversely triacylglycerol synthesis from fatty acid substrates
- Understand the physiological role of cholesterol and recognize the structure
- Outline cholesterol synthesis and regulation of this pathway
- Recognize the different lipoprotein particles and their various functions and characteristics
- Describe ketone synthesis and degradation, appreciating the role in metabolism of these pathways

LIPIDS: AN INTRODUCTION

Definition

Lipids are a large group of diverse molecules ranging from waxes to sterols. In this chapter the term 'lipids' is used synonymously with 'fats', i.e. referring to fatty acids and their derivatives. Lipid molecules all have the general structure shown in Fig. 5.1.

Lipid roles

Lipids have varied physiological roles; both structural and within metabolism. In anabolism, triacylglycerol (TAG, aka triglyceride) molecules are the major form of energy storage. TAGs consist of three fatty acids linked to a glycerol backbone by ester bonds. Figure 5.2 shows an example. In catabolism, lipid stores are mobilized, releasing fatty acids and glycerol, which enter the bloodstream and act as substrates for oxidation by distant tissues, generating energy.

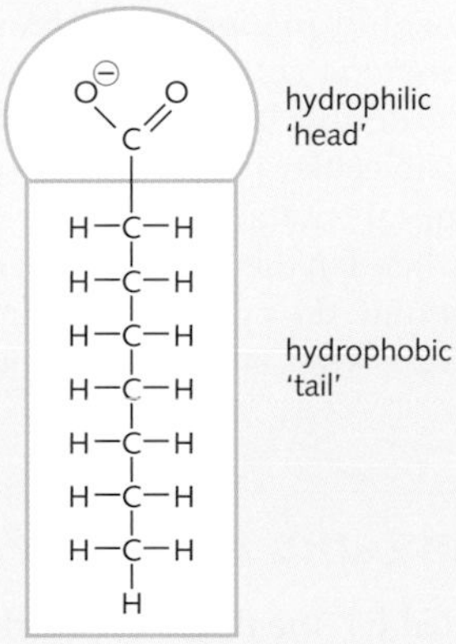

Fatty acids: archetype lipids

Fatty acids (FA) are excellent examples for illustrating lipid structure: a carboxylate ('head') linked to a long unbranched hydrocarbon chain ('tail') (Fig. 5.3).

Fatty acids in metabolism

Fatty acids are required as substrates for lipogenesis, i.e., synthesis of triacylglycerols; energy-dense storage molecules. FA are synthesized de novo from acetyl CoA. When acetyl CoA is abundant, i.e. the fed state, the energy intrinsic in acetyl CoA can be 'stored' by synthesis of triacylglycerols.

Conversely, FA can be released into the bloodstream from triacylglycerols (stored in adipose tissue) by lipolysis; once released they can be catabolized to release energy. The long hydrocarbon tails of FA molecules are incredibly efficient in terms of energy storage, because they contain fully reduced carbon and release maximal energy on oxidation (catabolism). FA catabolism is via β-oxidation, which both generates $FADH_2$ and $NADH+H^+$ and releases acetyl CoA. Acetyl CoA can enter the TCA cycle for oxidation, and reducing equivalents can undergo oxidative phosphorylation, releasing energy.

Fig. 5.1   General lipid structure; a hydrophobic 'tail' composed of a hydrocarbon chain (C and H) and a hydrophilic 'head' consisting of C, H and O.

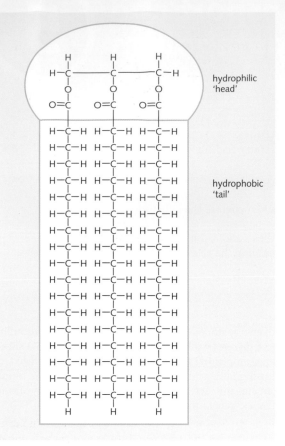

Fig. 5.2   Tristearin: a triacylglycerol (triglyceride).

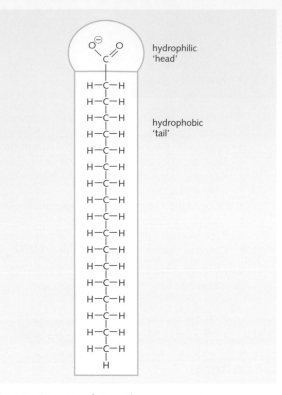

Fig. 5.3   Stearate: a fatty acid.

Fatty acids: the suffixes '-ic acid' and '-ate'

Note that fatty acids all have molecular formula 'R-COOH', i.e. 'something' carrying a carboxylic acid group. Therefore, fatty acids are weak acids:

$$R - COOH \longleftrightarrow R - COO^- + H^+$$

Due to the average pKa value (for FA) being ∼4.5, at physiological pH the equilibrium position lies to the right of the equation. FA exist in their anionic form under physiological conditions. This has the suffix '-ate' rather than '-ic acid', e.g. stear*ate* rather than stear*ic acid*. These terms are often incorrectly used synonymously. In this text the physiological anionic versions will be discussed, i.e. the suffix '-ate' is to be used.

Saturated vs. unsaturated

Fatty acids are described as 'saturated' or 'unsaturated'. Unsaturated FA contain a double bond at some location within the hydrocarbon tail, whilst saturated FA contain no double bonds. In saturated FA, there are no double

bonds within the hydrocarbon chain, and so no opportunity for any new bonds to be formed; the molecule is 'saturated' with hydrogen atoms. 'Polyunsaturated' FA have more than one double bond present, whereas monounsaturated FA have a single double bond (Fig. 5.4).

Stereoisomerism: *cis* and *trans* configurations of the C=C double bond

Double bonds within an unsaturated FA may adopt one of two stereoisomeric configurations: *cis* or *trans*. The nature of a C=C double bond can have significant consequences for molecular properties, for example structure and chemical characteristics. *cis* configurations impose a sharp bend in the hydrocarbon chain, whereas *trans* configurations do not. Most naturally occurring unsaturated FA possess C=C bonds in the *cis* configuration (Fig. 5.5).

Naming organic molecules

With unsaturated FA, the number of carbons as well as the number, position and nature of the double bonds must be communicated by the notation. This is illustrated using the example of palmitoleate (16:1cΔ9) and arachidonate (20:4cΔ5,8,11,14) in Fig. 5.6.

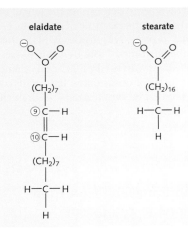

Fig. 5.4 Saturated and unsaturated fatty acids: stearate vs. elaidate. Note the ringed numbers illustrate the carbon number. Appreciate that stearate is the same molecule as in Fig. 5.3, however for brevity not every single carbon and bond has been drawn.

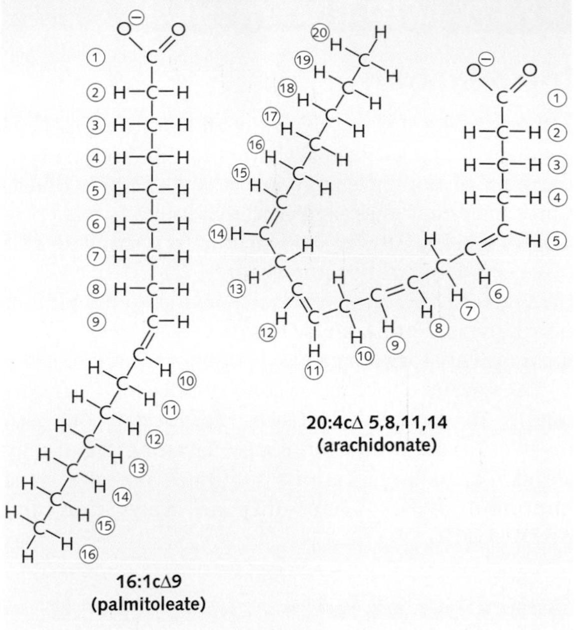

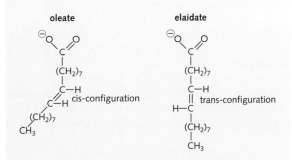

Fig. 5.5 Stereoisomerism: *cis* (oleate) and *trans* (elaidate) configuration of $CH_3(CH_2)_7CH = CH(CH_2)_7COO^-$.

Fig. 5.6 Fatty acid nomenclature: palmitoleate (16:1cΔ9) and arachidonate (20:4cΔ5,8,11,14). Ringed numbers indicate the carbon numbering.

The number before the colon describes the total number of carbons in the molecule (16), whilst the number directly after the colon describes the number of double bonds (1). The 'c' indicates that the configuration of that double bond is *cis* (as opposed to *trans*). The 'Δ' symbol is followed by a number representing the carbon atom at which the double bond starts.

HINTS AND TIPS

Carbon counting in chemistry begins from the carbon attached to the main functional group of the molecule (in FA this is the carboxyl group). The carbon bearing this functional group is carbon-1 (C1). C1 is also sometimes called the 'alpha' carbon, and C2 the 'beta' carbon. This explains why Greek letters are part of the names of biochemical molecules; for example α-ketoglutarate (this tells us that the keto (C=O) functional group originates from the alpha carbon of glutarate).

HINTS AND TIPS

Omega-3 fatty acids are a family of FA molecules with a common structural feature: a double bond between the 3rd and 4th carbon counted from the end of the hydrocarbon tail. The final carbon in the hydrocarbon tail is the "omega" carbon, irrespective of whether it is C5 or C25. This final carbon is at the opposite end of the molecule to the carboxyl group. Whilst confusing that this naming system counts from the other end to the functional group, it is used because the proximity of the first unsaturation (C=C double bond) to the terminal (omega) carbon has more influence upon molecular properties of the fatty acid than its proximity to the carboxylate group at the other end of the molecule.

FATTY ACID BIOSYNTHESIS

Introduction

Although fatty acids (FA) are accessible from dietary fats (hydrolysis of ingested triacylglycerols (TAG) releases FA) the bulk of human energy intake is via carbohydrates. Carbohydrate storage (as glycogen) is limited; thus a process for conversion of carbohydrate to fat is required. This process is fatty acid synthesis; acetyl CoA derived from pyruvate (a glycolysis product) is incorporated into new fatty acid molecules. These may then be esterified, forming TAG for storage in adipose tissue.

FA synthesis occurs in cell cytoplasm. It occurs mainly in specialised fat cells; **adipocytes**, but also in liver, kidney and of course lactating mammary glands. It requires various substrates but the most important ones to remember are **acetyl CoA** and **NADPH+H⁺**.

Overview of fatty acid synthesis

FA synthesis consists of a number of stages:

1. Transport of acetyl CoA to the cytoplasm, where the synthetic enzymes are located
2. 'Activation'; synthesis of malonyl CoA and localising at fatty acid synthase
3. A sequence of condensation, reduction, dehydration and a second reduction
4. Addition of a 2-carbon unit (derived from another malonyl CoA)
5. Repeat of [3] and [4].

The number of 'repeats' determines the length of the hydrocarbon chain. In the example of palmitate (16:0), after the initial process ([1] through [4]), this would repeat a further six times. Note that this process generates a saturated FA, with no double bonds (hence the '0' in 16:0). Synthesis of unsaturated fatty acids requires a saturated FA to first be synthesized and then enzymatically modified.

Details of fatty acid synthesis

1. Transport of acetyl CoA from mitochondria to cytoplasm

This is via a mechanism known as the 'citrate shuttle', aka the 'pyruvate-malate' cycle (Fig. 5.7).

- Acetyl CoA condenses with oxaloacetate (in the mitochondrial matrix) forming citrate, as in the TCA cycle. This is catalysed by citrate synthase
- Citrate is then exported from the matrix into the cell cytoplasm in exchange for malate
- Here it reacts with ATP and CoA to form oxaloacetate and acetyl CoA. This is catalysed by citrate lyase. The acetyl CoA is now in the cytoplasm and able to participate in fatty acid synthesis
- The oxaloacetate is reduced to malate by malate dehydrogenase, using NADH+H⁺ as a redox partner
- Malate is decarboxylated to pyruvate by malic enzyme, using NADP⁺ as a redox partner. This generates NADPH+H⁺, which is also required for FA

Fig. 5.7 The citrate shuttle mechanism for mitochondrial import of acetyl CoA. 1 = citrate synthase, 2 = citrate lyase, 3 = malate dehydrogenase, 4 = malic enzyme, 5 = pyruvate carboxylase.

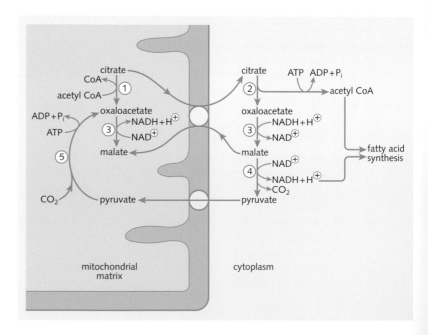

synthesis, or is returned to the mitochondrial matrix in exchange for citrate

- Pyruvate then re-enters the mitochondria, where it may either be used to regenerate oxaloacetate or acetyl CoA, completing the circuit. Figure 5.7 illustrates the entire process

2. Conversion of acetyl CoA to malonyl CoA

This is the irreversible rate-limiting step of FA synthesis. Carboxylation of acetyl CoA is mediated by acetyl CoA carboxylase (it requires biotin as a cofactor). The reaction is shown in Fig. 5.8.

Getting it together: assembly of malonyl and acetyl groups on ACP

ACP is 'acyl carrier protein', and is a component of fatty acid synthase (FAS). ACP accepts acyl groups, such as the acetyl and malonyl groups of acetyl CoA and malonyl CoA, thus anchoring them to the enzyme in preparation for FA synthesis. The CoA components are released and the acyl components bind to the terminal sulphur atom of the phosphopantetheine moiety (Fig. 5.9). This reaction is mediated by acetyl transacylase and malonyl transacylase. Note that

two ACP are present; this is because FAS exists as a homodimer.

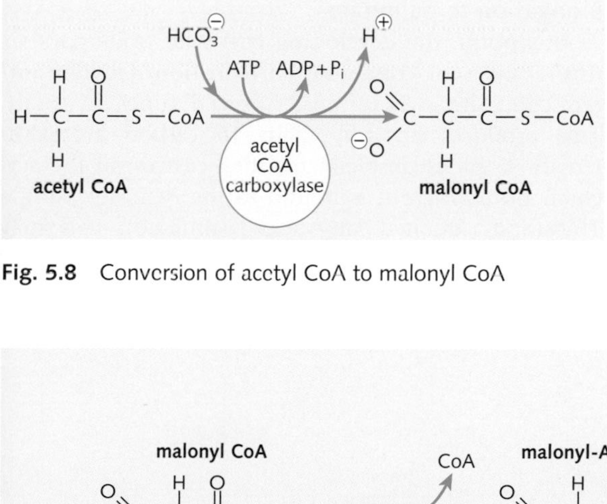

Fatty acid synthase (FAS)

This enzyme is a homodimer, consisting of two copies (a 'dimer') of identical ('homo') enzymatic units. The units themselves are also composed of a number of subunits, each fulfilling various enzymatic roles in the reactions of FA synthesis.

3. Condensation

The ACP-anchored acetyl group is cleaved off and transferred to the protruding end of the malonyl group (bound to the other ACP molecule). This transfer displaces the carboxyl group, liberating CO_2. This condensation reaction is catalysed by β-ketoacyl-ACP synthase and results in a saturated four-carbon chain, still attached to the ACP. This forms the basic skeleton of a fatty acid (Fig. 5.10).

Reduction, dehydration, reduction...

The nascent fatty acid has a C=O double bond at the C3 position, which is now removed. Two new bonds are created for C3; one with –H and one with –OH. $NADPH+H^+$ is oxidized as the redox partner for this reduction. This reduction reaction is mediated by β-ketoacyl-ACP reductase.

A double bond is then introduced between C2 and C3. This releases H_2O ('dehydration'), and is catalysed by 3-hydroxyacyl-ACP dehydrase.

Finally this double bond is removed, and C2 and C3 are fully saturated with H atoms. This second reduction reaction is mediated by enoyl-ACP reductase, and the redox partner again is $NADPH+H^+$. This has generated a four-carbon acyl-group, which remains attached to its ACP anchor (Fig. 5.11).

Fig. 5.8 Conversion of acetyl CoA to malonyl CoA

Fig. 5.9 Synthesis of acetyl-ACP and malonyl-ACP. FAS = fatty acid synthase.

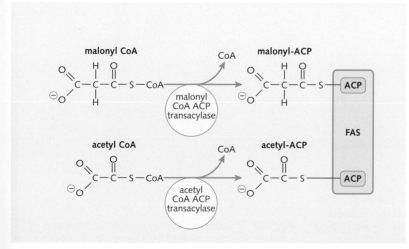

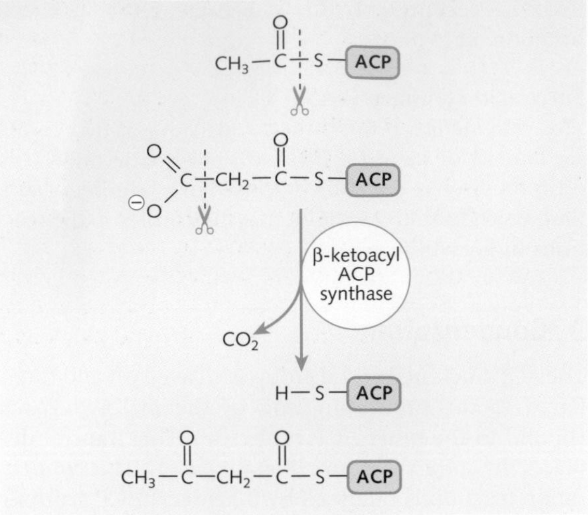

Fig. 5.10 Condensation: acetyl transfer to malonyl-ACP. The dotted lines indicate where β-ketoacyl synthase breaks bonds prior to transfer of the acetyl group.

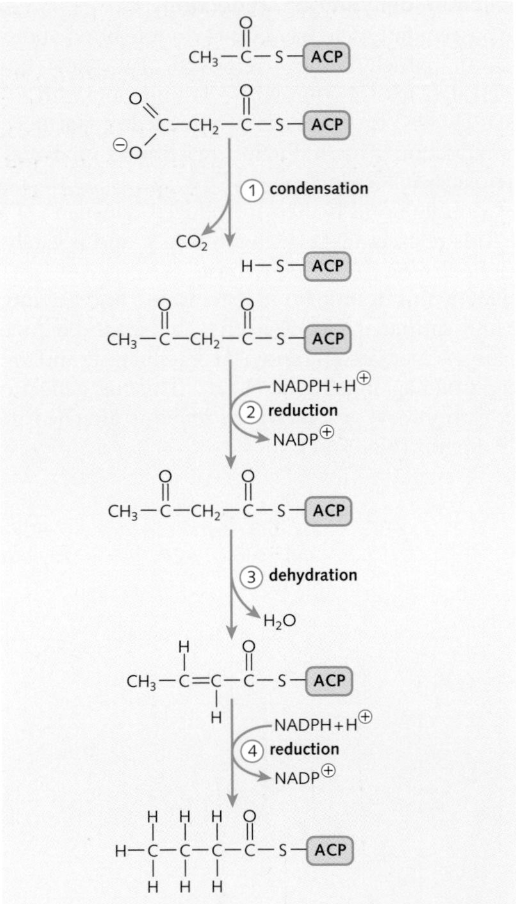

Fig. 5.11 The condensation, reduction, dehydration and reduction cycle. 1 = β-ketoacyl-ACP-synthase, 2 = β-ketoacyl reductase, 3 = 3-hydroxyacyl-ACP dehydrase, 4 = enoyl ACP reducase.

'Site switch' of the growing chain

β-ketoacyl-ACP synthase now transfers the four-carbon acyl chain from ACP onto one of its own cysteine residues (cysteine contains sulphur in its side-chain). This leaves the ACP free to receive further incoming malonyl CoA (Fig 5.12).

4. Addition of further malonyl CoA

Further malonyl CoA (produced by conversion of acetyl CoA) arrives, sheds its CoA and binds to the available ACP in a condensation reaction, forming malonyl-ACP (Fig. 5.9). Malonyl-ACP is now ready to receive the growing acyl chain, which is currently attached to a Cys residue within β-ketoacyl-ACP synthase.

Transfer of the lengthened acyl chain onto malonyl-ACP

The enzyme β-ketoacyl-ACP synthase catalyses the transfer (condensation) of the nascent acyl chain from itself onto the malonyl-ACP. This marks the start of a new cycle of fatty acid synthesis (Fig. 5.13).

Elongation to palmitate

At this point, the developing fatty acid undergoes six further cyles of condensation/reduction/dehydration/reduction/site switch/transfer (seven times in total). This produces an acyl chain 16 carbon atoms in length. A thioesterase enzyme then cleaves off the acyl chain from where it is bound to the ACP, releasing a 16-carbon saturated fatty acid (palmitate). This may later then be further elongated (via a different

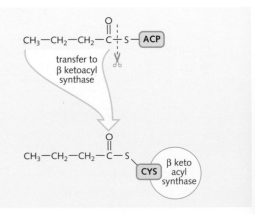

Fig. 5.12 Transfer of the growing chain to β-ketoacyl synthase. The chain binds to the S atom in the cysteine residue.

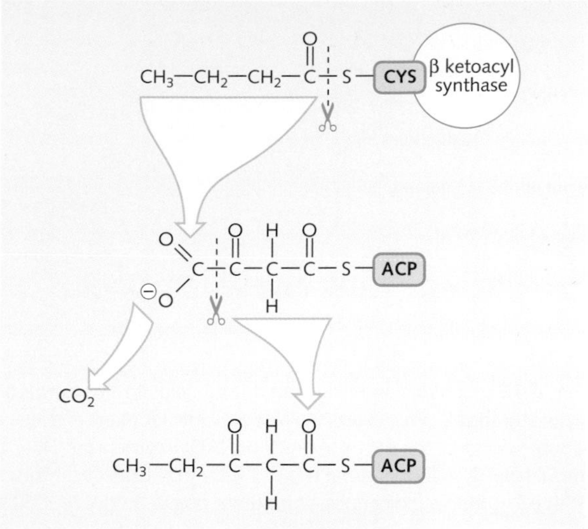

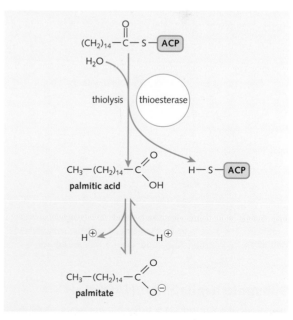

Fig. 5.13 Transfer from β-ketoacyl synthase to malonyl-ACP.

mechanism) or undergo further reactions to introduce double bonds, generating an unsaturated fatty acid (Figs 5.14A and 5.14B).

Elongation of fatty acids beyond 16 carbons

Fatty acid synthase can only manufacture fatty acids up to 16 carbons in length. Additional enzymes are required to lengthen 16-carbon FA. These are located within the **mitochondria** and the **endoplasmic reticulum**. The process is complex and is not addressed in this text; however it is important to be aware that further elongation occurs in the ER and in mitochondria.

Desaturation of fatty acids

This occurs in the smooth endoplasmic reticulum. A saturated fatty acyl CoA, oxygen and $NADH+H^+$ are required. A mono-unsaturated equivalent fatty acyl CoA is produced, along with NAD^+ and two H_2O (Fig. 5.15). Three enzymes are required:

- NADH-cytochrome b_5 reductase
- Cytochrome b_5
- Fatty acyl CoA desaturase.

Essential fatty acids

In mammals, double bounds can only be introduced at positions Δ4, Δ5, Δ6 and Δ9 due to enzyme availability: there are four subtypes of desaturase enzymes, each responsible for introduction of a double bond at these positions. However, FA with double bonds at the ω-6 and ω-3 positions, are also physiologically required, for example, for the synthesis of eicosanoids (such as prostaglandins). As these cannot be synthesised, they must be obtained in the diet and are termed 'essential fatty acids'. Linoleate (18:2 cΔ9,12 – double bond at the ω-6 carbon) and α-linolenate (18:3 cΔ9,12,15 – double bonds at ω-6 and ω-3) are the two unsaturated FA that cannot be endogenously synthesized in humans. Some plants possess desaturase enzymes capable of introducing the double bond at the ω-6 and ω-3 locations, hence the presence of ω-6 and ω-3 oils in plant seed oil.

Regulation of fatty acid synthesis

Substrate availability: malonyl CoA

Malonyl CoA availability is directly related to acetyl CoA availability. Acetyl CoA is abundant following carbohydrate intake (high glycolysis activity → high [pyruvate] → high [acetyl CoA]). Initially, elevated acetyl CoA fuels sustained high activity of the TCA cycle. Once TCA cycle products accumulate, they inhibit cycle activity. At this point acetyl CoA becomes available for FA synthesis. Citrate (a TCA cycle intermediate; Chapter 2) also allosterically activates the rate-limiting enzyme of FA synthesis, acetyl CoA carboxylase.

Fig. 5.14A Hydrolysis of the thioester linkage: release of palmitate.

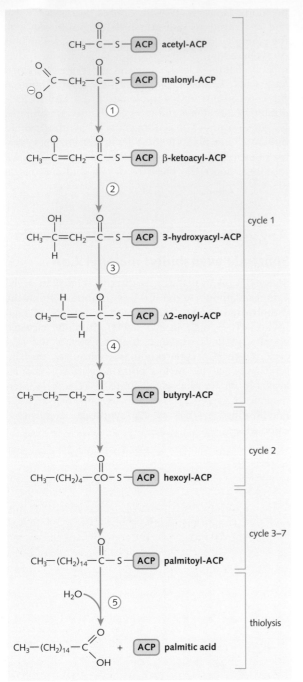

$$CH_3-(CH_2)_{14}-\overset{\overset{\displaystyle O}{\|}}{C}-S-CoA + O_2$$

$$CH_3-(CH_2)_5-\underset{\underset{\text{(10)}}{H}}{\overset{\overset{\text{H}}{|}}{C}}=\underset{\text{(9)}}{\overset{|}{C}}-(CH_2)_7-\overset{\overset{\displaystyle O}{\|}}{\underset{\text{(1)}}{C}}-S-CoA + 2H_2O$$

Fig. 5.15 Conversion of saturated fatty acids to unsaturated ('desaturation'). This example illustrates introduction of a *cis* double bond at the C9 position. 1 = NADH-cytochrome b_5 reductase, 2 = Cytochrome b_5, 3 = fatty acyl CoA desaturase. Ringed numbers indicate carbon numbering.

When FA synthesis occurs, $NADPH+H^+$ is oxidized to $NADP^+$, lifting the inhibition of glucose-6-phosphate dehydrogenase and increasing PPP activity. Thus FA synthesis activity promotes further $NADPH+H^+$ synthesis. Additionally, the citrate shuttle (which is highly active when [acetyl CoA] is high) also generates more $NADHP+H^+$ when acetyl CoA (and therefore malonyl CoA) is abundant.

Substrate availability: hormonal regulation

Acetyl CoA carboxylase is also subject to hormonal regulation. Insulin (a fed-state hormone) binding to its intracellular receptors activates a signalling cascade, including activation of a phosphatase enzyme (which dephosphorylates acetyl CoA carboxylase, activating it). Acetyl CoA carboxylase is re-phosphorylated (inactivated) in cells exposed to glucagon or adrenaline (epinephrine) (fasting-state hormones). The enzyme is of key regulatory importance because it mediates conversion of acetyl CoA to malonyl CoA, thereby controlling substrate provision for FA synthesis. Fatty acid synthesis is promoted by insulin, but inhibited by glucagon. Additionally, insulin promotes dephosphorylation (activation) of pyruvate dehydrogenase, which converts pyruvate to acetyl CoA (Fig. 5.16).

Fig. 5.14B Synthesis of palmitic acid. 1 = β-ketoacyl-ACP-synthase, 2 = β-ketoacyl reducatase, 3 = 3-hydroxyacyl-ACP dehydrase, 4 = enoyl ACP reductase, 5 = thioesterase.

Lipogenesis: triacylglycerol synthesis

Triacylglycerol (TAG) molecules, in medicine more commonly called 'triglycerides', consist of three FA linked to glycerol by ester bonds. TAG synthesis allows fatty acid storage in adipocytes (specialized fat storage cells). Synthesis from glycerol and FA occurs in three stages, and is illustrated in Fig. 5.17.

Substrate availability: NADPH+H$^+$

Recall that $NADPH+H^+$ inhibits glucose-6-phosphate dehydrogenase, and in doing so slows flux through the pentose phosphate pathway (PPP) (Chapter 4).

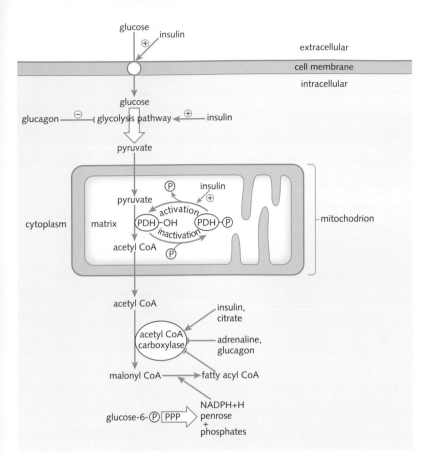

Fig. 5.16 Adipocyte: regulation of fatty acid synthesis. For simplicity, no shuttle mechanisms are shown, but recall that acetyl CoA leaves the mitochondria via the citrate shuttle (Fig. 5.7). PPP = pentose phosphate pathway, PDH = pyruvate dehydrogenase.

- Formation of glycerol-3-phosphate via one of two mechanisms. Either glycerol is phosphorylated at C3 by glycerol kinase using ATP as the phosphate donor, or the glycolytic intermediate dihydroxyacetone phosphate (DHAP, Chapter 4) is reduced by glycerol-3-phosphate dehydrogenase
- Fatty acid activation. FA must be linked to CoA in order to undergo lipogenesis. Fatty acyl CoA synthetase performs this reaction
- The three activated FA are esterified to glycerol-3-phosphate in stages.

LIPID CATABOLISM

The major physiological identity of lipids is as energy-dense molecules, which can be rapidly mobilized. Lipid degradation releases FA for energy provision during prolonged exercise or when energy utilization exceeds dietary energy intake. Lipid breakdown includes the following stages:

1. Lipolysis (splitting triacylglycerol into FA and glycerol)
2. FA activation (molecular modification of liberated FA necessary to obtain access to the mitochondria)
3. FA entry into mitochondria (from the cytoplasm)
4. β-oxidation (oxidation, releasing energy).

1. Lipolysis

This occurs in the cytoplasm, where TAG are stored in droplets. A hormone-sensitive lipase hydrolyzes the ester bonds at C1 or C3, liberating one FA, leaving a di-acyl glycerol (DAG) comprising the glycerol backbone with two remaining FA attached. Next, di-acyl glycerol lipase removes a second FA, leaving mono-acyl glycerol (MAG). Mono-acyl glycerol lipase then cleaves off the remaining FA, freeing glycerol (Fig. 5.18).

Fate of liberated fatty acids

The newly freed fatty acids are released into the bloodstream, where they bind to proteins. They are taken up by muscle or liver cells and oxidized. They may also

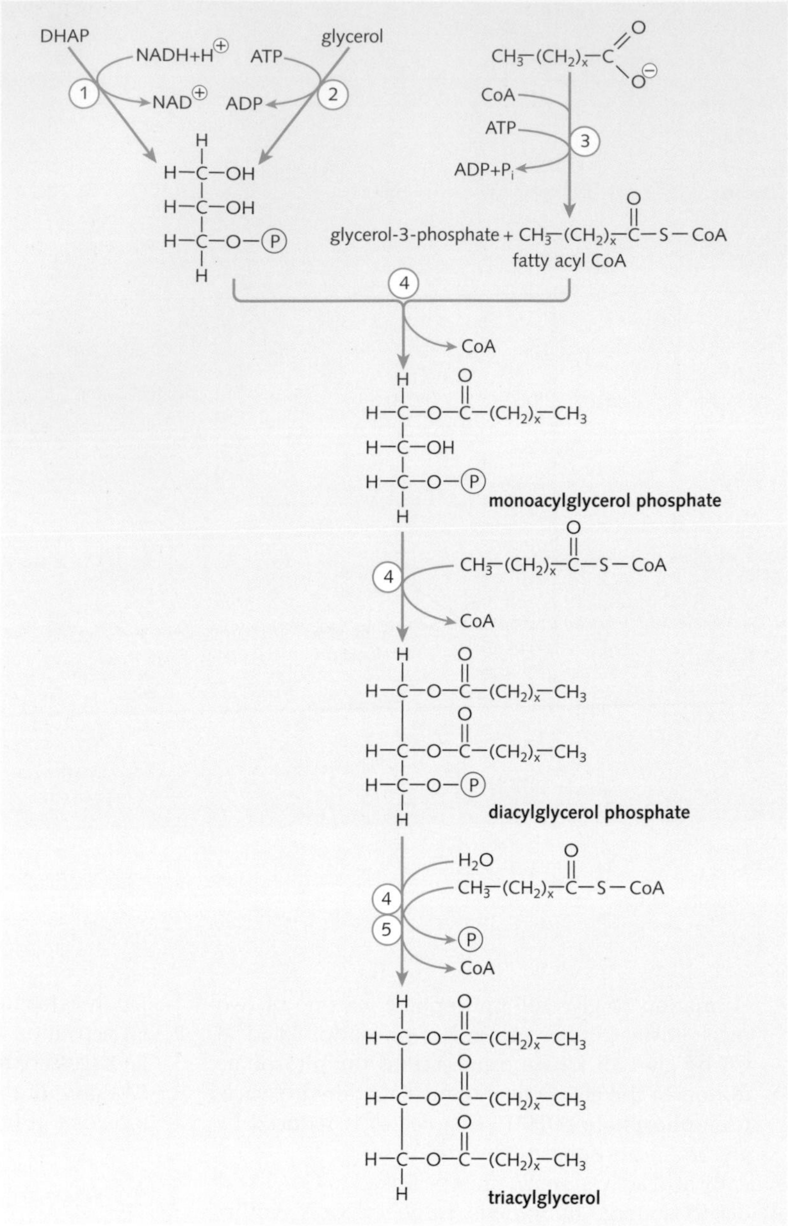

Fig. 5.17 Triacylglycerol synthesis. The 'x' is to emphasize that the fatty acid varies in tail length and saturation. Also note that DHAP forms glycerol-3-phosphate in adipocytes since they lack glycerol kinase. DHAP = dihydroxyacetone phosphate. 1 = glycerol-3-phosphate dehydrogenase, 2 = glycerol kinase, 3 = fatty acyl CoA synthase, 4 = acyltransferase, 5 = phosphatase.

Fate of liberated glycerol

Intracellular glycerol is phosphorylated and oxidized to DHAP, which is then isomerized to glyceraldehyde-3-phosphate (GAP, Chapter 4). This may then enter glycolysis. Alternatively, glycerol may be released into the bloodstream and enter hepatocytes, where it may be taken up again by adipocytes and re-esterified to triacylglycerols.

participate in glycolysis or gluconeogenesis, depending on cellular energy status.

2. Fatty acid activation

Thiokinase enzymes convert FA to fatty acyl-CoA. This reaction requires ATP for generation of an adenylyl intermediate (Fig. 5.19). The second high-energy phosphoanhydride bond is also hydrolyzed. Thus the equivalent of *two* ATP is consumed during fatty acid

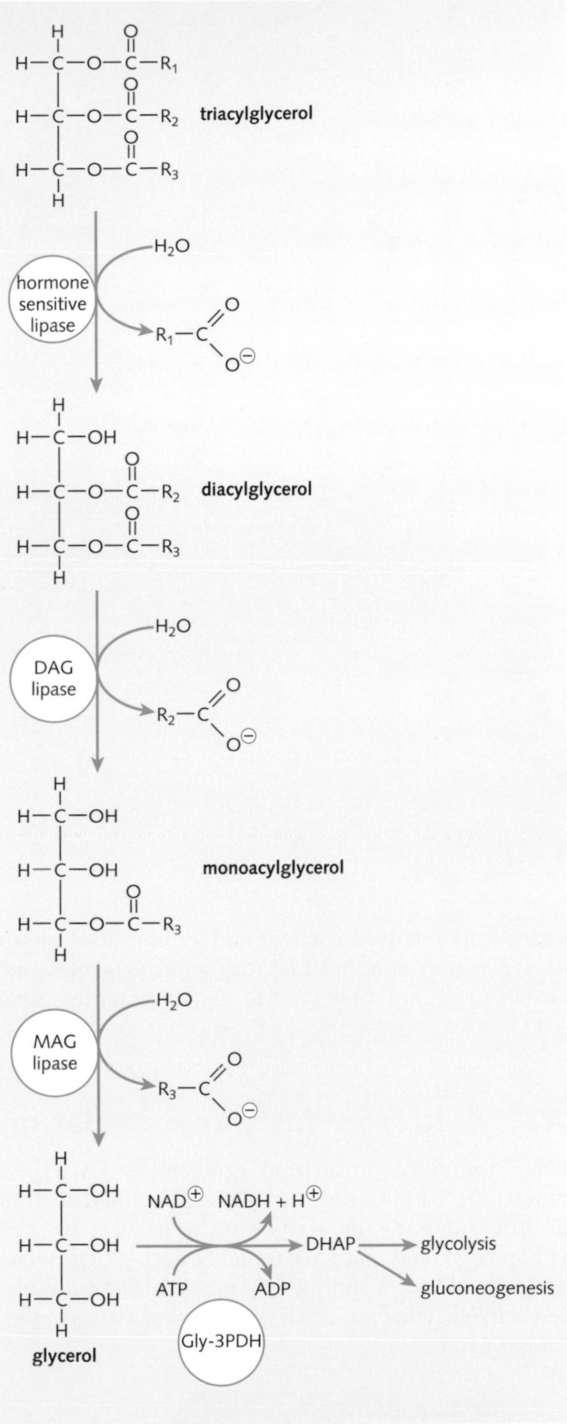

Fig. 5.18 Lipolysis of triaclyglycerols. Please note that 'R' represents any acyl chain, for example –(CH$_2$)x–CH$_3$. DAG lipase = diacylglycerol lipase, MAG lipase = monoacylglycerol lipase, Gly-3-PDH = glycerol-3-phosphate dehydrogenase.

activation. Now activated, fatty acyl CoA is then ready to enter the mitochondrial matrix via the carnitine shuttle.

3. Accessing the mitochondrial matrix: the carnitine shuttle

Due to mitochondrial membrane impermeability to fatty acyl CoA, a specialized mechanism exists to allow these molecules to access their site of catabolism (the matrix). This is the carnitine shuttle, which is best illustrated diagrammatically (Fig. 5.19).

4. β-oxidation of fatty acids

This occurs in the mitochondrial matrix and is a four-stage process which repeats itself until the fatty acid molecule is completely consumed.

(1) Oxidation by FAD

The fatty acyl CoA is oxidized by fatty acyl-CoA dehydrogenase. This enzyme exists in various isoforms, each specific for different length FA (long, medium and short). Oxidation converts the single bond between C2 (the 'β' carbon) and C3 to a double bond. The H atoms are accepted by the redox partner FAD, which reduces to FADH$_2$. This can enter the ETC, generating ~ 1.5 ATP.

(2) Hydration

Enoyl-CoA hydratase introduces an O atom and two H atoms to the newly formed double bond between C2 and C3.

(3) Oxidation by NAD$^+$

β-Hydroxyacyl CoA dehydrogenase mediates oxidation of the –OH group at C3, converting it to a C=O (ketone) functional group. This molecule is 3-ketoacyl-CoA. The two H atoms removed are transferred to NAD$^+$ (the redox partner) generating NADH+H$^+$. This may enter the electron transport chain (ETC), generating ~ 2.5 ATP.

(4) Thiolysis: release of acetyl CoA

Thiolase enzyme cleaves off C1 and C2 from 3-ketoacyl CoA, releasing acetyl CoA. This shortens the fatty acyl chain by two carbons. Another CoA is required to 'cap' the newly shortened molecule. This molecule is a fatty acyl CoA, but with two fewer carbons than the molecule in step 1.

Fig. 5.19 Fatty acid activation and entry to the mitochondria: the carnitine shuttle. OMM = outer mitochondrial membrane, IMM = inner mitochondrial membrane, CAT = carnitine acyltransferase – note the two isoforms – CAT I at the OMM and CAT II at the IMM.

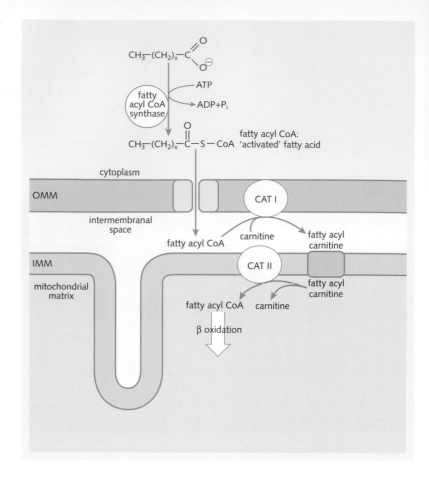

Reiteration of 1→4

Steps 1 to 4 are repeated until the fatty acid is almost completely degraded. The penultimate repeat leaves a four-carbon fatty acyl CoA, which is then undergoes steps 1→4 as previously; however this final 'round' of β-oxidation differs in that produces two acetyl CoA rather than one. Note that this final step is only the case for FA with an even number of carbons (Fig. 5.20).

Odd-chain fatty acids

This final step differs for FA with an odd number of carbons; the penultimate repeat leaves a five-carbon fatty acyl CoA. This undergoes a final round of steps 1→4, but the final two products are one acetyl CoA molecule and one three-carbon propionyl CoA molecule (instead of two acetyl CoA) (Fig. 5.21).

Propionyl CoA

This molecule may be converted to succinyl CoA in three steps. This requires 1 ATP and a bicarbonate ion (HCO_3^-). One of the requisite enzymes requires a vitamin B12-derived cofactor and another uses biotin as a cofactor. Succinyl CoA oxidation generates one $NADH+H^+$ and one $FADH_2$, together representing 4 ATP.

ATP yield from fatty acid oxidation

Every round of β-oxidation generates 1 $FADH_2$, 1 $NADH+H^+$, and 1 acetyl CoA. Recall that full oxidation of one molecule of acetyl CoA generates 10 ATP (Chapter 2), and that $FADH_2$ and $NADH+H^+$ generate approximately 1.5 and 2.5 ATP per oxidized molecule, respectively. Therefore, each round of β-oxidation represents 14 ATP.

> **HINTS AND TIPS**
>
> To calculate the number of rounds of β-oxidation an even-numbered fatty acid must undertake, divide the number of carbons by two, and then minus 1. In the example of the sixteen-carbon palmitate: $(16 \div 2) - 1 = 7$, so palmitate undergoes seven cycles of β-oxidation.

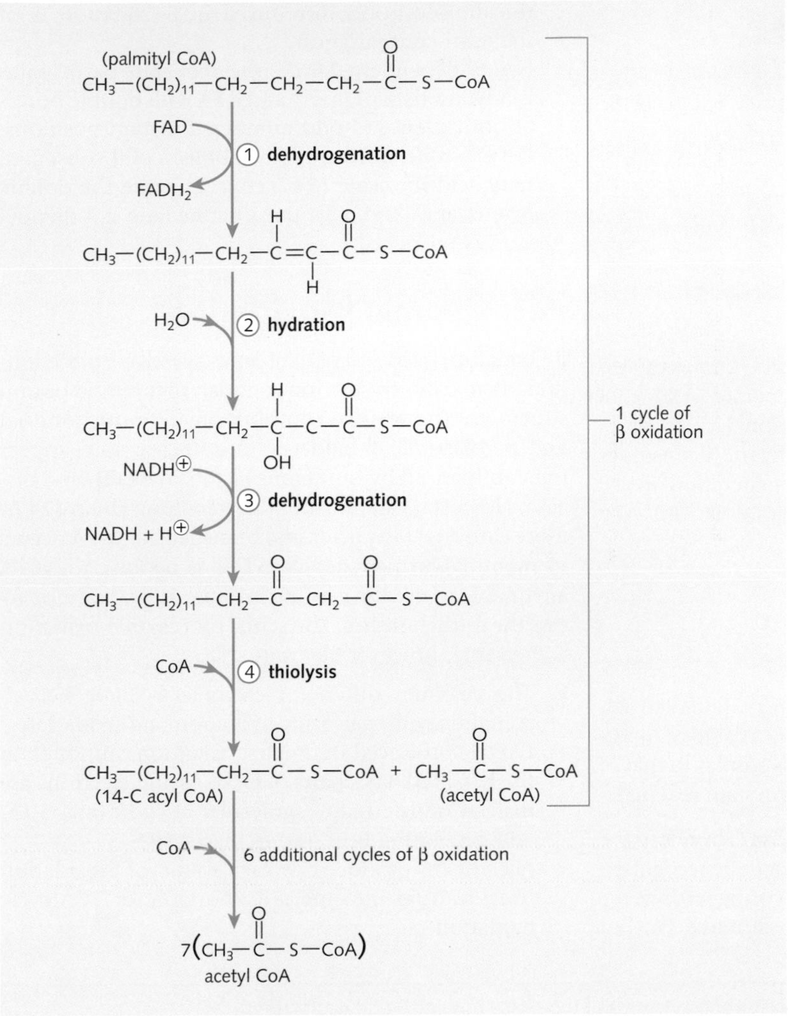

Fig. 5.20 β-Oxidation of fatty acids. Palmitate is used for illustration.
1 = fatty acyl-CoA dehydrogenase,
2 = enoyl-CoA hydratase,
3 = 3-hydroxyacyl-CoA dehydrogenase, 4 = thiolase.

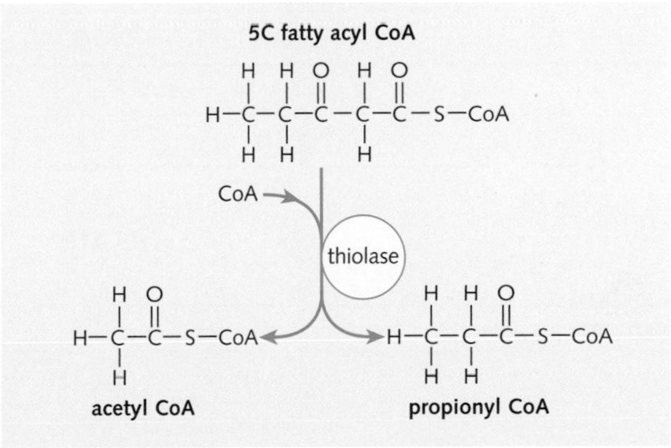

Fig. 5.21 Final round of β-oxidation of odd-numbered fatty acids.

Palmitate (16C) undergoes seven rounds of β-oxidation. Therefore, $14 \times 7 = 98$ ATP are produced from these seven rounds. However, remember that the final round generates an extra acetyl CoA, representing an additional 10 ATP; $98+10 = 108$ ATP. Also, remember that 2 ATP are consumed during fatty acid activation. The net generation of ATP from the complete oxidation of palmitate is $108 - 2 = 106$ ATP.

ATP yield from β-oxidation of odd-numbered fatty acids

The final round of β-oxidation for an odd-numbered FA generates a propionyl CoA rather than an acetyl CoA. Propionyl CoA is metabolized to succinyl CoA, a TCA cycle intermediate (Chapter 4). Entry to the TCA cycle and complete oxidation to oxaloacetate yields one each of GTP, $FADH_2$ and $NADH+H^+$. This equates to 5 ATP; however, 1 ATP is consumed during conversion of propionyl CoA to succinyl CoA, so the energy yield represented by propionyl CoA is 4 ATP.

To calculate the number of rounds of β-oxidation an odd-numbered fatty acid must undertake, first minus 1 from the number of carbons and then divide by two and then minus 1 as with even-numbered FA. In the example of the seventeen-carbon margarate: $17 - 1 = 16$. $(16 \div 2) - 1 = 7$, so margarate undergoes seven cycles of β-oxidation.

Bearing this in mind, using margarate (C17) as an example, seven rounds of β-oxidation generate $14 \times 7 = 98$ ATP. The final round generates propionyl CoA, representing 4 ATP: $98+4 = 102$. Also, activation consumes 2 ATP: $102 - 2 = 100$. Therefore, total generation of ATP from complete oxidation of margarate is 100 ATP (Fig. 5.22).

Oxidation of unsaturated fatty acids

This process is slower than oxidation of saturated FA, since the carnitine shuttle is retarded by a cargo of unsaturated FA. The process of catabolism is similar to that of saturated FA, however two extra enzymes are required:

- Enoyl CoA isomerase converts *cis* C = C bonds to the *trans* configuration, allowing the FA to be recognised by the enzymes of β-oxidation. *cis* configurations are present in naturally occurring unsaturated FA, but the double bond introduced in β-oxidation is of the *trans* configuration

- NADP-dependent 2,4-dienoyl reductase participates in metabolism of unsaturated FA with double bonds at both even and odd-numbered carbon positions. For example, during the metabolism of the essential fatty acid linoleate (18:2 cΔ9,12) (note the double bonds at 9 and 12), the intermediate 2,4-dienoyl CoA is produced.

Peroxisomal β-oxidation

β-Oxidation occurs in peroxisomes as well as mitochondria. Peroxisomes are intracellular membrane-bound structures. The relative contributions of mitochondrial and peroxisomal β-oxidation are unclear and appear to be influenced by numerous factors in health and disease. However, catabolism of all very-long-chain (24 or more carbons) fatty acids and branched chain FA occurs in mammalian peroxisomes. This is because these FA are unable to use the carnitine shuttle and so cannot access the mitochondria. The actual process of β-oxidation is the same; however be aware that:

- The enzymes differ, for example a single peroxisomal enzyme performs hydration and oxidation
- $FADH_2$ produced in the first oxidation cannot enter the ETC; $FADH_2$'s pairs of H^+ ions and electrons are instead transferred to molecular O_2, forming H_2O_2 and generating heat, rather than ATP
- Acetyl CoA produced by each round of β-oxidation must transfer into the mitochondria for TCA cycle oxidation

Fig. 5.22 Comparison of ATP yields of six-carbon glucose and the six-carbon fatty acid caproiate	
Caproiate: 6 carbons	
Cycles of β-oxidation	$(6 \div 2) - 1 = 2$ cycles
Per cycle, 14 ATP are generated	$2 \times 14 = 28$ ATP
Final acetyl CoA represents	ATP
Cost of FA activation	$- 2$ ATP
Total ATP	$28+10 - 2 = $ **36 ATP**
Glucose: 6 carbons	
Glycolysis: 2 ATP	2 ATP
Glycolysis: 2 NADH+H$^+$	$2 (2.5) = 5$ ATP
Glycolysis: 2 Pyruvate 2 (Pyruvate →acetyl CoA conversion yield = 1 NADH+H$^+$), and since 1 NADH+H$^+\sim$ 2.5 ATP:	$2 (2.5) = 5$ ATP
2 (acetyl CoA)	$2 (10) = 20$ ATP
Total	$2+5+5+20 = $ **32 ATP**

- Once the fatty acyl CoA is shortened to medium length (6–12 carbons), it is esterified with carnitine, and then diffuses out from the peroxisome to the cytoplasm. It must enter the mitochondria via the carnitine shuttle for further β-oxidation.

Regulation of lipid breakdown

Control of lipid degradation operates at three levels. These are described below.

Regulation of lipolysis

Lipolysis controls oxidation of fatty acids by virtue of regulating FA availability. Hormone-sensitive lipase (HSL) is a major control point: remember, this enzyme catalyses the first step of TAG degradation, where the first FA is cleaved off the TAG. It is activated by phosphorylation, mediated by a cAMP-dependent protein kinase. Increase in intracellular cAMP increases phosphorylation of HSL. cAMP is synthesized from AMP by adenylate cyclase. This enzyme is activated by hormones adrenaline and glucagon – released in context requiring mobilization of energy reserves. Insulin lowers cAMP levels by activation of a phosphodiesterase that degrades cAMP. Therefore, insulin ultimately inhibits phosphorylation (activation) of HSL, inhibiting lipolysis (Chapter 8).

Regulation of mitochondrial access

Oxidation of fatty acids is limited by the rate they can access their oxidation site, i.e. the mitochondria, where β-oxidation of all short- and medium-chain FA occurs. Malonyl CoA, which increases when fatty acid synthesis is active, inhibits carnitine acyl transferase I and therefore FA import. This prevents simultaneous synthesis and oxidation occurring (a 'futile cycle').

Availability of NAD$^+$ and FAD

Both NAD$^+$ and FAD are required to function as redox partners in β-oxidation reactions. When these are scarce, due to cellular energy status being high (i.e. all the NAD$^+$ and FAD have been converted to NADH+H$^+$ and FADH$_2$), FA catabolism is inhibited due to lack of substrate availability. Conversely, when NAD$^+$ is plentiful, indicating low cellular energy status, FA catabolism is promoted.

Abnormalities of fatty acid metabolism

Deficiencies of the enzymes catalysing the first step of β-oxidation result in inability to successfully oxidize fatty acids. This imposes reliance upon catabolism of glucose, and can cause life-threatening hypoglycaemia when glycogen reserves and ultimately gluconeogenic substrates become exhausted. Individuals recovering from such metabolic crises may still suffer developmental delay. Clinical severity varies depending on how severely β-oxidation is impaired. Severe phenotypes can cause sudden unexplained death in infants, leading to this being a valid clinical differential for sudden infant death syndrome ('cot death').

Medium-chain acyl-CoA dehydrogenase deficiency is the most common disorder of β-oxidation and with an incidence of 1/14 600 is one of the most common inborn errors of metabolism. Newborn screening aims to identify individuals prior to clinical symptom development.

CHOLESTEROL METABOLISM

Cholesterol is a 27-carbon molecule. It is an integral structural component of all cell membranes, conferring permeability and regulating fluidity, as well as being a precursor of a wide range of hormones and other signalling molecules. There is continuous demand for this molecule, which is synthesized endogenously, but is also obtained in the diet from animal fat.

Cholesterol is transported in the vascular system as a component of lipoprotein particles. Long-term elevation of plasma cholesterol above a certain level has potentially serious pathological consequences for cardiovascular health. Excessive consumption of high-cholesterol foods contributes to development of high cholesterol, but, interestingly, ingested saturated fats contribute more to blood cholesterol levels than actual cholesterol intake.

Molecular features

Cholesterol is classed as a steroid because it contains a 17-carbon sterane core, a feature of all steroid molecules. Cholesterol contains 27 carbon atoms in total, all of which are derived from acetyl CoA. It contains four fused ring structures, two cyclohexane and one cyclopentane (Fig. 5.23). Different steroids vary by virtue of different functional groups attached to these rings, and also via the oxidation state of the rings themselves.

Physiological roles of cholesterol

Cholesterol is a precursor of various important physiological molecules, including:

- Bile acids, which mediate fat solubilization in the gut
- All steroid hormones, e.g. glucocorticoids, mineralocorticoids and sex hormones

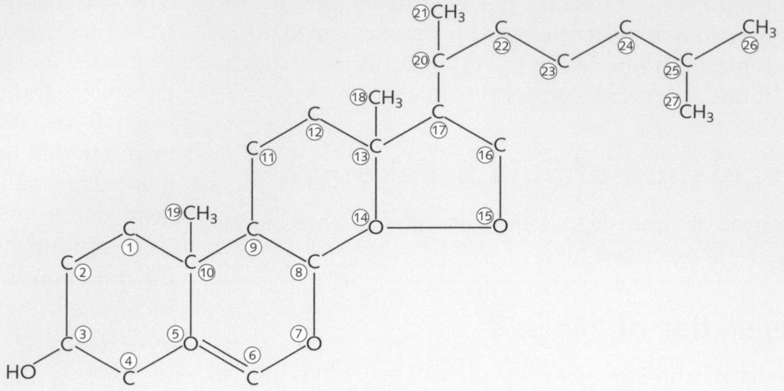

Fig. 5.23 Structure of cholesterol. Note that the hydrogen atoms are not detailed; appreciate that each C atom is fully saturated. If it is bonded to three other C atoms, one hydrogen atom fulfils the valence requirement. If bonded to two C atoms, two hydrogen atoms likewise fulfil the valence requirement, and so on.

- Vitamin D metabolites, which are mandatory for bone health and intact immune system function amongst their numerous diverse roles.

Cholesterol synthesis

This occurs in the cytoplasm, particularly the liver. The process comprises three stages:

- Stage I: formation of the basic isoprene unit
- Stage II: progressive assimilation of isoprene units to form squalene
- Stage III: conversion of squalene to lanosterol, and then lanosterol to cholesterol.

Stage I: formation of isopentyl pyrophosphate (IPP)

The 3-hydroxy-3-methylglutaryl-CoA (HMG-CoA) is first synthesized. This involves:

- Condensation of a pair of acetyl CoA molecules, generating the 4 C acetoacetyl CoA
- HMG-CoA synthase catalyses incorporation of a third acetyl CoA, generating HMG-CoA. This molecule is also an intermediate in ketogenesis, but the enzymes underpinning ketogenesis are mitochondrial, so cytoplasmic HMG-CoA cannot be diverted to ketogenesis.

HMG-CoA is then converted to isopentenyl pyrophosphate (IPP) in a two-step process:

- HMG-CoA is reduced to mevalonate by HMG-CoA reductase. $NADPH+H^+$ is the redox partner, undergoing oxidation to $NADP^+$. This is the irreversible, rate-limiting step of cholesterol synthesis
- Mevalonate is then phosphorylated and decarboxylated, forming IPP (the basic 5 C isoprene unit).

Stage II: Progressive assimilation of isoprene units to form squalene

- IPP units are first isomerized to dimethylallyl pyrophosphate (DMAP)
- DMAP combines with another IPP, forming geranyl pyrophosphate (GPP), a 10-carbon molecule
- GPP combines with another IPP unit, forming farnesyl pyrophosphate (FPP), a 15-carbon unit
- Two FFP now unite in a condensation reaction catalysed by squalene synthase. This generates squalene, a 30-carbon molecule. This reaction requires $NADPH+H^+$ as a redox partner.

HINTS AND TIPS

Ergosterol, a vital component of fungal cell membranes, is a useful antifungal drug target, particularly since it is absent in animal (including human) cell membranes. For example, allylamines such as terbinafine inhibit squalene epoxidase, blocking synthesis of ergosterol (which is derived from lanosterol). Imidazole antifungals such as clotrimazole inhibit fungal synthesis of ergosterol from lanosterol, whilst amphotericin B physically associates with ergosterol forming a monovalent ion channel.

Stage III: Further conversions: squalene → cholesterol

- Squalene epoxidase recruits molecular oxygen and $NADPH+H^+$, oxidizing squalene to squalene epoxide

- Lanosterol synthase converts squalene epoxide to lanosterol
- Finally, lanosterol is converted to cholesterol. This conversion involves a complex series of reactions, many of have yet to be characterized. In essence, three methyl ($-CH_3$) functional groups are removed, the double bond between C8 and C9 of lanosterol is found (in cholesterol) between C5 and C6 and the double bond between C24 and C25 is opened (Fig. 5.24).

Regulation of cholesterol synthesis

Product-mediated inhibition

Cholesterol, the pathway product, allosterically inhibits the synthesis pathway's rate-limiting enzyme, HMG-CoA reductase. Furthermore, HMG-CoA reductase synthesis is inversely proportional to intracellular cholesterol. Abundant intracellular cholesterol inhibits cholesterol synthesis by decreasing availability of the pathway's rate-limiting enzyme.

Hormonal regulation

The insulin:glucagon ratio regulates cholesterol synthesis activity; the greater this ratio the greater pathway activity. To understand the mechanism, it is important to recognise that HMG-CoA reductase is activated by dephosphorylation and inactivated by phosphorylation. Insulin and glucagon influence phosphorylation in the following ways:

- Insulin lowers intracellular cAMP (by up-regulation of a cAMP-degrading phosphodiesterase). Recall that cAMP activates a cAMP-dependent protein kinase, which is responsible for phosphorylation of a wide range of intracellular enzymes. Insulin also upregulates HMG-CoA reductase expression. Similarly, it down-regulates expression of HMG-CoA reductase kinase, which would otherwise phosphorylate and inactivate the enzyme. These factors contribute to insulin stimulation promoting endogenous cholesterol synthesis
- Glucagon and adrenaline activate adenylyl cyclase, increasing intracellular cAMP and consequently activity of the cAMP-dependent protein kinase (Chapter 8). This phosphorylates (inactivates) HMG-CoA reductase, inhibiting endogenous cholesterol synthesis in situations where these hormones are elevated, such as fasting. Glucagon also increases expression of HMG-CoA reductase kinase, thus promoting phosphorylation (inactivation) of HMG-CoA reductase.

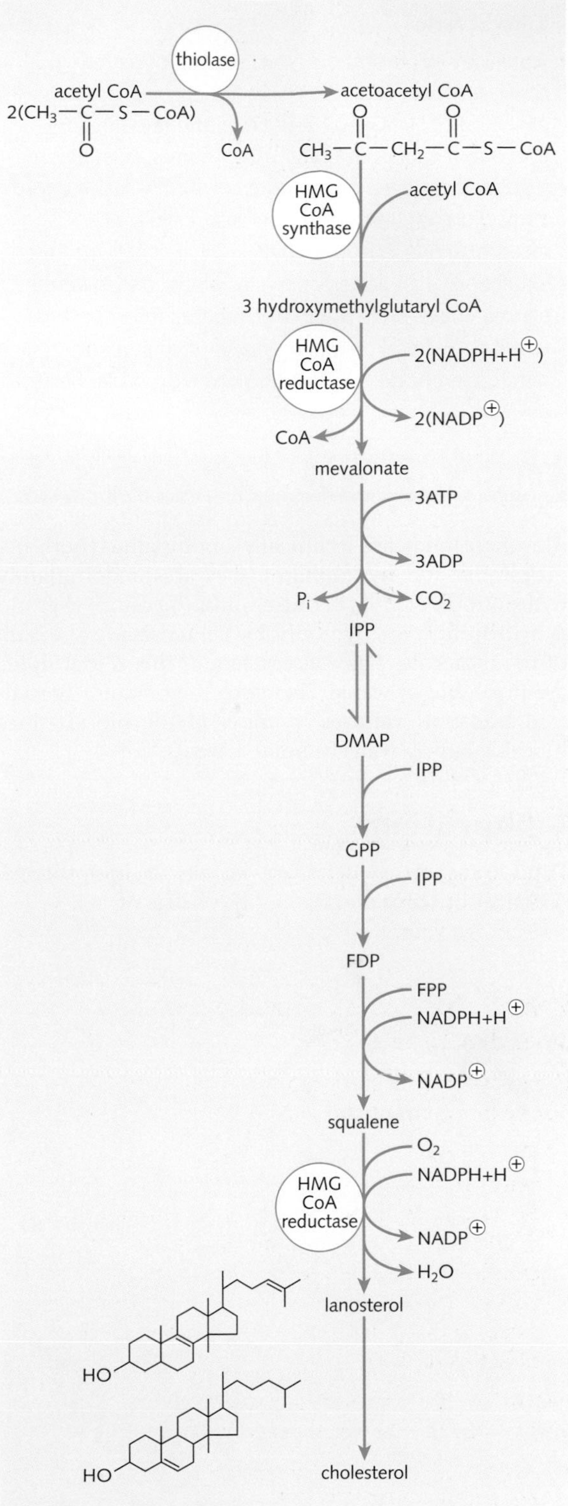

Fig. 5.24 Cholesterol synthesis.
IPP = isopentylpyrophosphate, DMAP = dimethylallyl pyrophosphate, GPP = geranyl pyrophosphate, FPP = farnesyl pyrophosphate.

LIPID TRANSPORT

Although lipids are technically amphipathic (both hydrophobic and hydrophilic), they are predominantly hydrophobic. This is because whilst the carboxyl group is hydrophilic, the hydrophobic tail represents the bulk of the molecule. The consequence of this is that lipids are insoluble in water. Therefore, they require specialized transport vehicles to travel in the blood, since blood is largely water, a polar solvent.

Lipoproteins

Lipid transport vehicles are known as lipoproteins. A typical lipoprotein (Fig. 5.25) consists of:

- A hydrophilic surface shell, typically composed of a phospholipid monolayer (hydrophilic head groups orientated outwards)
- Cholesterol. This is present in both the surface shell as free cholesterol and the lipoprotein interior as cholesterol esters
- Apoproteins; specialized proteins of lipoproteins (Fig. 5.26). They function as structural components, enzyme cofactors, and receptor binding sites for the lipoproteins
- Hydrophobic interior, consisting of the lipid cargo. This includes triacylglycerol and esterified cholesterol.

Lipoprotein classes

The different classes of lipoprotein are characterized by density, size, origin of lipid cargo, specific array of apoprotein and physiological role. The main properties are illustrated in Fig. 5.27.

Lipid processing

There are two main routes by which lipids are processed and access peripheral tissues, and these are differentiated by the origin of the lipid; exogenous (from the diet) or endogenous (synthesized physiologically).

Exogenous lipids

This describes the physiological digestion, absorption and transport of ingested lipids to tissue destination.

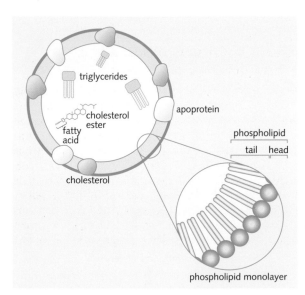

Fig. 5.25 Basic lipoprotein structure. Note phospholipid orientation; hydrophilic head groups orientated to the exterior of the structure, hydrophobic tail groups to the interior.

Fig. 5.26 Functions of major apoproteins.	
Apoprotein	**Characteristics**
AI	HDL shell protein. Activates LCAT. Interacts with ABCA1
AII	HDL shell protein
B48	Structural in CM
B100	Major VLDL, IDL and LDL shell protein
CI	CM apoprotein. Activates LCAT and LPL
CII	Present in mature VLDL, Acquired by CM. Cofactor for LPL
CIII	Found in HDL particles. Inhibits LPL
D	HDL apoprotein, also called cholesterol ester transfer protein
E	Present in mature VLDL, IDL HDL and mature CM particles

LCAT = lecithin : choline acetyltransferase, LPL = lipoprotein lipase, ABCA1 = ATP-binding cassette transporter-1

Fig. 5.27 Lipoprotein classes.

Lipoprotein	Density	Cargo origin	Apoproteins	Role
Chylomicron (CM)	Lowest	Dietary fatty acids and glycerol absorbed from intestinal cells	AI, AII, **B48**, CI, CII (mature CM), CII, E (mature CM)	Transport of lipids absorbed from ingested fats to the liver and rest of body
VLDL (very low density lipoprotein)	Very low	Assembled in the liver	**B100**, CI, CII, CIII, E	Distribution of lipids from the liver to the rest of the body
IDL (intermediate density lipoprotein)	Intermediate	VLDL particles	B100, CI, CII, CIII, **E**	IDL are a consequence of VLDLs progressively offloading lipid cargo and thus increasing in density. They continue in the same fashion, distributing lipids peripherally
LDL (low density lipoprotein)	Low	IDL particles	B100	LDL are a consequence of IDL progressively offloading lipid cargo and thus increasing in density. They continue in the same fashion, distributing lipids peripherally
HDL (high density lipoprotein)	High	Assembled in the liver	**AI, AII**, CI, CII, CIII, D, E	Transport peripheral cholesterol and other lipids to the liver for biliary excretion

1. Chylomicron formation

Lipases in the gastrointestinal (GI) tract hydrolyse dietary triacylglycerol, generating free fatty acids and 2-monoacylglycerol. These are absorbed across the lumenal face of enterocytes (epithelial cells lining the gut). Once in the enterocyte cell cytoplasm, products of lipid hydrolysis are assembled, along with apoprotein B-48, into chylomicrons (CM) (refer to Fig. 5.27).

2. Chylomicron circulation

CM are extruded from enterocytes into lacteals by exocytosis. Lacteals are blind-ending projections of the lymphatic system that protrude into intestinal villi. CM travel in the lymphatic system to the main vascular circulation via the thoracic duct. Once in the bloodstream, CM 'steal' apoproteins CII and E from HDL particles they encounter, and integrate them into the structure of their own surface shells.

3. Peripheral hydrolysis of chylomicron triacylglycerol cargo

Once chylomicrons (CM) have acquired surface CII apoproteins, their role can now switch from transport mode to delivery mode. This is because the newly acquired surface CII apoproteins allow CM to react with the enzyme lipoprotein lipase (LPL), since CII functions as a cofactor for this enzyme. LPL is sited at the surface of endothelial cells throughout the entire vascular system. On contact with CII (CM), LPL is activated and becomes able to perform its hydrolytic function on triacylglycerols in the CM interior. These are hydrolyzed to their fatty acid and glycerol components.

FA and glycerol diffuse across the vascular lumenal surface into endothelial cells. From here they are able to access the body tissues, such as adipocytes or muscle cells. They may be re-assembled into TAG for storage or catabolized to produce energy.

4. Loss of CII apoproteins: remnant generation

Now the triacylglycerol cargo has been delivered, the chylomicron is greatly reduced in size. The CM now thoughtfully returns CII apoproteins to any passing HDL it encounters. It does not, however, return the 'stolen' E apoproteins. These smaller structures, with E but not CII apoproteins, are known as chylomicron remnants. Note that at no point have the CM lost their B-48 apoproteins; these have been present throughout and maintain the CM remnant structure. When the remnants next traverse the hepatic circulation, they are endocytosed and degraded by hepatocytes (i.e. removed from the circulation) (Fig. 5.28).

Endogenous lipids

This describes transport of hepatically synthesized triacylglycerols from the liver to peripheral tissues.

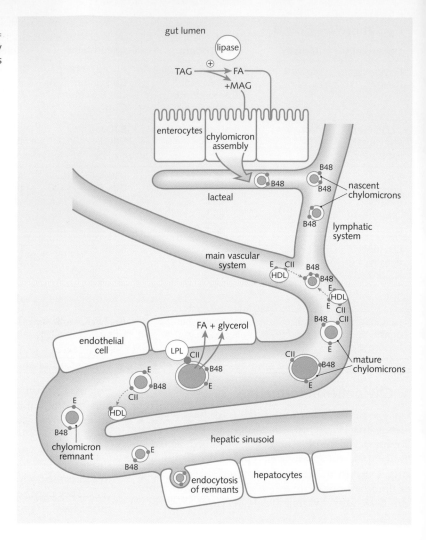

Fig. 5.28 Chylomicron life cycle: distribution of exogenous lipids. LPL = lipoprotein lipase, HDL = high-density lipoprotein. Endothelial LPL hydrolyzes CM TAG cargo to FA and glycerol which enters the endothelial cells. Please note this diagram is schematic not anatomically precise.

1. VLDL assembly

Very low-density lipoproteins (VLDL) are assembled in hepatocytes from triacylglycerol, cholesterol and apoprotein B100, and released into the circulation. Like chylomicrons, VLDL 'steal' apoproteins CII and E from HDL particles they encounter in the bloodstream. Once these are acquired, VLDL are termed 'mature'; prior to acquisition of CII and E, they are termed 'nascent'.

2. LPL hydrolysis of VLDL cargo

Just as with chylomicrons, CII functions as a cofactor for endothelial LPL, allowing hydrolysis of VLDL triacylglycerol cargo and release of fatty acids and glycerol. The only difference is that the triacylglycerol cargo of the VLDL is endogenously synthesized rather than acquired from the diet (as in chylomicrons).

3. IDL and LDL formation

Progressive offloading of cargo leaves the VLDL reduced in size. IDL now return CII (but not apoprotein E) to HDL they encounter in the circulation, just like triacylglycerol-depleted chylomicrons. During this encounter, HDLs also donate cholesterol esters (mediated by plasma cholesterol ester transfer protein), and in exchange receive phospholipids and triacylglycerols from the VLDL. The resulting lipoprotein is now known as VLDL remnants (a term pretty much equivalent to intermediate-density lipoprotein (IDL)).

HINTS AND TIPS

'Intermediate density' in this context refers to density intermediate to 'very low density' and 'low density', rather than intermediate between 'high density' and 'low density'.

Some remnants are endocytosed and dismantled by the liver, but those remaining in the circulation are further depleted of their TAG cargo, progressively reducing in size (and increasing in density). Further encounters with HDL results in further depletion of TAG, further loss of CII and increase in cholesterol ester load. This results in remnants (IDL) progressively transforming into LDL.

4. Cholesterol offloading at periphery

LDL apoprotein E binds to endothelial LDL-receptors, mediating internalization of the entire particle by endocytosis. Internalized LDL fuse with lysosomes, lysosomal enzymes dismantling the LDL and releasing cholesterol intracellularly. This may enter various synthetic pathways, or may be esterified with fatty acids to form cholesterol esters. This esterification is mediated by acyl-CoA: cholesterol acyl transferase (ACAT) (Fig. 5.29).

HDL metabolism

HDL (the smallest, densest lipid transport vehicle) are assembled in the liver and intestine from apoproteins AI, AII, E and phospholipids. HDL donate apoproteins to chylomicrons and VLDL particles. HDL also play a very important role in cholesterol metabolism; by transporting excess cellular cholesterol through the bloodstream to the liver for excretion in bile.

> **HINTS AND TIPS**
>
> Remember that intracellular cholesterol inhibits HMG-CoA reductase, inhibiting endogenous synthesis and reducing intracellular cholesterol. Statins also inhibit this enzyme, with the same effect. Note also that reduced intracellular cholesterol enhances transcription of the LDL-receptor, increasing the amount of cholesterol the cell can assimilate via LDL. This up-regulation of LDL-receptor expression is the main physiological mechanism for lowering plasma cholesterol, and is also the mechanism by which statins exert their therapeutic effects.

Cholesterol: modification for transport

Prior to integration into HDL, cholesterol undergoes esterification. The polar hydroxyl group at C3 (see Fig. 5.23) is hydrophilic, and cholesterol tends to locate itself superficially in lipid phases, such as the phospholipid monolayer. However, molecular 'shielding' of this hydroxyl group allows cholesterol to be packaged in the hydrophobic interior of lipoproteins, allowing for increased transport capacity.

'Shielding' involves covering the –OH group with a fatty acid acyl group. This is an esterification reaction and the reaction product is a cholesterol ester. This may occur intracellularly, in which case it is catalysed by acyl CoA:cholesterol acyl transferase (ACAT). It may also be performed by HDL, in which case it is catalysed by plasma lecithin:cholesterol acyl transferase (LCAT). In the case of HDL, the fatty acid used to modify cholesterol is sourced from the phospholipid phosphatidylcholine, which is present within the HDL shell.

Excess cellular cholesterol elimination

HDL apoprotein AI interacts with the ATP-binding cassette transporter 1 (ABCA1), aka cholesterol efflux regulatory protein. ABCA1 is a cellular cholesterol efflux pump, ejecting excess cholesterol from cells into blood plasma. This free cholesterol is then esterified by plasma LCAT, and internalized to HDL interior.

Cellular cholesterol clearance

HDL interacts with (and removes cholesterol from) peripheral cells such as macrophages, which may contribute to the well-established association between higher HDL levels and reduced atheromatous disease.

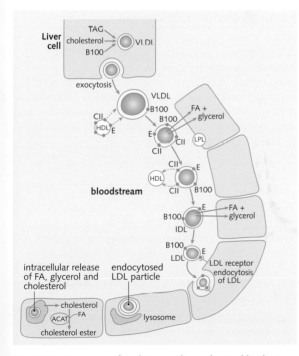

Fig. 5.29 Transport of endogenously synthesized lipids via VLDL, IDL and LDL particles. VLDL CII acts as a cofactor for endothelial LPL, allowing hydrolysis of the TAG cargo and offloading the products FA and glycerol. ACAT = acyl-CoA: cholesterol acyltransferase.

Clinical Note

Atheromata (atherosclerotic plaques) are arterial wall deposits, which may be fibrous or lipid-rich. Lipid-rich atheromata consist of cells, connective tissue elements, lipids and debris. They are medically significant since they narrow arterial lumens and, if they rupture, promote thrombus formation and rapid occlusion. In the coronary arteries, complete occlusion results in ischaemia and necrosis of downstream heart muscle; a myocardial infarction.

Genetic dyslipidaemias

Dyslipidaemia is elevation of plasma triglycerides or total cholesterol (or both) resulting from an abnormality of lipid metabolism or uptake. This can be due to a deficiency in either:

- An enzyme (e.g. LPL)
- An apoprotein (e.g. CII, E)
- A receptor (e.g. the LDL-receptor).

HINTS AND TIPS

The term 'triglycerides' is used synonymously with 'triacylglycerol', however as 'triglycerides' is used in clinical biochemistry and medicine, this term will be used in this section.

Inappropriately high cholesterol or triglycerides result in equally inappropriate deposition of lipid in multiple locations, including the skin, connective tissue, the corneal limbus and arterial walls. This results in development of palmar and tendon xanthomata, periorbital xanthelasma, corneal arcus and atheromata respectively. These features comprise the clinical phenotype of dyslipidaemia. Severe hypertriglyceridaemia may also cause acute pancreatitis.

Two clinically important examples of genetic dyslipidaemia are discussed below, but be aware that there are many; consult a reference textbook for more detail.

Familial hypercholesterolaemia

Familial hypercholesterolaemia is the most common inherited dyslipidaemia. This condition results from an absent or dysfunctional LDL-receptor (95%) or defective B100 apoproteins (remaining 5%). This results in reduced (heterozygotes) or absent (homozygotes) cellular uptake of circulating LDL, resulting in increased plasma LDL.

Homozygotes have extreme hypercholesterolaemia, exhibit all the clinical features of the hyperlipidaemias phenotype and experience childhood onset of symptomatic coronary atherosclerosis. In heterozygotes the hypercholesterolaemia is less pronounced, since half the receptor population is functional, but individuals are still at increased susceptibility of cardiovascular disease.

Familial chylomicronaemia

This is a very rare, autosomal recessive condition. It is defined by gross elevation of plasma chylomicrons. This occurs because of deficiency or absence of either the enzyme LPL or its cofactor, apoprotein CII. This results in hypertriglyceridaemia from the extremely high plasma chylomicron. This causes frequent pancreatitis, and strict avoidance of dietary fat and alcohol is mandatory to manage symptoms.

Fig. 5.30 Lipid-lowering drugs.

Drug	Mechanism of action
Statins, e.g. rosuvastatin, pravastatin atorvastatin, simvastatin, etc.	Inhibit HMG-CoA reductase, resulting in reduced endogenous synthesis of cholesterol
Fibrates, e.g. bezafibrate, fenofibrate, etc.	Potentiate the hepatocyte PPAR-α receptor signaling cascade. Amongst the many effects, hepatic β-oxidation of FA is enhanced and increased synthesis of HDL particles ensues
Bile acid sequestrants, e.g. colesevelam, colestipol, etc.	These bind and 'sequester' bile acids in the gut lumen, preventing their reabsorption. Their subsequent loss reduces the total capacity for lipid absorption. Now rarely used
Cholesterol absorption attenuators (Ezetimibe)	Localizes to enterocyte apical membranes (within the gut lumen). Here it inhibits absorption of dietary cholesterol. Decreased cholesterol absorption results in up-regulation of LDL receptors, increasing LDL clearance from the blood

Acquired hypercholesterolaemia

This is raised total plasma cholesterol (>5.0 mmol) in the absence of an inherited disorder of lipid metabolism. It is typically accompanied by raised LDL (>3.0 mmol). It is at least partially attributable to a high intake of saturated fat, and is partially correctable by diet and lifestyle modification.

However, since elevated plasma cholesterol has such serious implications for cardiovascular health, a number of therapeutic drugs have been developed to manage this risk (Fig. 5.30). Statins are by far the most commonly used preparations.

KETONES AND KETOGENESIS

In biochemistry, the term 'ketones' (also called 'ketone bodies') refers to three particular molecules. They are all acetyl CoA-derived, and function as substrates for ATP generation. The three biologically significant ketones are:

- Acetoacetate
- 3-Hydroxybutyrate
- Acetone.

They are continuously synthesized in the liver at low levels, but when intracellular glucose is low, their synthesis is up-regulated.

Ketone synthesis

Ketone synthesis, or 'ketogenesis', occurs in the mitochondrial matrix of hepatocytes. Acetyl CoA is the substrate of the synthesis pathway. It may derive from:

- β-Oxidation of fatty acids
- Catabolism of the ketogenic amino acids leucine, tryptophan and isoleucine
- Pyruvate dehydrogenase-mediated oxidative decarboxylation of pyruvate.

The pathway is illustrated in Fig. 5.31.

Formation of acetoacetate

Three acetyl CoA molecules condense to form HMG-CoA, just as in the cholesterol synthesis pathway (Fig. 5.24). However, cholesterol synthesis occurs in the cytoplasm, and ketogenesis in the mitochondria, so HMG-CoA can only participate in one of these pathways, determined by its location. HMG-CoA then releases acetyl CoA (mediated by HMG-CoA lyase), forming **acetoacetate**.

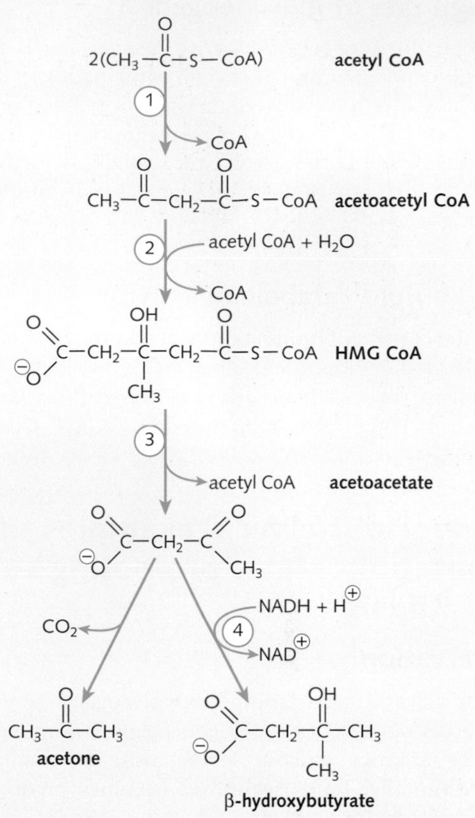

Fig. 5.31 Ketone synthesis. HMG-CoA = 3-hydroxy-2-methylglutaryl-CoA. 1 = β-ketothiolase, 2 = HMG-CoA synthase, 3 = HMG-CoA lyase, 4 = β-hydroxybutyrate-dehydrogenase.

Acetoacetate conversion to acetone or 3-hydroxybutyrate

Note that catabolism of the amino acids tyrosine, phenylalanine, leucine and lysine generates acetoacetate, which may integrate into the ketogenesis pathway at this point. Acetoacetate may spontaneously decarboxylate, forming acetone, or may be reduced by 3-hydroxybutyrate dehydrogenase to 3-hydroxybutyrate. This latter reaction requires NADH+H$^+$ as a redox partner and represents the main fate of acetoacetate.

Regulation of ketone synthesis

Regulation of ketone synthesis is primarily by substrate (acetyl CoA) availability. There are two main metabolic contexts in which ketogenesis is particularly active; high lipid catabolism activity and high rate of gluconeogenesis.

High rate of gluconeogenesis

When gluconeogenesis is active, oxaloacetate is diverted to gluconeogenesis, rather than participating in the TCA cycle. Reduced oxaloacetate availability has the consequence of less acetyl CoA consumption by the TCA cycle. This increases acetyl CoA availability for ketogenesis. A high rate of gluconeogenesis results in increased ketogenesis.

High lipid catabolism activity

In the context of lipid catabolism, plasma FA is elevated. This provides abundant substrate for β-oxidation by numerous tissues. In the liver, increased β-oxidation increases hepatocyte mitochondrial acetyl CoA. This increases acetyl CoA availability for ketogenesis.

Important clinical examples of metabolic states promoting ketone synthesis

Starvation

During prolonged fasting, once glycogen reserves have been exhausted, hepatic gluconeogenesis is up-regulated, since plasma glucose levels must be maintained. Additionally, lipid catabolism becomes predominant. Therefore, in starvation, both metabolic scenarios promoting ketone synthesis are present. This explains the observed rise in plasma ketones (Chapter 8).

Type 1 diabetes: diabetic ketoacidosis

Untreated or inadequately treated (insufficient insulin replacement) type 1 diabetic patients are insulin-deficient. This insulin insufficiency is accompanied by elevation of hormones such as glucagon and adrenaline (epinephrine). These promote widespread lipid mobilization, leading to an increase in plasma FA level and ultimately increased ketogenesis via the mechanisms discussed previously. In addition, hepatic gluconeogenesis is highly active during insulin insufficiency (even though blood glucose is elevated), due in part to the low insulin:glucagon ratio (Chapter 4). Insulin insufficiency promotes ketogenesis (leading to increased plasma ketones) by both mechanisms. Metabolic acidosis and elevation of plasma ketones secondary to insulin insufficiency is known as diabetic ketoacidosis (DKA). DKA is uncommon in type 2 diabetes.

Ketoacidosis

Ketoacidosis results from ketone accumulation. Acetoacetate and 3-hydroxybutyrate are chemically carboxylic acids; at physiological pH they are in the anionic form,

dissociated from their H^+ ions. If ketones production is excessive and prolonged, these H^+ ions cause acidosis (plasma pH < 7.35, or $[H^+] > 10^{-7.35}$) once normal physiological buffering systems are overwhelmed. This scenario is known as ketoacidosis; acidosis due to pathological ketone elevation.

It is important to understand the difference between the terms 'ketosis' and 'ketoacidosis'. 'Ketosis' describes an elevated level of ketones in the blood, and is a normal consequence of ketone synthesis. 'Ketoacidosis' is a pathological state occurring when ketones accumulate to the extent they cause significant metabolic acidosis. Ketoacidosis is a feature of decompensated diabetes mellitus (particularly type 1; see Chapter 8).

Ketone catabolism

Ketones are oxidized in mitochondria, generating acetyl CoA. In this way, ketones may be thought of as 'alternatives' to glucose, since their oxidation generates acetyl CoA to fuel TCA cycle oxidation, ultimately generating ATP to meet the cell's energy requirements.

In starvation, once glycogen reserves are exhausted, plasma glucose is maintained at the expense of muscle protein breakdown. This provides amino acids to sustain hepatic gluconeogenesis, but with the unhelpful side-effect of further weakening the starving individual.

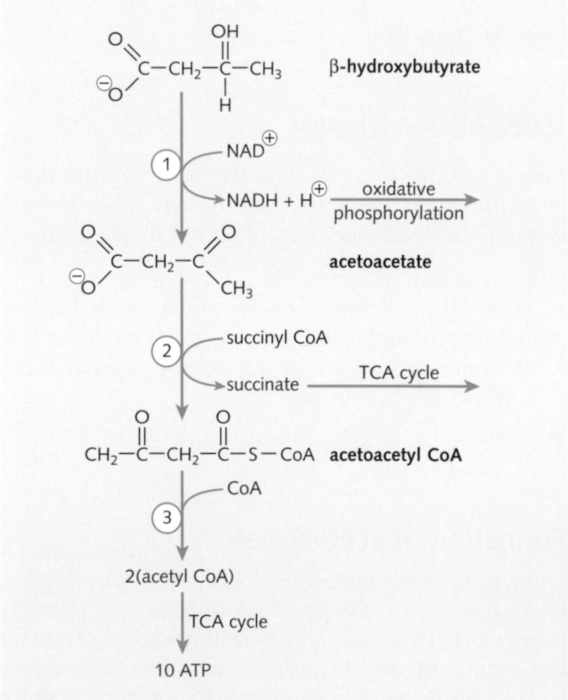

Fig. 5.32 Ketone catabolism. 1 = β-hydroxybutyrate dehydrogenase, 2 = β-ketoacyl-CoA transferase, 3 = β-ketothiolase.

Existence of ketones as 'back-up' oxidation substrate reduces the demand placed on gluconeogenesis to produce glucose for cellular oxidation in the various tissues.

Ketone catabolism can occur in all mitochondria-containing cells (except hepatocytes, since the enzyme 3-ketoacyl-CoA transferase is absent in the liver). The pathway is shown in Fig. 5.32. NAD^+ is required as a redox partner for oxidation of 3-hydroxybutyrate to acetoacetate, producing $NADH+H^+$; however since the reverse of this reaction occurs during original synthesis of 3-hydroxybutyrate from acetoacetate, there is no net generation of $NADH+H^+$.

Ketone utilization in the CNS

In hypoglycaemic states, the CNS is forced to partially switch from glycolysis to ketone oxidation for acetyl CoA production. Fatty acids cannot cross the blood–brain barrier and so are of no use to the CNS for acetyl CoA generation; thus the CNS relies on glucose and ketones to meet its metabolic demands. The CNS is able to gradually increase ketone utilization relative to glycolysis during sustained hypoglycaemia, but unable to make a complete transition. This persistent reliance on glucose accounts for why blood glucose levels must be always maintained.

Ketone utilization in cardiac myocytes

Surprisingly, cardiac myocytes preferentially catabolize fatty acids in all metabolic contexts except starvation. This means that these cells utilize β-oxidation of fatty acids (rather than glycolysis) to generate acetyl CoA for TCA cycle oxidation and energy generation. In starvation, when plasma FA gradually diminishes, cardiac myocytes are able to switch to ketone catabolism to meet their energy requirements.

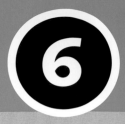
Objectives

After reading this chapter you should be able to:

- Reproduce the basic amino acid structure
- Appreciate the role of amino acids in metabolism
- Describe amino acid import via the γ-glutamyl transport cycle
- Outline the synthesis of certain amino acids
- Understand transamination and oxidative deamination
- Describe amino acid catabolism, including transdeamination
- Appreciate the need for and outline the mechanism of the urea cycle
- Briefly detail protein degradation and synthesis

PROTEIN STRUCTURE

Amino acids link with each other via peptide bonds, forming a polymer ('polypeptide'). The name 'protein' is reserved for polypeptides containing 50 or more amino acid residues. A protein may also consist of a single polypeptide, or may be a number of closely associated polypeptides. The linear order of the amino-acid sequence in a polypeptide (protein) is termed the primary structure.

Amino acids also associate with each other via a second type of bond. They form hydrogen bonds between the oxygen atom of the C=O component of the carboxyl group of one amino acid and the amino N atom of another (see Fig. 6.1). These hydrogen bonds are responsible for the spontaneous formation of protein 'secondary structure'. These are ubiquitous architectural features, such as α-helices and β-pleated sheets.

Protein 'tertiary structure' describes the three-dimensional structure that a polypeptide adopts, whilst retaining the secondary structure features. Finally, 'quaternary structure' describes the interaction between different polypeptide chains – how they associate with each other to form the complete protein.

AMINO ACIDS

Proteins are composed of amino acids. Amino acids all share a common structural 'skeleton', which includes an amino group (the N-terminus of the protein molecule) and a carboxyl group (the C-terminus) (Fig. 6.1). Individual amino acids have different side-chains ('R-groups'), which confer them with different properties (Fig. 6.2). Amino acids form bonds with each other via peptide bonds (Fig. 6.3).

KEY REACTIONS IN AMINO ACID METABOLISM

There are two types of reaction that one must appreciate before understanding amino acid metabolism. These are transamination and oxidative deamination. Both perform the same function; removal of the amino group $(-NH_2)$ from the carbon skeleton of the amino acid.

Transamination: conversion of any amino acid into alanine, glutamate or aspartate

The amino group of any amino acid is transferred to α-ketoglutarate, converting it to glutamate. The deaminated molecule is now structurally a keto-acid. This is catalysed by the aminotransferase enzymes (Fig. 6.4), all of which use pyridoxal phosphate (PLP) as a co-factor. The second reaction converts the newly formed glutamate into alanine, aspartate or glutamate, depending on whether the glutamate reacts with pyruvate,

Fig. 6.1 Molecular structure of an amino acid. 'R' represents the R-group.

One letter code	Three letter code	Amino acid	Essential or non-essential	Side group	Additional information
R	ARG	Arginine	Essential	$-CH_2-CH_2-CH_2-C{\overset{NH_2}{\underset{NH_2}{+}}}$	Precursor for nitric oxide. Role in the urea cycle. Basic R-group
H	HIS	Histidine	Essential	$-CH_2-$ (imidazole ring) N—H	Basic R-group
I	ILE	Isoleucine	Essential	$-CH{\overset{CH_3}{\underset{CH_2-CH_3}{}}}$	Hydrophobic R-group; hence normally located in the interior of protein structures
L	LEU	Leucine	Essential	$-CH_2-CH{\overset{CH_3}{\underset{CH_3}{}}}$	Like isoleucine, leucine has a hydrophobic R-group; hence normally located in the interior of protein structures
K	LYS	Lysine	Essential	$-CH_2-CH_2-CH_2-CH_2-NH_3^+$	Basic R-group
M	MET	Methionine	Essential	$-CH_2-CH_2-S-CH_3$	Cysteine precursor
T	THR	Threonine	Essential	$-CH{\overset{OH}{\underset{CH_3}{}}}$	-OH group in the R-group is a site for post-translational modification such as O-linked glycosylation
W	TRP	Tryptophan	Essential	$-CH_2-$ (indole ring)	Precursor to serotonin and melatonin
F	PHE	Phenylalanine	Essential	$-CH_2-$ (benzene ring)	Precursor to catecholamine hormones noradrenaline, adrenaline and dopamine, and also the pigment melanin. Tyrosine precursor
V	VAL	Valine	Essential	$-CH{\overset{CH_3}{\underset{CH_3}{}}}$	Hydrophobic R-group; hence normally located in the interior of protein structures
A	ALA	Alanine	Non-essential	$-CH_3$	In muscle, via the glucose-alanine cycle, alanine fulfils the role glutamine performs in all other tissues, i.e. transport of nitrogen to the liver for urea synthesis
N	ASN	Asparagine	Non-essential	$-CH_2-C{\overset{NH_2}{\underset{O}{}}}$	Few metabolic roles aside component of proteins
D	ASP	Aspartate	Non-essential	$-CH_2-C{\overset{O^-}{\underset{O}{}}}$	Amino group donor of the urea cycle. Role in purine and pyrimidine synthesis. Acidic R-group. Precursor of threonine
C	CYS	Cysteine	Non-essential	$-CH_2-SH$	Sulphur-containing R-group allows important structural role in proteins (disulphide bridges). Component of glutathione
E	GLU	Glutamate	Non-essential	$-CH_2-CH_2-C{\overset{O^-}{\underset{O}{}}}$	Operates as in intermediate linking nitrogen metabolism with carbon metabolism. Central neurotransmitter. Acidic R-group
Q	GLN	Glutamine	Non-essential	$-CH_2-CH_2-C{\overset{NH_2}{\underset{O}{}}}$	Able to cross the blood-brain barrier. Functions to transport nitrogen from most tissues to the liver for urea synthesis
G	GLY	Glycine	Non-essential	$-H$	'Imino' amino acid. Central neurotransmitter. Important structural component of collagen. Role in synthesis of purines, porphyrins, creatine and glutathione. Participation in drug metabolism. Component of glutathione

Fig. 6.2   Amino acid reference table.

Continued

One letter code	Three letter code	Amino acid	Essential or non-essential	Side group	Additional information
P	PRO	Proline	Non-essential	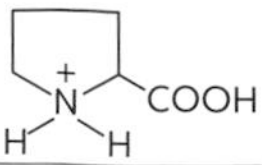	Also an 'imino' amino acid. This is the only amino acid where the side chain incorporates the α-amino group of the amino acid skeleton
S	SER	Serine	Non-essential	CH_2-OH	Contribution of activated one-carbon units required for tetrahydrofolate conenzymes. Required for biosynthesis of cysteine and phospholipids
Y	TYR	Tyrosine	Non-essential	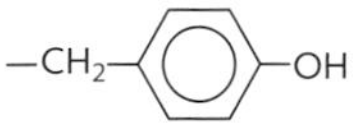	Precursor in synthesis of catecholamines, melanin and thyroxine

Fig. 6.2—cont'd

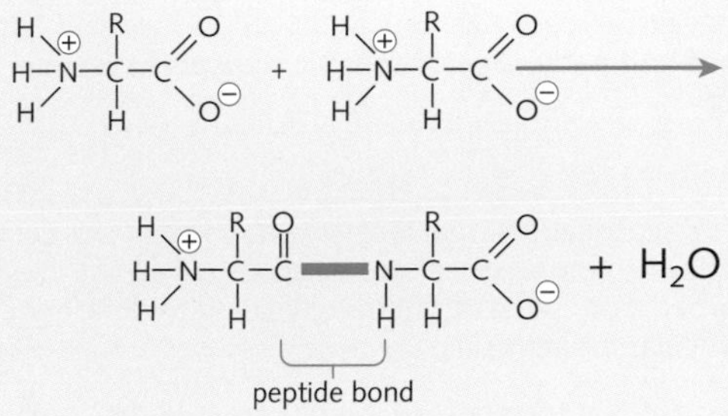

Fig. 6.3 Formation of a peptide bond between two amino acids.

oxaloacetate or α-ketoglutarate respectively. The transaminase enzyme catalysing this second reaction is named according to the end product; e.g. alanine transaminase (ALT) or aspartate transaminase (AST).

Oxidative deamination: removal of the amino group

In these reactions, the amino group of an amino acid is removed (resulting in the formation of α-ketoglutarate) and released as ammonia (NH_3). This enters the urea cycle for excretion. The redox partner for this oxidation is NAD^+ (Fig. 6.5). The main substrate for oxidative deamination is glutamate, since most amino acids are degraded (as described previously) by the transamination generating glutamate.

Amino acid transport

Since amino acids are present at much higher concentrations intracellularly than extracellularly, amino acid import requires energy. Transporters exist that couple ATP

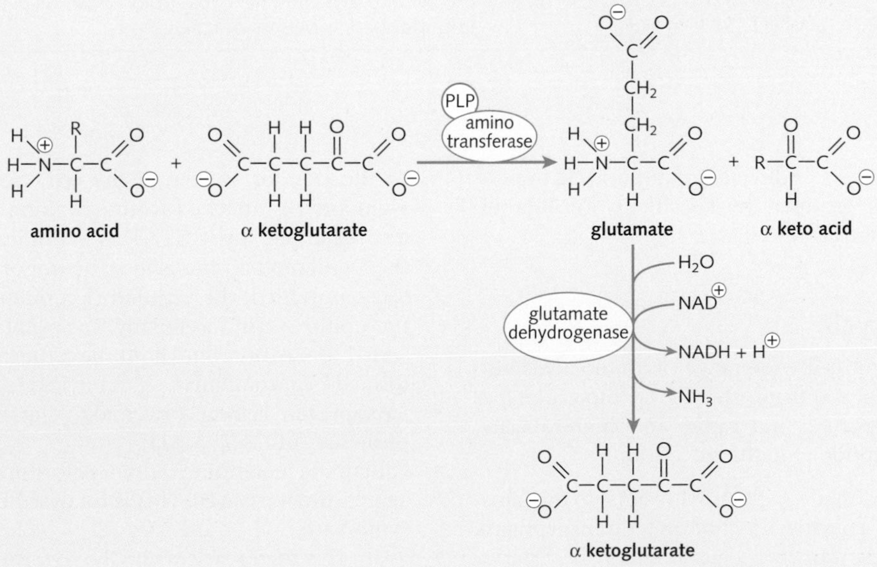

Fig. 6.4 Transamination reactions. The example illustrates the glutamate → α-ketoglutarate transamination.

Fig. 6.5 Oxidative deamination of glutamate.

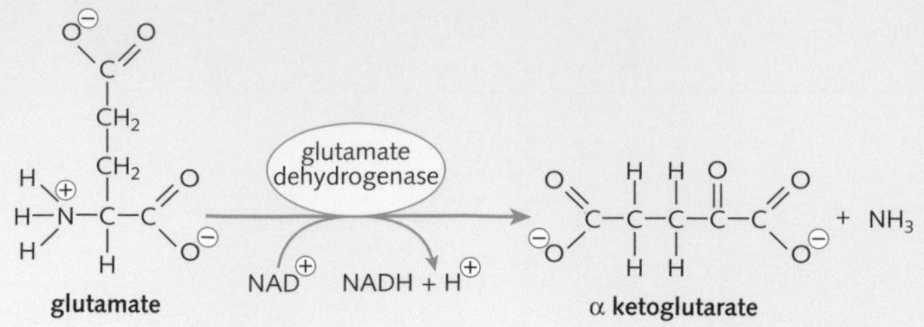

Fig. 6.6 Amino acid transporters.

R-group properties	Specific amino acids transported	Inheritance and pathology of specific transport system deficiency
Small and neutral	ALA, SER, THR	–
Large and neutral/Aromatic	ILE, LEU, VAL, TYR, TRY, PHE	Hartnup's disease: autosomal recessive absence of this carrier system. These amino acids cannot be absorbed across the gut or reabsorbed from renal ultrafiltrate, leading to deficiency of these particular amino acids
Basic (positively charged) and cysteine	ARG, LYS, HIS, CYS	Cystinuria: autosomal recessive condition resulting from absence of this carrier system. This causes inability to reabsorb cysteine from renal ultrafiltrate, leading to crystallisation of cysteine and stone formation in the renal tract
Negatively charged (acidic)	GLU, ASP	–
Neutral large/Neutral small	ALA, SER, THR, GLY, CYS, GLN, ASN	–
'Imino' acids: proline and glycine	PRO, GLY	Iminoglycinuria: autosomal recessive illness resulting from the carrier deficiency, causing failure of both absorption of dietary proline and glycine and reabsorption from renal ultrafiltrate. Important components of collagen

hydrolysis (directly or indirectly) to amino acid import. Transporters are grouped by specificity for R-group properties (Fig. 6.6).

γ-glutamyl cycle

This process imports a wide range of amino acids into cells. It is active, requiring three ATP molecules per amino acid imported, but rapid and high-capacity. It utilizes the peptide glutathione

- Glutathione donates γ-glutamyl residue to the transmembrane enzyme γ-glutamyl transpeptidase (GGT), which transfers γ-glutamyl to the exterior face of the membrane. The glutathione Cys-Gly 'remnant' remains intracellular

- At the exterior surface of the cell membrane, the γ-glutamyl is attached to the awaiting amino acid, also catalysed by GGT. This modification allows the γ-glutamyl-amino acid to be imported by GGT
- Once imported, the γ-glutamyl component releases the amino acid intracellularly. The γ-glutamate is converted to 5'oxoproline. Both these functions are performed by intracellular γ-glutamyl cyclo-transferase
- 5'oxoproline is then converted to glutamate by oxoprolinase, utilizing 1 ATP
- Glutamate recombines with Cys forming γ-Glu-Cys, again utilizing 1 ATP. This is catalysed by γ-Glu-Cys synthetase
- γ-Glu-Cys then reacts with Gly, re-forming glutathione. This is catalysed by glutathione synthetase, again utilizing 1 ATP (Fig. 6.7).

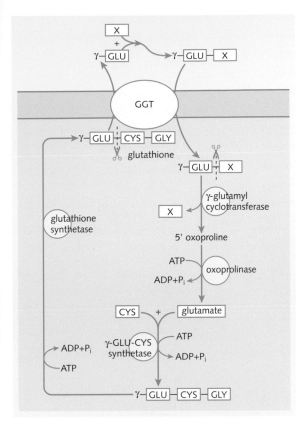

Fig. 6.7 General amino acid import: the γ-glutamyl cycle.
GLU = glutamate, CYS = cysteine, GLY = glycine.

'Essential' and 'non-essential' amino acids

Essential amino acids are mainly those that humans cannot endogenously synthesize de novo and thus required in the diet. However, arginine, phenylalanine and methionine are considered essential although they can be synthesized endogenously. This is for the following reasons:

- Arginine is not synthesized at a fast enough rate to meet physiological demand, mainly because the majority of arginine synthesis occurs in the context of nitrogen excretion during the urea cycle
- Phenylalanine likewise is not synthesized sufficiently rapidly for normal requirements, since a large amount is diverted towards tyrosine synthesis
- Methionine, similarly, is required in high quantities to synthesize cysteine, and is considered 'essential' since maximal endogenous synthesis still requires dietary supplementation.

The non-essential amino acids are those that can be synthesized endogenously. Their synthesis is described below.

Glutamate, glutamine, proline and arginine biosynthesis

These are grouped together since glutamate is used as a substrate for synthesis of the other three.

Glutamate biosynthesis

α-Ketoglutarate is converted to glutamate by transamination. This is, as described earlier, mediated by glutamate dehydrogenase (Fig. 6.4).

Glutamine biosynthesis

Glutamine is synthesized by amidation of glutamate by glutamine synthetase (Fig. 6.8). This combines NH_3 (ammonia) with glutamate, and requires ATP hydrolyzis.

Proline biosynthesis

This is a three-step pathway (Fig. 6.8):

- Reduction of glutamate to glutamate γ-semialdehyde (redox partner is $NADPH + H^+$)
- Glutamate γ-semialdehyde spontaneously undergoes molecular rearrangement to lower-energy pyrroline-5-carboxylate
- Pyrroline-5-carboxylate is reduced to proline (reaction redox partner is $NADPH + H^+$).

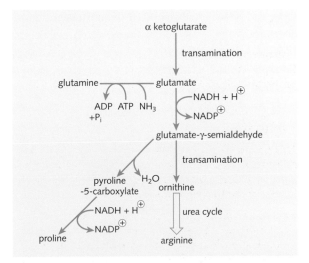

Fig. 6.8 Synthesis of glutamate, glutamine, proline and arginine.

Arginine biosynthesis

Like proline synthesis, glutamate is first reduced to glutamate γ-semialdehyde (redox partner $NADPH + H^+$). This is then transaminated, forming ornithine. Ornithine enters the urea cycle, ultimately forming arginine.

Aspartate and asparagine biosynthesis

Asparagine is a derivative of aspartate.

- Aspartate is formed by transamination of oxaloacetate. This is catalysed by aspartate-aminotransferase, and the amino group is helpfully provided by glutamate (which is converted to α-ketoglutarate)
- Aspartate is then converted to asparagine by asparagine synthetase. The amide group is donated by glutamine. This reaction consumes an ATP (Fig. 6.9).

Serine, glycine and cysteine biosynthesis

Serine biosynthesis

The majority of serine synthesis occurs in cell cytoplasm. This utilizes 3-phosphoglycerate (a glycolytic intermediate; Chapter 4). The pathway involves three steps: oxidation, transamination and hydrolysis (Fig. 6.10).

Glycine biosynthesis

This occurs mitochondrially, via two routes. One is the generation of glycine from serine (serine hydroxymethyltransferase). The other (not illustrated) is catalysed by glycine synthase, uses $NADH + H^+$ as a redox partner and requires the ammonium ion (NH_4^+), CO_2, and N^5N^{10}-methylene-THF as substrates.

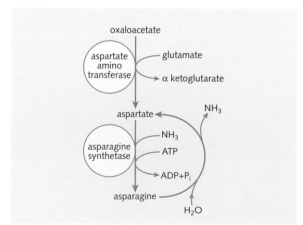

Fig. 6.9   Aspartate and asparagine synthesis.

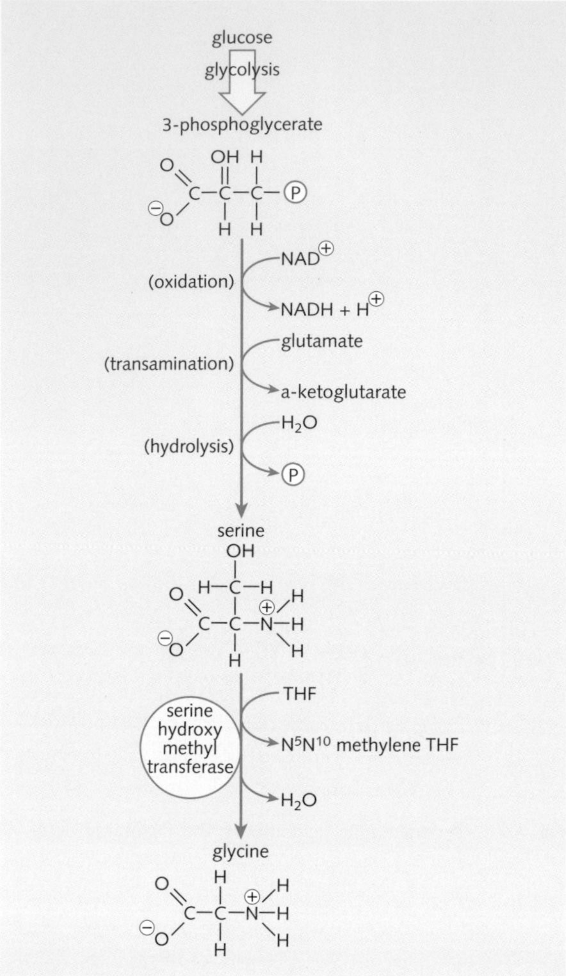

Fig. 6.10   Serine and glycine synthesis. As many of the enzymes in serine synthesis have not yet been conclusively identified, some names are omitted.

Cysteine biosynthesis

Cysteine is formed from methionine and serine in the cytoplasm. The synthesis pathway is not yet fully identified; however, the main steps are shown in Fig. 6.11. Deficiency of the enzyme cystathionine-β-synthase results in accumulation of the intermediate homocysteine. This causes homocystinuria; a multisystem disorder characterized by elevated serum and urinary homocysteine.

Tyrosine biosynthesis

Tyrosine synthesis is simply hydroxylation of phenylalanine (Fig. 6.12). The reaction is highly exergonic, explaining why phenylalanine cannot be synthesized from tyrosine. The reaction is catalysed by phenylalanine hydroxylase and requires tetrahydrobiopterin as a cofactor.

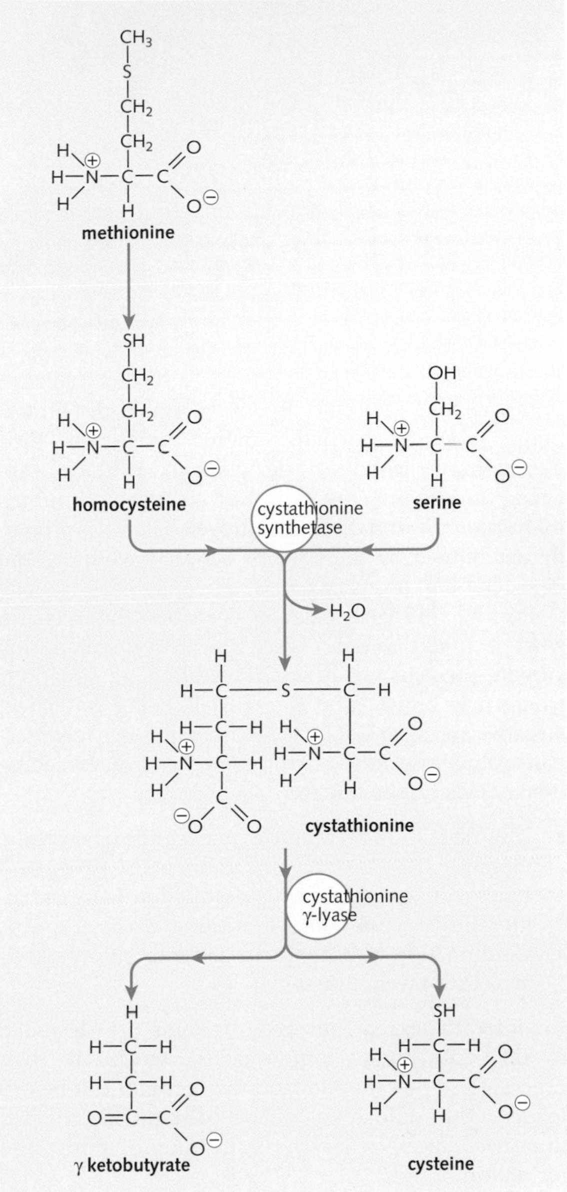

Fig. 6.11 Cysteine synthesis.

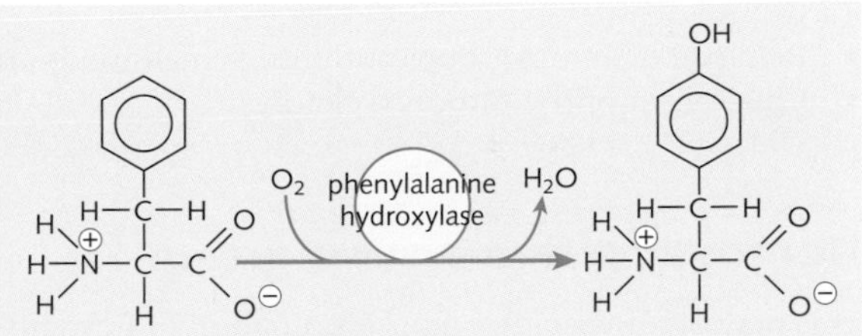

The autosomal recessive disease phenylketonuria (PKU) arises from deficiency or absence of phenylalanine hydroxylase. Tyrosine cannot be synthesized endogenously, making it an essential amino acid in individuals with PKU. Phenylalanine accumulates, saturating the large-neutral R-group/aromatic R-group amino acid transporter at the blood–brain barrier. This denies other molecules relying on this transporter access to the developing CNS. This manifests with progressive brain damage and seizures. Treatment is by strict dietary exclusion and tyrosine supplementation.

Clinical Note

Tyrosine is oxidized by the enzyme tyrosinase to produce the pigment melanin. Tyrosinase deficiency results in failure of melanogenesis, leading to oculocutaneous albinism type 1. Ocular complication arising from iris translucency and reduced retinal pigmentation are common.

Alanine biosynthesis

Alanine is synthesized by transamination of pyruvate to alanine (Fig. 6.13). This is catalysed by alanine aminotransferase (cofactor PLP), and requires glutamate to donate the amino group.

BIOLOGICAL DERIVATIVES OF AMINO ACIDS

Amino acids are essential as the building blocks of proteins; however they also fulfil important functions as individual molecules; for example, the majority of central neurotransmitters are derived from amino acids.

Fig. 6.12 Tyrosine synthesis.

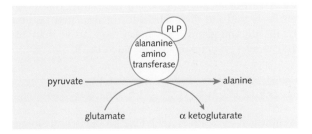

Fig. 6.13 Alanine synthesis.

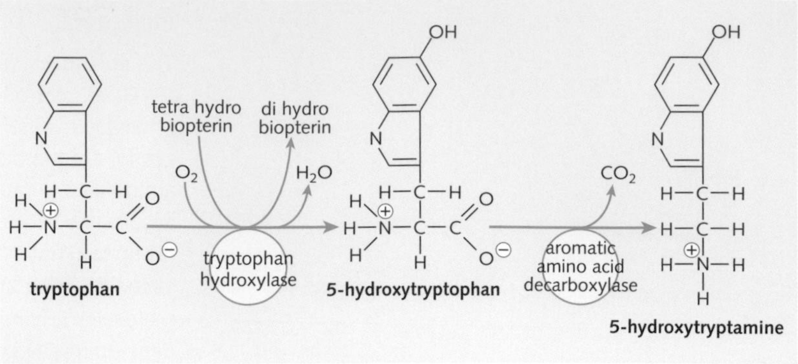

Fig. 6.14 Serotonin (5-HT) synthesis.

Serotonin synthesis from tryptophan

Serotonin (5-hydroxytryptamine, 5-HT) is synthesized from tryptophan. This is a two-step pathway (Fig. 6.14): tryptophan is hydroxylated to 5-hydroxytryptophan, by tryptophan hydroxylase (cofactor tetrahydrobiopterin). 5-OH-tryptophan is then decarboxylated by amino acid decarboxylase (cofactor PLP) to form 5-HT.

Adrenaline, noradrenaline and dopamine synthesis from tyrosine

These three neurotransmitters ('catecholamines') are all derived from tyrosine. The pathway is best shown as a diagram (Fig. 6.15).

Thyroid hormone synthesis from tyrosine

Two tyrosine residues in the same polypeptide (the glycoprotein thyroglobulin) are iodinated at their R-groups, forming mono-iodotyrosine or di-iodotyrosine depending on whether iodination occurs at one or two sites. These two iodinated tyrosine residues react with each other. This forms T3 (tri-iodothyronine) when one di-iodotyrosine combined with another mono-iodotyrosine, and T4 (thyroxine) if two di-iodotyrosines combined with each other. Generation of T3 and T4 (both termed 'thyroid hormones') is catalysed by thyroid peroxidase. The newly formed thyroid hormones are excised from their thyroglobulin scaffold by lysosomal enzymes and are then released in a regulated fashion by the thyroid gland. T3 is much more active than T4; T4 can also be peripherally converted to T3.

NITROGEN BALANCE

As nitrogen breakdown yields toxic products, and biological availability of nitrogen is limited, the balance between synthesis and breakdown of nitrogen-containing ('nitrogenous') molecules is closely regulated. Nitrogenous molecules include amino acids and their derivatives, nucleotides, nucleic acids and, of course, proteins. Nitrogen presence in the body is largely accounted for by proteins, and therefore nitrogen balance is primarily determined by the balance between synthesis and degradation of proteins.

Positive nitrogen balance describes the scenario where N intake exceeds N excretion. This is seen during growth, pregnancy, and wound healing; all situations where new body tissue (protein) is being generated. Negative nitrogen balance describes the converse scenario; a net loss of N occurs due to excretion exceeding intake. This can be due to:

- Insufficient nitrogen intake: malnutrition, anorexia, dieting
- Excess nitrogen loss: tissue destruction (surgery, injury burns, sepsis), muscle wasting
- Combination of both: cachexia (emaciation associated with severe illness).

In order to excrete nitrogen, proteins are degraded to their constituent amino acids, which are then processed so that the nitrogen they contain can be off-loaded. This offloading can be conceptually divided into two stages; removal of the amino group and formation of urea.

AMINO ACID CATABOLISM

There are two components of amino acid catabolism:

- Removal of amino groups and nitrogen elimination
- Catabolism of the carbon skeletons.

Removal of the amino group

This may occur via either trans*de*amination or transamination. Each route generates different products, but both are able to enter the urea cycle.

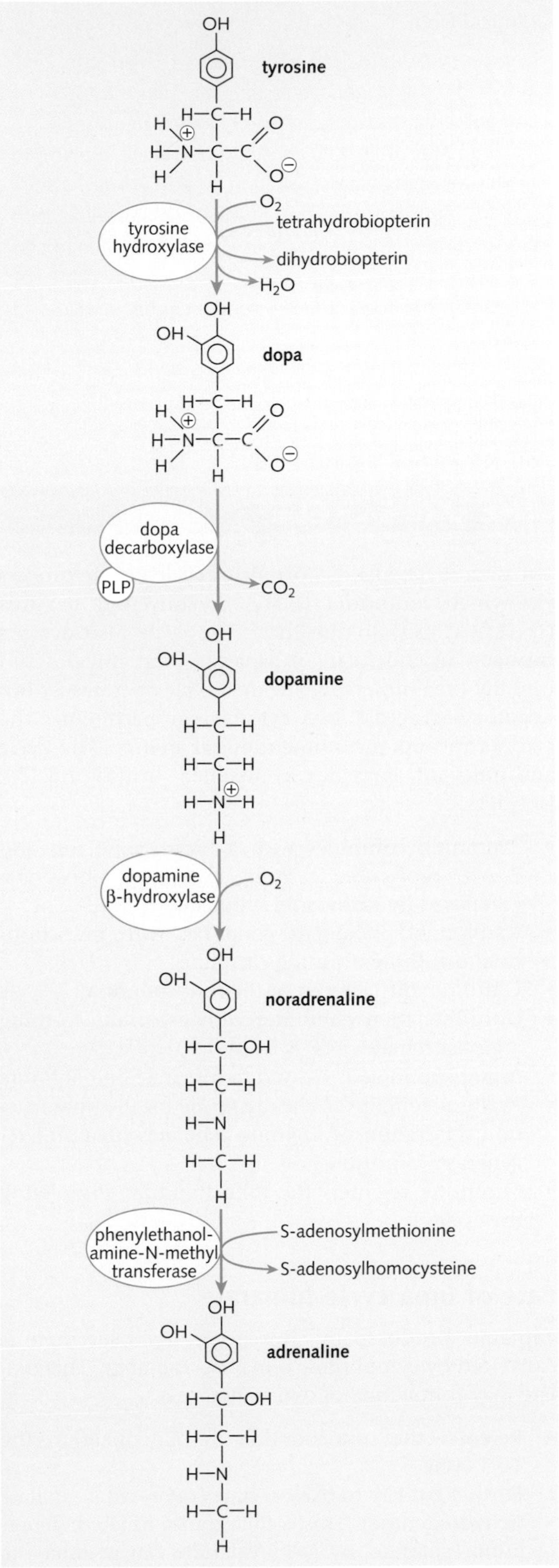

Transdeamination: removal of the amino group as NH$_3$

'Transdeamination' is where amino acids are converted to their corresponding keto acid (which is further metabolized) and NH$_3$ is released, entering the urea cycle. It involves sequential transamination and oxidative deamination:

- Cytoplasmic transamination, where aminotransferases 'convert' the amino acid to glutamate; in reality the amino group is transferred to α-ketoglutarate, generating glutamate, whilst the amino acid skeleton is released as the corresponding keto acid
- This is followed by mitochondrial oxidative deamination of glutamate (Fig. 6.5) releasing α-ketoglutarate and NH$_3$ (Fig. 6.16).

Transamination: incorporation of the amino group into aspartate

Transamination was described earlier in the chapter (Fig. 6.4). In the context of nitrogen excretion, the second transaminase reaction generates aspartate and is mediated by AST. This aspartate is then able to enter the urea cycle (Fig. 6.19).

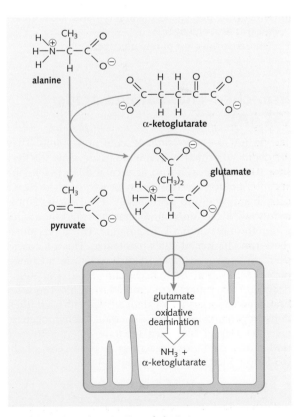

Fig. 6.16　Transdeamination of alanine.

Fig. 6.15　Catecholamine synthesis.

Catabolism of carbon skeletons

Once the amino group has been removed (from an amino acid), the carbon 'skeleton' remains. This skeleton (the corresponding keto-acid) will vary in structure according to the individual amino acid. Each structure is further catabolized to form intermediates of the TCA cycle or ketogenesis pathways. Figure 6.17 provides further detail.

The terms 'glucogenic' and 'ketogenic'

Amino acids whose skeletons are ultimately processed into TCA cycle intermediates are termed 'glucogenic'. This term is used since all TCA cycle intermediates ultimately form oxaloacetate, which can be converted to glucose via gluconeogenesis. Some amino acid catabolism products, however, do not correspond to any of the TCA cycle intermediates, instead becoming intermediates of the ketogenesis pathway; acetoacetate and acetyl CoA (Chapter 5). These are termed 'ketogenic' amino acids. Some amino acids are able, depending on their route of catabolism, to generate intermediates of both ketogenesis and the TCA cycle. Others are only able to ultimately produce intermediates of one or other pathways:

- Leucine, lysine and tryptophan are purely ketogenic
- Isoleucine, phenylalanine and tyrosine are both ketogenic and glucogenic
- The remainder are purely glucogenic.

Branched-chain amino acids (BCAA)

The BCAA are isoleucine, leucine and valine. They are degraded primarily in muscle tissue, since the liver (the usual site for amino acid catabolism) lacks the specific aminotransferase enzyme required to cleave off the amino group from BCAA. Their catabolism is as follows: BCAA aminotransferase transfers the amino group from BCAA to α-ketoglutarate. This forms glutamate and a branched-chain α-ketoacid. This α-ketoacid then undergoes oxidative decarboxylation, mediated by mitochondrial branched-chain α-ketoacid dehydrogenase complex (cofactor PLP). This produces branched-chain acyl-CoA derivatives, which are then dehydrogenated by two separate dehydrogenase enzymes (Fig. 6.18). Each separate BCAA derivative undergoes oxidation reactions reminiscent of β-oxidation, ultimately producing:

- (Leucine $\rightarrow$) acetyl CoA and acetoacetate
- (Isoleucine $\rightarrow$) acetyl CoA and succinyl CoA
- (Valine $\rightarrow$) succinyl CoA.

Clinical Note

Deficiency of mitochondrial branched-chain α-ketoacid dehydrogenase results in a failure to catabolise all three branched-chain amino acids. Plasma levels of Ile, Leu and Val accumulate, leading to severe neurological dysfunction. The BCAA are also seen at high concentration in the urine as well as the blood, 'branched-chain ketoaciduria'. This gave rise to the name 'maple-syrup urine disease', as the odour of affected individuals' urine is reminiscent of maple syrup.

THE UREA CYCLE

The urea cycle, aka the 'ornithine cycle', is the process via which ammonia (NH_3) is converted to urea ($(NH_2)_2 C=O$) in the liver. The cycle also accepts nitrogen in the form of aspartate and integrates it into the urea molecule. The urea cycle operates within hepatocytes across two cellular compartments; the cytoplasm and the mitochondrial matrix. The cycle and relevant enzymes is detailed in (Fig. 6.19). In brief:

- Ammonia combines with a bicarbonate ion and 2 ATP molecules, forming carbamoyl phosphate (catalysed by carbamoyl synthetase-I)
- Carbamoyl phosphate combines with mitochondrial ornithine, forming citrulline
- Citrulline diffuses out of the mitochondria
- Citrulline then combines with aspartate, forming arginosuccinate. ATP is hydrolyzed
- Arginosuccinate is cleaved to fumarate and arginine
- Arginine remains in the urea cycle for the final reaction; hydration of arginine generates urea and regenerates ornithine
- Ornithine re-enters the mitochondria, completing the cycle.

Fate of urea cycle fumarate

Fumarate produced by cleavage of arginosuccinate is converted by cytoplasmic fumarase to malate. This malate may follow one of two routes:

- Re-enter the mitochondria to participate in the TCA cycle
- Further oxidize to oxaloacetate (catalysed by malate dehydrogenase). This is then transaminated, generating aspartate, by AST. Aspartate can re-enter the urea cycle, as shown in Fig. 6.19.

Fig. 6.17 Catabolism of individual amino acid carbon skeletons.

Amino acid	TCA cycle/ ketogenesis pathway intermediate	Deaminated carbon skeleton processing	Glucogenic	Ketogenic
GLU	α-ketoglutarate	Undergoes oxidative deamination (Fig. 6.5), forming α-ketoglutarate, NH_3 and $NADH + H^+$	√	
GLN	α-ketoglutarate	Hydrolyzed by glutaminase to form glutamate	√	
CYS	Pyruvate	Cysteine aminotransferase converts cysteine into glutamate	√	
ARG	α-ketoglutarate	Cleaved to form ornithine and urea in the urea cycle. Ornithine is transaminated to form glutamate γ-semialdehyde, which converts to glutamate	√	
PRO	α-ketoglutarate	Proline dehydrogenase and Δ1-pyrroline-5-carboxylate dehydrogenase oxidize proline to glutamate	√	
HIS	α-ketoglutarate	Histidine catabolism involves a complex, seven-enzyme pathway culminating in formation of glutamate. Initial de-amination is mediated by histidase: deficiency of this enzyme causes histidinaemia	√	
ALA	Pyruvate	Transamination of alanine generates pyruvate (and glutamate)	√	
GLY	Pyruvate	Glycine is converted to serine (which is catabolized ultimately to pyruvate) by serine hydroxymethyltransferase	√	
SER	Pyruvate	Serine-threonine dehydratase converts serine to pyruvate	√	
VAL	Succinyl CoA	Branched chain amino acid catabolism: see following section	√	
MET	Succinyl CoA	Methionine donates its methyl group to various acceptors via the intermediate S-adenosyl-methionine (SAM). This generates propionyl CoA, which is metabolised to succinyl CoA by the odd-chain fatty acid oxidation pathway	√	
THR	Succinyl CoA	Serine-threonine dehydratase coverts threonine to α-ketobutyrate, which is converted to propionyl CoA and CO_2. Propionyl CoA is metabolized to succinyl CoA by the odd-chain fatty acid oxidation pathway	√	
ASP	Fumarate/ oxaloacetate	Transaminated by aspartate aminotransferase to produce oxaloacetate	√	
ASN	Oxaloacetate	Converted first to aspartate by asparaginase	√	
TYR	Fumarate/ acetoacetate	Tyrosine aminotransferase catalyses the first step in this 5-step pathway, culminating in fumarate and acetoacetate. Deficiency of homogentisic acid dioxygenase, one of the tyrosine catabolism enzymes, causes alkaptonuria (accumulation of the intermediate homogentisate)	√	√
PHE	Fumarate/ acetoacetate	Converted first to tyrosine by phenylalanine hydroxylase	√	√
ILE	Acetyl CoA/ succinyl CoA	Branched chain amino acid catabolism: see following section. Catabolism yields acetyl CoA and succinyl CoA	√	√
TRY	Acetyl CoA	The complex catabolism of tryptophan has not yet been fully elucidated; however the TRY catabolism pathway culminates with acetyl CoA		√
LEU	Acetyl CoA + Acetoacetate	Branched chain amino acid catabolism: see following section		√
LYS	Acetoacetate	De-aminated lysine undergoes a complex pathway which ultimately produces acetoacetate		√

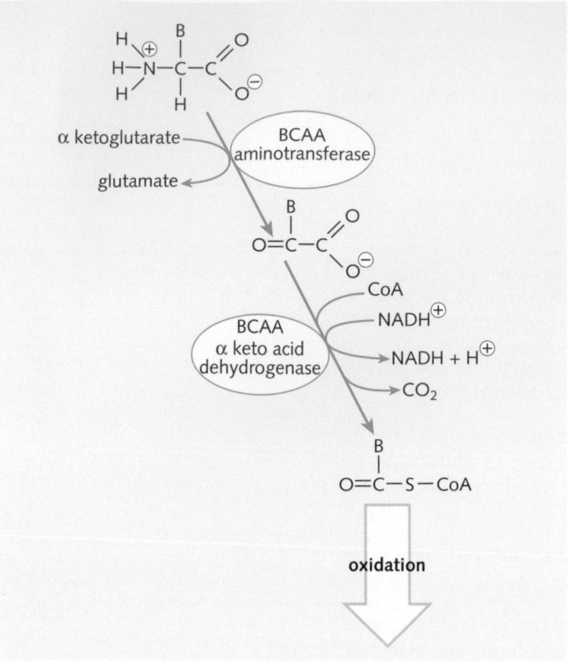

Fig. 6.18 Branched-chain amino acid (BCAA) catabolism. 'B' indicates a branched-chain 'R' group.

Sources of urea cycle aspartate

Aspartate may be derived from urea cycle fumarate (as described previously). Alternatively, it may originate from transaminated oxaloacetate. Any amino acid can be transaminated (first via the relevant aminotransferase, and then via AST) to generate aspartate.

Vital metabolic role of the urea cycle

The urea cycle is the main physiological mechanism for nitrogen elimination. Produced in the liver, urea is excreted from the body via specialized mechanisms in the kidney. The urea is nearly 50% nitrogen by molecular weight and is an efficient nitrogen transport molecule. It diffuses freely across cell membranes and is highly soluble in plasma; therefore, it is easily transported from the liver to the kidneys via the bloodstream. It is electrically neutral and does not affect blood pH.

Regulation of the urea cycle

Sustained increases in nitrogen intake result in increased expression of urea cycle enzymes. Therefore, the cycle can operate at a faster rate, processing more NH_3 and aspartate and thus eliminating more nitrogen.

Sustained high-protein intake is the most common context in which the urea cycle is up-regulated, since more ingested protein results in more nitrogen requiring processing for elimination.

Short-term regulation of the urea cycle is mainly via modulation of mitochondrial carbamoyl-phosphate synthase-I (CPS-I) activity, the enzyme that uses ATP, NH_3 and HCO_3^- to form carbamoyl phosphate. This enzyme is allosterically activated by N-acetyl glutamate, itself formed by the combination of acetyl CoA and glutamate. This is appropriate, since intracellular glutamate will rise following catabolism of ingested protein. Remember that the amino group of amino acids undergoing catabolism is transferred to α-ketoglutarate, forming glutamate – this is why this amino acid in particular is a sensitive indicator of amino acid catabolism.

Abnormalities of the urea cycle

Deficiencies of each urea cycle enzyme and carriers have been identified. These are rare, and inheritance varies according to enzyme. For example, the most common inborn error of metabolism of the urea cycle, ornithine trancarbamoylase deficiency, follows an X-linked recessive pattern of inheritance. However, all disorders of the urea cycle result in a failure to synthesize urea and accumulation of NH_3: 'hyperammonaemia'.

> **Clinical Note**
>
> Ammonia toxicity manifests initially with decreased level of cognition, tremors and blurred vision, progressing with increasing $[NH_3]$ to seizures, brain damage, coma and death. This occurs soon after birth with inborn enzyme deficiencies, or develops gradually with progressive failure of a previously functioning urea cycle, e.g. in liver failure. In this scenario progressive loss of functioning hepatocytes results in failure of the urea cycle to function at a rate sufficient to prevent accumulation of NH_3, resulting in hyperammonaemia.

PROTEIN SYNTHESIS AND DEGRADATION

Protein turnover

Proteins, both structural and functional, undergo continuous synthesis and degradation. If these processes

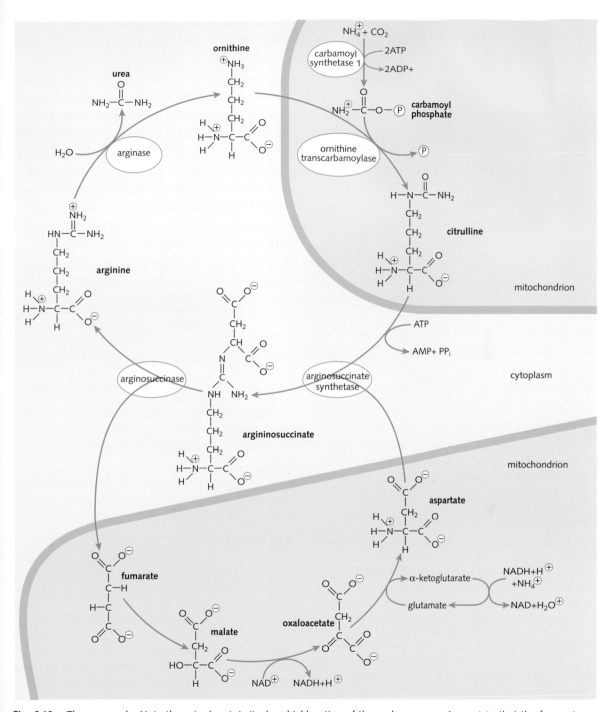

Fig. 6.19 The urea cycle. Note the cytoplasmic/mitochondrial location of the cycle enzymes. Appreciate that the fumarate → malate → oxaloacetate stages are part of the TCA cycle; for simplicity the enzymes are not shown in this illustration.

occur at equal rates, the total protein quantity remains constant. Since proteins are comprised of amino acids (nitrogen-containing molecules), protein intake and excretion broadly approximates to nitrogen balance (see above).

Protein degradation

This section describes enzymatic breakdown of proteins to their constituent amino acids. Enzymes that hydrolyse peptide bonds (between amino acids) are called proteases. There are two major routes of

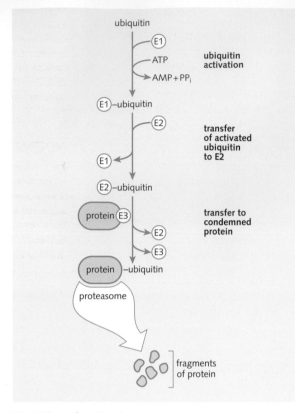

Fig. 6.20 Ubiquitination.

protease-mediated protein degradation: ubiquitination and the lysosomal pathway.

Ubiquitination

This is an ATP-dependent cytoplasmic mechanism of protein destruction. Ubiquitin, a small protein present in all cells, is attached to proteins by ubiquitin ligase. This is called 'ubiquitination'. It functions as a molecular label, identifying proteins destined for destruction by the 25S proteosome. The proteosome is a large cylindrical protease complex with a central access pore. Ubiquitinated proteins enter the pore, possibly due to ubiquitin acting as a recognition element, and are proteolytically degraded to their component amino acids. Ubiquitination is a four-step process (Fig. 6.20) that includes:

- Production of an active adenylated ubiquitin intermediate and covalent binding of activated ubiquitin to enzyme E1 (ubiquitin-activating enzyme)
- Transfer of ubiquitin to enzyme E2 (ubiquitin-conjugating enzyme)
- Association of E2-ubiquitin with substrate-bound E3 (ubiquitin ligase). E3 'reads' the N terminus of a protein

- If the N-terminus is unstable, a peptide bond is generated between ubiquitin and the E3-bound substrate. E2 and E3 then dissociate.

Lysosomal proteolysis

Lysosomes are intracellular organelles. Intralysosomal protease enzymes ('cathepsins') mediate lysosomal proteolysis. Proteins gain access to lysosomal interior by either endocytosis (extracellular proteins) or intracellular autophagy. Autophagy is when endoplasmic reticulum wraps around intracellular organelles (e.g. mitochondria), forming an 'autophagosome'.

Intracellular degradation signals

There are various structural features that decrease the lifespan of proteins by conferring susceptibility to various cellular degradation processes. Appreciate that exposure of such features during conformational change also renders a protein vulnerable to degradation.

N-terminus components

High density of the amino acids Met, Gly, Ala and Ser promotes N-terminus stability, since these are not readily ubiquitinated. Thus dense presence of these amino acids at the N-terminus of a protein renders it relatively insensitive to ubiquitin-mediated destruction. Conversely, Phe, Try, Asp, Asn and Lys destabilize the N-terminus. These amino acids are an N-terminal feature of short-lived proteins, since they are readily ubiquitinated by E3.

'PEST' regions

These are features of a protein's primary structure; regions with high density of Pro, Glu, Ser and Thr (P, E, S and T according to the one-letter amino acid code) residues are common in proteins with short lifespans. PEST regions are examples of a 'degradation motif'; their presence condemns a protein to a rapid turnover. The mechanism of PEST-mediated susceptibility is not yet clarified but may be due to caspase or proteasome action.

Protein synthesis: translation

Proteins are synthesized in the cytoplasm by ribosomes. Ribosomes assemble amino acids in the correct order to form individual polypeptides. This order is determined, or 'coded for' by the ribonucleotide sequence of the particular messenger RNA (mRNA). Ribosomes are structures composed of protein and ribosomal RNA (rRNA). Ribosomes associate with mRNA strands in the cytoplasm and function as 'assembly stations' for in-coming amino acids.

These amino acids arrive bound to individual trans-fer RNA molecules (tRNA). Amino acids are integrated into growing polypeptides by ribosomes if, and only if, the anticodon on their tRNA is complementary to the next codon in the ribonucleotide sequence of the mRNA strand. So, if the mRNA strand sequence is A–U–G, only a tRNA with anticodon U–A–C can 'dock' at the ribo-some for incorporation into the growing protein.

Clinical Note

A codon is three sequential nucleotides representing ('coding for') a particular amino acid. For example; the mRNA sequence 'A–U–G' (adenine, uracil and guanine) codes for methionine. The nuclear DNA sequence encoding methionine is however 'A–T–G', since RNA contains uracil (U) in place of thymine (T).

Protein synthesis: transcription

mRNA is 'messenger' RNA. This is an RNA sequence reflecting the DNA sequence of a gene, except that RNA cannot incorporate thymine, so utilizes uracil in its place. The DNA sequence 'A–C–T–T–T–C–G' would be represented in mRNA by 'A–C–U–U–U–C–G'. Every three ribonucleotides (a 'codon') represents an amino acid.

The mRNA sequence codes for the gene from which it was originally transcribed. This gene lies within chromosomal DNA, in the nucleus. A base sequence on one strand (the 'sense' strand) of the double-stranded DNA helix codes for a gene. The complemen-tary strand (the 'antisense' strand) acts as a template for mRNA. RNA polymerase catalyses the assembly of a ribonucleotide polymer (mRNA) complementary to the antisense strand. This means the new mRNA strand has a base sequence identical to the gene sequence, except that 'U' is substituted for 'T' in the mRNA sequence.

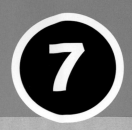

After reading this chapter you should be able to:
• Discuss the roles of one-carbon units in amino acid synthesis
• Describe the processes involved in purine and pyrimidine metabolism
• Discuss the clinical features, causes and management of gout
• Discuss the main features of haem and bilirubin metabolism

ONE-CARBON POOL

One-carbon units

Single carbon units exist in a number of oxidation states; for example, methane, formaldehyde and methanol. They are used in the synthesis and elongation of many organic compounds. To do this, carbon units require a carrier to activate them and to enable their transfer to the molecule being synthesized. The main carriers used are folate and S-adenosyl methionine. The term 'one-carbon pool' refers to single-carbon units attached to these carriers.

I.e. One carbon pool = single carbon units
+S-adenosyl methionine
(SAM) or Folate (THF)

S-adenosyl methionine

S-adenosyl methionine (SAM) is a high-energy compound formed by the condensation of the amino acid methionine with ATP. It contains an activated methyl group, which can be transferred easily to a variety of molecules. SAM is the major donor of methyl groups for biosynthetic reactions; for example, the methylation of norepinephrine to epinephrine.

Folate

The active form of folate is 5,6,7,8-tetrahydrofolate (THF). THF is a carrier of one-carbon units, which bind to its nitrogen atoms at positions N^5, N^{10} or both, to form the compounds shown in Fig. 7.1. THF receives these one-carbon fragments from donor molecules such as serine, glycine or histidine, and transfers them to intermediates in the synthesis of other amino acids, purines and thymidine. These THF compounds are all interconvertible except the N^5-methyl group.

Folate metabolism

Formation of THF

THF is formed by the two-step reduction of folate by dihydrofolate reductase (DHFR) (Fig. 7.2). DHRF is competitively inhibited by methotrexate, a folic acid analogue used in the treatment of certain cancers. Methotrexate decreases THF synthesis and its availability for purine and pyrimidine formation, which decreases DNA and RNA synthesis in cells.

Fig. 7.1 Compounds formed by the binding of THF to various one-carbon compounds.

One-carbon unit	Compound
—CH=NH	N^5-formimino THF
—CHO	N^5-formyl THF
—CHO	N^{10}-formyl THF
=CH—	N^5, N^{10}-methenyl THF
—CH$_2$—	N^5, N^{10}-methylene THF
—CH$_3$	N^5-methyl THF

and requires vitamin B_{12} as an essential cofactor (methylcobalamin).

Amino acids and the one-carbon pool

The synthesis and breakdown of certain amino acids produce THF carriers that can be used in the synthesis of other amino acids and nucleotides. The following reactions demonstrate the use of the one-carbon pool.

Formation of SAM from methionine (numbers refer to Fig. 7.3)

1. Condensation of ATP and methionine to form SAM
2. SAM contains an activated methyl group that can be donated to a number of acceptor molecules, while SAM transforms into S-adenosyl homocysteine
3. Hydrolysis of S-adenosyl homocysteine releases adenosine to form homocysteine
4. Homocysteine can be used either for the synthesis of the amino acid cysteine, or for point 5 below
5. Regeneration of methionine (and THF) in the methionine salvage pathway.

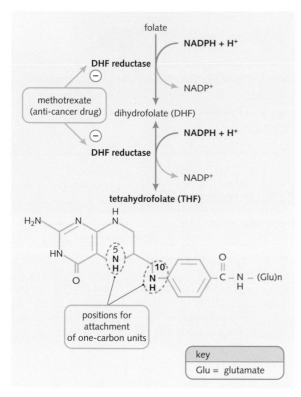

Fig. 7.2 Formation of tetrahydrofolate (THF). THF is formed by the two-step reduction of folate by dihydrofolate (DHF) reductase.

Methyl-folate trap (Fig. 7.3)

Reactions involving transfer of methyl groups result in the formation of N^5-methyl THF. Unlike other THF compounds, N^5-methyl THF is not interconvertible further, therefore THF cannot be released and remains trapped as N^5-methyl THF. However, the methionine salvage pathway is present. Methionine is formed by methylation of homocysteine using N^5-methyl THF as the methyl group donor, therefore releasing THF. This reaction is catalysed by homocysteine methyltransferase

PURINE METABOLISM

Structure and function of purines

Purines are the nitrogenous bases adenine, guanine and hypoxanthine. They have a double-ring structure, consisting of a six-carbon ring and a five-carbon ring. They can either exist as free bases or with a pentose sugar (5 C), usually ribose or deoxyribose, attached at the N9 position to form a nucleoside (i.e. adenosine). Phosphorylation of the sugar at the C5 position leads to the formation of mono-, di- and tri-nucleotides as shown in Fig. 7.4. The phosphate groups cause these molecules to be negatively charged. The main functions of purines are listed in Fig. 7.5.

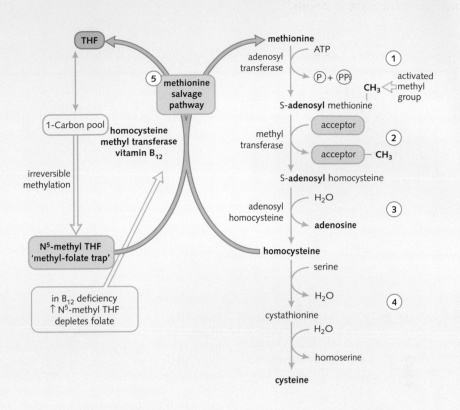

Fig. 7.3 Formation of S-adenosyl methionine (SAM) and the methionine salvage pathway. (Numbers refer to the text.)

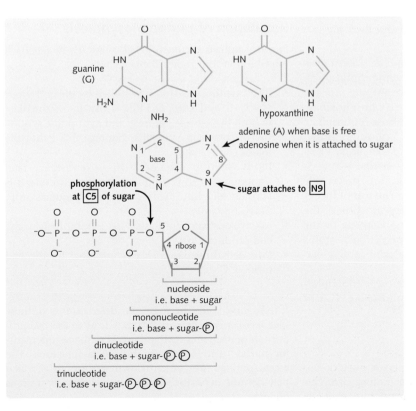

Fig. 7.4 Structure of purines, nucleosides and nucleotides.

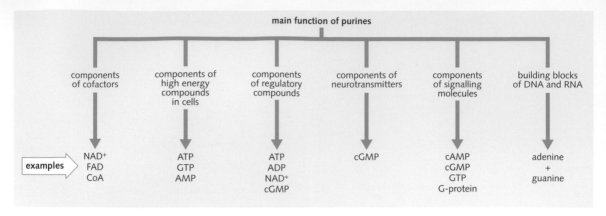

Fig. 7.5 Main functions of purines [this is old fig 6–5 converted to diagram]

An overview of purine metabolism

Diet provides negligible amounts of purines because they are broken down in the gut to form uric acid. Two pathways are concerned with the formation of purine nucleotides (Fig. 7.6).

I. De novo synthesis of purines

The purine ring is assembled on a molecule of ribose-5-phosphate; therefore, the purines are synthesized as mononucleotides instead of as free bases. This process occurs in the cytosol of hepatocytes and there are two stages:

- Formation of inosine monophosphate. Eleven reactions are necessary to form inosine monophosphate (IMP), the nucleotide of hypoxanthine. In the first reaction, ribose phosphate pyrophosphokinase catalyses the phosphorylation of ribose-5-phosphate at the C1 position, forming 5-phosphoribosyl-1-pyrophosphate. In the second reaction, PRPP amidotransferase catalyses the synthesis of 5-phosphoribosylamine, which is an irreversible rate-limiting step of the pathway. The rest of the reactions are concerned with the construction of the purine ring of the inosine monophosphate by the addition of five carbon and four nitrogen atoms from amino acids (aspartate, glycine and glutamine), CO_2 and THF derivatives
- Conversion of IMP to AMP (adenosine monophosphate) and guanosine monophosphate (GMP) (Fig. 7.7).

II. Salvage pathways

When nucleic acids and nucleotides are broken down, free bases are released. The salvage pathway recycles these free bases by re-attaching ribose-5-phosphate to them (Fig. 7.8). It is a one-step pathway where the ribose-5-phosphate is transferred to the free bases from PRPP. The release of pyrophosphate makes the reactions irreversible. Only two enzymes are necessary: adenine phosphoribosyl transferase (APRT) and hypoxanthine guanine phosphoribosyl transferase (HGPRT). The pathway is simple and requires much less ATP than de novo synthesis because the bases do not have to be made first.

Regulation of purine biosynthesis

Purine synthesis is controlled allosterically by feedback inhibition at four major control sites:

- PRPP synthetase. This is inhibited by the end products GMP and AMP. As PRPP is also an intermediate in both the salvage pathway and pyrimidine synthesis (discussed later in this chapter), this is not the major control site
- PRPP amidotransferase. This irreversible, rate-limiting reaction is unique to purine synthesis. It is allosterically inhibited by the end products IMP, AMP and GMP
- Adenylsuccinate synthase. This is inhibited by the end product AMP
- IMP dehydrogenase. This is inhibited by the end product GMP.

If regulation is lost because of a defect in one of these four regulatory enzymes, this may lead to the overproduction of AMP and GMP, in excess of the requirements for nucleic acid synthesis and other functions. The excess purines are broken down to uric acid, which may become deposited in tissues, leading to symptoms of gout.

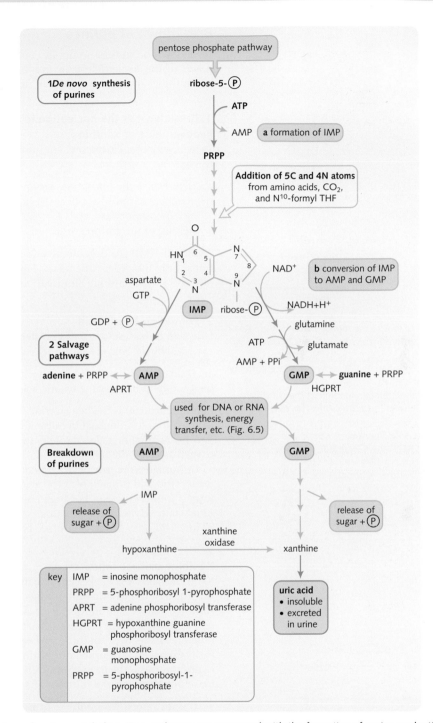

Fig. 7.6 Overview of purine metabolism. Two pathways are concerned with the formation of purine nucleotides:
1. De novo synthesis of purines, where the purine ring is assembled on a molecule of ribose-5-phosphate. The pathway consists of two stages:
   a. Formation of IMP, which occurs in 11 reactions. The purine ring is constructed by addition of C and N atoms from a number of sources: amino acids, CO_2 and THF derivatives
   b. IMP is then converted to either GMP or AMP
2. Salvage pathways 'recycle' free purines released during nucleic acid turnover by re-attaching a sugar phosphate unit to them. There is only one pathway for purine breakdown, which converts the purines to the free bases hypoxanthine and xanthine; these are then oxidized to uric acid for excretion by the kidney.

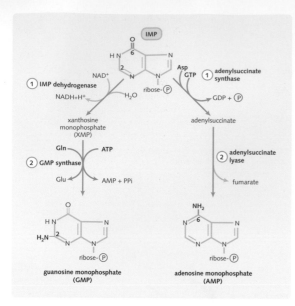

Fig. 7.7 Conversion of inosine monophosphate (IMP) to AMP and GMP. Both conversions involve two steps. Conversion of IMP to GMP involves:
1. Oxidation at the C2 position by IMP dehydrogenase, forming xanthosine monophosphate
2. The amino group of glutamine insertion at the C2 position by GMP synthase to form GMP. This reaction requires ATP.

Conversion of IMP to AMP involves:
1. Addition of aspartate at the C6 position to form adenylsuccinate. This reaction requires GTP
2. Adenylsuccinate lyase then eliminates the C-skeleton of aspartate as fumarate, leaving behind the amino group at C6 to form AMP.

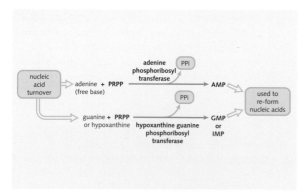

Fig. 7.8 Salvage pathways. When nucleic acids and nucleotides are broken down, free bases are released. The salvage pathway recycles these free bases by re-attaching ribose-5-phosphate to them by transfer from PRPP.

Breakdown of purines

Breakdown of purines occurs in two stages: the breakdown of the nucleotide to a free base hypoxanthine or xanthine, and the formation of uric acid (Fig. 7.9).

1. Breakdown of the nucleotide to a free base: hypoxanthine or xanthine

Three reactions are necessary (numbers and letters refer to Fig. 7.9):

a. Removal of the phosphate group by a nucleotidase
b. Removal of ribose as ribose-1-phosphate by nucleoside phosphorylase
c. Release of the amino group.

AMP and GMP are degraded by the same three reactions; only the order differs (see Fig. 7.11). AMP and IMP form hypoxanthine and GMP forms xanthine.

2. Formation of uric acid

Uric acid formation requires two steps, which are both catalysed by the enzyme xanthine oxidase (see Fig. 7.9):

a. Oxidation of hypoxanthine to xanthine
b. Oxidation of xanthine to uric acid.

Xanthine oxidase is the key enzyme involved in purine degradation. It is unusual because it is a molybdenum- and iron-containing flavoprotein that uses molecular oxygen as an oxidizing agent.

In humans, the uric acid formed is excreted in the urine. Uric acid is insoluble. The acidic pH of urine allows it to precipitate out at high concentrations as sodium urate. Hyperuricaemia, that is, high serum levels of uric acid, may lead to gout (see below).

Xanthine oxidase inhibitors

Xanthine oxidase is the key enzyme involved in controlling the amount of uric acid produced. Treatment with xanthine oxidase inhibitors decreases the amount of uric acid formed and increases the amounts of the soluble precursors hypoxanthine and xanthine, which are easily excreted in the urine. Allopurinol, an analogue of hypoxanthine, is the most commonly used xanthine oxidase inhibitor. It has a number of actions:

- It is a competitive inhibitor of xanthine oxidase
- The salvage enzyme can catalyse addition of ribose-5-phosphate to allopurinol, forming allopurinol ribonucleotide. This can inhibit the rate-limiting enzyme of de novo purine synthesis, namely by PRPP amidotransferase, leading to a decrease in the level of purines and also of the PRPP pool
- Allopurinol can be metabolized by xanthine oxidase to oxypurinol, an even stronger inhibitor of xanthine oxidase.

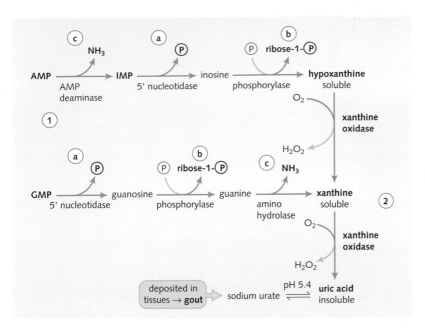

Fig. 7.9 Breakdown of purines. Breakdown of purines occurs in two stages:
1. The breakdown of the nucleotide to a free base, hypoxanthine or xanthine. For both AMP and GMP, three reactions are necessary, although the order differs:
   a. Removal of the phosphate group
   b. Removal of ribose as ribose-1-phosphate
   c. Release of amino group
2. Formation of uric acid by the oxidation of hypoxanthine and xanthine by xanthine oxidase.

Gout

The prevalence of gout varies from about 0.1–0.2% in Europe to as high as 10% in the Maori population of New Zealand. It is caused by an abnormality of uric acid metabolism, resulting in hyperuricaemia and the deposition of sodium urate crystals in joints (first metatarsal phalangeal (MTP)), soft tissues and the kidney (Fig. 7.10).

Gout predominantly affects men in middle life. It does not occur before puberty (unless it is part of Lesch-Nyhan syndrome). In women, it only occurs after menopause (the male to female ratio is 8:1). It is an inherited condition in some families.

Symptoms of gout

Gout intitially presents as recurrent, acute attacks of arthritis, usually affecting only one joint (monoarthropathy). Presenting complaint: A warm swollen and very tender joint, (usually the first meta-tarsophalangeal joint of the big toe). The most common differential diagnoses for the acute symptoms of gout are trauma and aseptic arthritis (Fig. 7.11). After repeated attacks occur and resolve, symptoms may start to persist due to permanent urate crystal deposition, leading to chronic tophaceous gout. Further complications can develop including calcium oxalate kidney stones causing dysuria and renal colic.

Causes of gout

Genetic
- Decreased HGPRT levels to 2–5% of normal. Similar to Lesch-Nyhan syndrome but not as severe
- Overactive PRPP synthetase, involved in the regulation of purine biosynthesis. Overactivity causes release from normal control, leading to increased rates of de novo synthesis of purines
- Insensitive PRPP amidotransferase, the rate-controlling enzyme of purine synthesis. A mutant form has full activity but no regulatory sites, therefore feedback control is lost, causing overproduction of purines
- The excess purines produced in these conditions are broken down to uric acid, leading to hyperuricaemia and gout.

Fig. 7.10 Clinical features and diagnosis of gout.	
Clinical features	**Diagnosis**
Hyperuricaemia Recurrent attacks of acute arthritis caused by deposition of sodium urate crystals in joints; usually only one joint is affected (big toe > 90%) Kidney stones and ↑ risk of renal disease Tophi under skin and around joints	Synovial fluid examination: affected joint is aspirated and fluid examined under polarized light microscopy for long, needle shaped, negatively birefringent crystals (detected in 85% of cases of gout) Hyperuricaemia does not necessarily cause gout

Fig 7.11 Simplified diagnostic approach to gout.

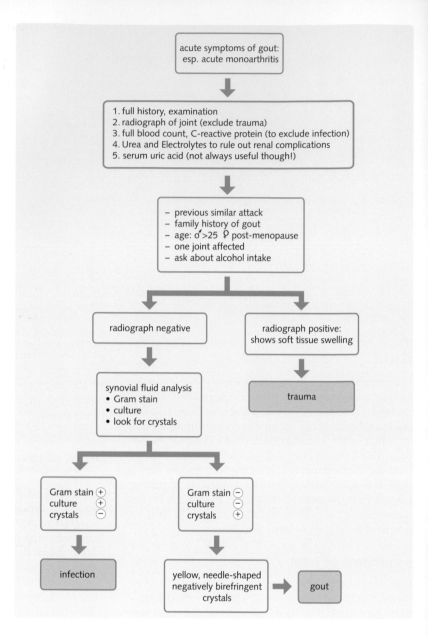

Secondary causes

- Increased purine turnover, for example in leukaemia, myeloproliferative disorders, and due to the use of cytotoxic drugs in the treatment of cancers
- Decreased excretion of uric acid, for example drug therapy (thiazides, low-dose aspirin), lead toxicity, excess alcohol.

HINTS AND TIPS

Aspirin is contraindicated in gout because it impairs the excretion of uric acid by the renal tubules, thus aggravating hyperuricaemia.

Treatment of gout

Acute attacks are treated with anti-inflammatory drugs: colchicine or non-steroidal anti-inflammatory drugs (e.g. *indometacin*) provide relief within 24–48 hours.

Long-term prevention is aimed at decreasing uric acid levels.

- Simple measures are weight reduction (reduce energy intake especially of saturated fats), decreased alcohol intake and withdrawal of drugs such as salicylates and thiazides
- Allopurinol, a xanthine oxidase inhibitor, is the main drug used for the prevention of gout not to be initiated as a treatment during an acute attack of gout

- Probenecid, a uricosuric drug, is an alternative to allopurinol. It has a direct action on the renal tubule, preventing the reabsorption of uric acid in the kidney, causing it to be excreted.

Lesch-Nyhan syndrome

Lesch-Nyhan syndrome is a very rare, X-linked disorder caused by an almost complete absence of the salvage enzyme hypoxanthine guanine phosphoribosyl transferase (HGPRT). HGPRT catalyses the addition of 5-phosphoribosyl-1-pyrophosphate (PRPP) to the purine bases, guanine and hypoxanthine, in the salvage pathway (see Fig. 7.12). In Lesch-Nyhan syndrome, a decreased level of HGPRT results in:

- Excess guanine and hypoxanthine, which are broken down to form large amounts of uric acid, leading to severe hyperuricaemia (causing kidney stones, arthritis) and gout.
- Increased PRPP, which is therefore used for the de novo synthesis of purines, causing purine overproduction and severe neurological disturbances (spasticity and mental retardation).

These symptoms begin at 3 months, which can lead to diagnosis, or this may be detected by an orange nappy, or HGPRT activity. Treatment is also with allopurinol to control gout and arthritis. The prognosis is very poor; with irreversible neurological impairment, and death by the age of 5 years; usually from kidney failure (especially in boys).

PYRIMIDINE METABOLISM

Structure and function of pyrimidines

Structure

There are three main pyrimidines: thymine, cytosine and uracil. Like purines, the pyrimidines are mostly found associated with a five-carbon sugar attached at N1 to form the nucleosides thymidine, cytidine and uridine (Fig. 7.13). The sugar may be mono-, di- or tri-phosphorylated to form the corresponding nucleotides.

Fig. 7.12 Clinical features and treatment of Lesch-Nyhan syndrome.

Clinical features	Diagnosis and treatment
Hyperuricaemia causing: • Kidney stones • Arthritis • Gout Severe neurological disturbances: • Spasticity and mental retardation • Self-mutilation (bite fingers and lips to the bone) Symptoms begin at about 3 months	**Diagnosis:** • Orange nappy (urine) can be suggestive • Hypoxanthine guanine phosphoribosyl transferase activity • Symptoms **Treatment:** • Allopurinol lowers uric acid levels and helps to control gout and arthritis • With time, high purine levels result in worsening of neurological symptoms because no treatment is possible • Boys usually die from kidney failure because of high sodium urate deposits causing kidney stones

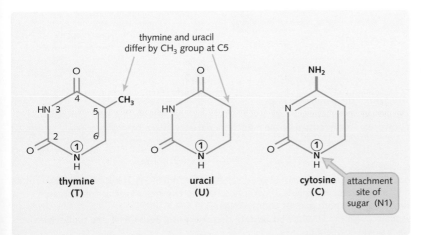

Fig. 7.13 Structure of pyrimidines. Like purines, the pyrimidines are mostly found associated with a five-carbon sugar attached at N1 to form nucleosides.

Functions

Pyrimidines are the building blocks of DNA and RNA: thymine and cytosine are present in DNA and cytosine and uracil are present in RNA.

Pyrimidine nucleotide derivatives are activated intermediates in a number of synthetic reactions; for example, UDP-glucose, the precursor of glycogen (see Chapter 4).

Biosynthesis of pyrimidines

There are three main stages in the biosynthesis of pyrimidines (see Fig. 7.14 and 7.16). All of the three stages take place in the cell cytosol.

a. Construction of the pyrimidine ring to form uridine monophosphate (UMP). Unlike purine synthesis, the pyrimidine ring is synthesized before attachment to ribose-5-phosphate, that is, it is formed as a free base. The ring is derived from glutamine, aspartate and CO_2 (Fig. 7.15). There are six steps in the reaction sequence (Fig. 7.14). In the first three steps, the enzymes involved are present as a single polypeptide chain, forming a multifunctional enzyme (CAD), which consists of carbamoyl phosphate synthase II, aspartate trans carbamoylase and dihydroorotase. In a way similar to fatty acid synthase, the enzymes are linked together to minimize side reactions and loss of substrate

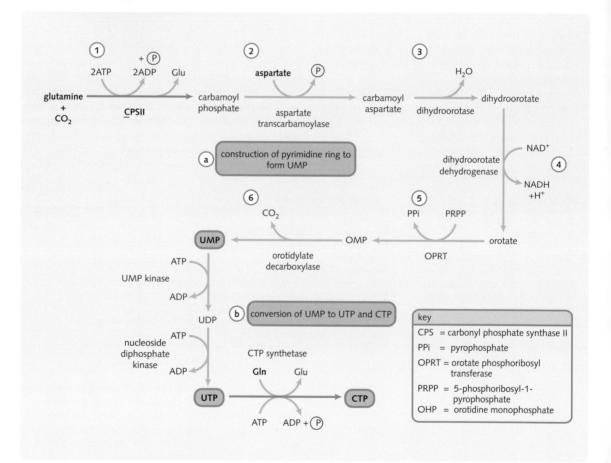

Fig. 7.14 Pyrimidine synthesis. (A) Construction of the pyrimidine ring.

1. Synthesis of carbamoyl phosphate by carbamoyl phosphate synthase II (CPSII). This is the rate-limiting step. Carbamoyl phosphate is also the precursor of urea; however, urea is formed by the mitochondrial enzyme, carbamoyl phosphate synthase I
2. Addition of aspartate
3. Closure of the ring by dihydroorotase
4. Oxidation of dihydroorotate to orotate using NAD^+
5. Conversion of the free pyrimidine to a nucleotide by the addition of ribose-5-phosphate from PRPP. This is catalysed by orotate phosphoribosyl transferase (OPRT) and is driven by the hydrolysis of pyrophosphate to two free molecules of inorganic phosphate. PRPP is thus required for the synthesis of both purines and pyrimidines
6. Decarboxylation of orotidine monophosphate (OMP) to UMP by orotidylate decarboxylase. Both OPRT and orotidylate decarboxylase are also found together as a single polypeptide.

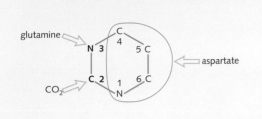

Fig. 7.15 The pyrimidine ring. The ring is derived from glutamine, aspartate and CO_2.

b. Conversion of UMP to uridine triphosphate (UTP) and cytidine triphosphate (CTP), the ribonucleotides found in RNA. UMP is phosphorylated to UDP and UTP as shown in Fig. 7.14. CTP is formed from UTP by amination, that is, the addition of an NH_2 group from glutamine to position 4 of the pyrimidine ring. Both UTP and CTP are used for RNA synthesis

c. Formation of the deoxyribonucleotides dCTP and dTTP found in DNA (Fig. 7.16).

Regulation of pyrimidine synthesis

The rate-limiting step is the formation of carbamoyl phosphate by carbamoyl phosphate synthase II. CPSII is inhibited by the end products of pyrimidine

synthesis, namely UDP and UTP. The reaction is activated by ATP and PRPP.

Regulation of deoxyribonucleotide synthesis

The regulatory enzyme of deoxyribonucleotide synthesis is ribonucleotide reductase, which catalyses the irreversible reduction of all four nucleoside diphosphates (ADP, GDP, CDP and UDP) to their corresponding deoxy forms. The enzyme has four subunits (two B1 and two B2). Each B1 subunit has two allosteric sites distinct from the active site: an activity site and a substrate specificity site. The binding of the product dATP to the activity site inhibits the enzyme. The binding of the substrate, a ribonucleotide, e.g. ATP, to the substrate specificity site, activates the enzyme.

Salvage pathways

The salvage pathways for pyrimidines are similar to those for purines (Fig. 7.17). The breakdown of nucleotides releases free pyrimidines, thymine and uracil. These pyrimidines are salvaged by the enzyme uracil/thymine phosphoribosyl transferase (UTPRT), which transfers a ribose-5-phosphate from PRPP to the free pyrimidines to re-form the mononucleotides. However, the enzyme UTPRT cannot salvage cytosine. Therefore cytidine (nucleoside) is deaminated to uridine; this is then converted to uracil, which can be salvaged.

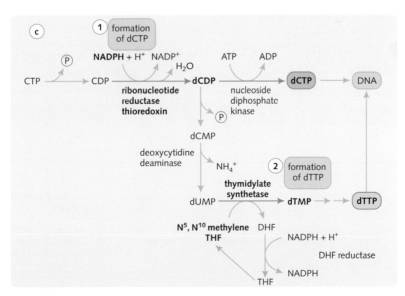

Fig. 7.16 Third stage of pyrimidine synthesis: the formation of deoxyribonucleotides.
1. Ribonucleotide reductase reduces CDP to deoxyCDP by removal of the C2 hydroxyl group on ribose, converting it to deoxyribose. The dCDP formed is phosphorylated to dCTP
2. dTTP is formed by the methylation of dUMP. Thymidylate synthetase transfers a methyl group from N^5,N^{10}-methylene THF to position 5 of the pyrimidine ring, forming dTMP, which can be phosphorylated to dTTP (numbers refer to text here). DHF, dihydrofolate; THF, tetrahydrofolate.

Fig. 7.17 Salvage pathways.

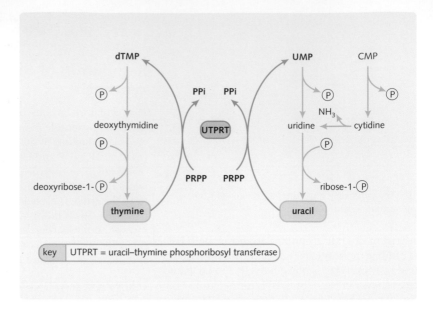

key | UTPRT = uracil–thymine phosphoribosyl transferase

Breakdown of pyrimidines

Purines are excreted with their ring still intact as uric acid. The pyrimidine ring, however, can be split and broken down to soluble structures. Uracil and cytosine are broken down to β-alanine, which forms acetyl CoA. Thymine is degraded to β-amino-isobutyrate, which forms succinyl CoA. The carbon skeletons of the pyrimidines, namely acetyl CoA and succinyl CoA, can be oxidized by the TCA cycle.

Anti-cancer drugs

These drugs inhibit the formation of nucleotides, leading to a decrease in DNA synthesis and cell growth. Cancer cells divide rapidly and have an increased demand for DNA synthesis. These drugs help to slow down the growth of cancer cells. However, they also affect normal cell replication, leading to serious side effects (Fig. 7.18).

HINTS AND TIPS

Most anti-cancer drugs affect normal cell replication and proliferation, especially cells of the bone marrow, gastrointestinal tract, gonads, skin and hair follicles. This results in severe side effects such as anaemia, neutropenia (making patients susceptibile to infection), hair loss, vomiting, infertility, impaired wound healing and stunting of growth.

Fig. 7.18 Action of anti-cancer drugs.

Drugs	Action	Effects on pyrimidine and purine synthesis
Glutamine antagonists: azaserine, diazo-oxonorleucine	Analogues of glutamine: competitively inhibit enzymes that use glutamine as substrate	↓ pyrimidine synthesis: inhibits CPS II ↓ purine synthesis: inhibits PRPP amidotransferase and reaction 5 (Fig. 7.13)
Folate antagonists: methotrexate	Inhibits DHF reductase leading to decreased available THF for transfer of one-carbon units	Inhibits methylation of dUMP to dTMP causing ↓ dTMP synthesis ↓ pyrimidine synthesis (Fig. 7.15)
5-fluorouracil	Analogue of dUMP: irreversibly inhibits thymidylate synthetase	Inhibits synthesis of dTMP; no effect on purine synthesis

HAEM METABOLISM

Structure and function of haem

Structure

Haem is a complex structure containing an iron atom (as Fe^{2+}) placed in the centre of a tetrapyrrole ring of ferroprotoporphyrin (formerly protoporphyrin IX) (Fig. 7.19).

- The basic structure is a four-ringed cyclic structure called a porphyrin
- Each ring is called a pyrrole ring and the rings are linked together via methenyl bridges
- Three types of side chains can be attached to the pyrrole ring – methyl, vinyl or propionyl – and the arrangement of these is important to the activity
- Porphyrins bind metal ions to form metalloporphyrins.

Functions

Haem is the prosthetic group found in a number of proteins. The function of haem in each group can vary (Fig. 7.20). The Fe^{2+} atom (ferrous form) at the centre of the haem structure can undergo oxidation to Fe^{3+} (ferric form); this is important for its function in cytochromes and enzymes, enabling it to act as a recyclable electron carrier. However, in haemoglobin and myoglobin, Fe^{3+} cannot bind oxygen, and its function as an oxygen transporter is impaired (it forms methaemoglobin, see Chapter 3).

Haemoglobin and myoglobin are oxygen-binding proteins with different mechanisms of action.

Fig. 7.20 Functions of haem in different proteins.

Protein	Function of haem
Haemoglobin and myoglobin	Reversibly binds O_2 for transport
Peroxidases and catalase	Forms part of the active site of enzyme
Cytochromes (a, b, c, and P450)	Electron carrier: continually oxidized and reduced, enhancing electron flow

Haemoglobin–oxygen binding is described as being co-operative, and follows a sigmoidal curve; compared to the hyperbolic curve which myoglobin exhibits. The sigmoidal curve means that haemoglobin becomes highly saturated at high oxygen partial pressures, and releases a significant amount of oxygen at pressures which are fairly low, but not extremely so. This cooperative binding mechanism is more efficient at collecting oxygen where it is in high concentration, and supplying it where it is needed. In contrast, low partial pressures of oxygen can almost totally saturate myoglobin. As a result, haemoglobin is described as having a lower affinity for oxygen than myoglobin.

Haem biosynthesis

The main locations of haem biosynthesis are:

- Bone marrow erythroid cells, where haem is used to form haemoglobin
- Hepatocytes, where haem is used for cytochrome synthesis, particularly cytochrome P450 which is involved in drug metabolism.

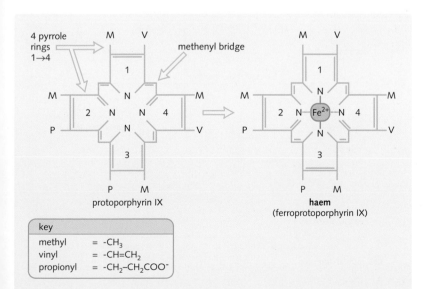

Fig. 7.19 Structure of haem. Haem consists of an Fe $2+$ atom placed in the centre of protoporphyrin IX.

The human body makes 40–50 mg/day of haem, about 80–85% of which is used for haemoglobin synthesis. Mature erythrocytes lack mitochondria and therefore cannot make haem.

Site

Haem biosynthesis is partitioned between mitochondria and the cytosol (Fig. 7.21).

An overview of the pathway

- There are eight reactions; the first and last three occur in the mitochondria, the rest are in the cytosol
- The substrates for haem synthesis are glycine and succinyl CoA
- Eight moles of each are required to form eight moles of δ-aminolevulinic acid (ALA), which condenses to form four moles of porphobilinogen (PBG). These, in turn, condense to form one mole of uroporphyrinogen I (UROgen I)
- The rest of the reactions modify the side chains.

Protoporphyrinogen IX is a colourless, unstable and easily oxidized precursor of porphyrin. Porphyrins are highly coloured (red), stable compounds that characteristically absorb ultraviolet light at a wavelength of 400 nm.

Regulation of haem synthesis

The rate-limiting enzyme of haem synthesis is ALA synthase. It is a good control point because the enzyme undergoes rapid turnover (has a half-life of 60–70 minutes). ALA synthase is inhibited by high levels of the end product haem (Fe^{2+}) and also haemin (ferriprotoporphyrin; Fe^{3+}), formed by the oxidation of haem.

In the liver, control of ALA synthase by haem is considered at three levels (numbers refer to Fig. 7.22):

1. Allosteric inhibition of the enzyme by haem. However, high concentrations of haem are necessary (10^{-5} M) and, therefore, this is not an important control mechanism
2. Haem also inhibits the transport of newly synthesized enzyme from cytosol into mitochondria

Fig. 7.21 Haem synthesis.
1. The synthesis of ALA. ALA synthase catalyses the condensation of glycine and succinyl CoA in the mitochondria. The reaction requires pyridoxal phosphate (PLP) as a cofactor. This is the irreversible, rate-limiting step of haem synthesis
2. The formation of porphobilinogen (PBG). ALA dehydrase catalyses the dehydration of two molecules of ALA to form PBG. The enzyme is inhibited by heavy metals such as lead
3. Formation of uroporphyrinogen I (UROgen I). UROgen I synthase catalyses the condensation of four molecules of PBG to form UROgen I (inactive)
4. UROgen III cosynthase produces the asymmetrical active uroporphyrinogen III (UROgen III). The rest of the reactions alter the side chains and the degree of unsaturation of the porphyrin ring
5. The first decarboxylation results in the formation of coproporphyrinogen III
6. The second decarboxylation forms protoporphyrinogen IX in the mitochondria
7. Oxidation to protoporphyrin IX
8. Ferrochelatase inserts the Fe^{2+} ion into the ring to form haem.

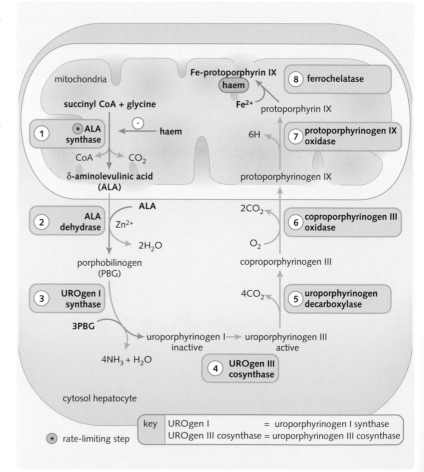

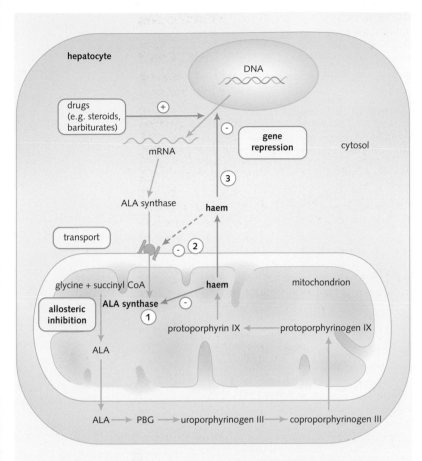

Fig. 7.22 Control of haem synthesis in the hepatocyte.

3. Repression of transcription of the ALA synthase gene by haem. This is probably the most effective regulation because it works at low concentrations (10^{-7} M).

In erythroid tissue, the same regulatory mechanisms apply as in the liver but additionally, under certain conditions such as chronic hypoxia or anaemia, erythropoietin production is stimulated, leading to an increase in red cell production and, therefore, an increase in haem.

Induction of ALA synthase in the liver

A number of drugs, such as steroids and barbiturates, cause an increase in the amount of hepatic ALA synthase. The mechanism proceeds as follows:

- Drugs are metabolized by microsomal cytochrome P450 enzymes, which are haem-containing proteins themselves
- Certain drugs induce the synthesis of cytochrome P450, leading to an increase in the consumption and breakdown of haem
- This leads to an overall decrease in the concentration of haem in the liver cells, which in turn stimulates or induces the transcription of ALA synthase and haem synthesis (Fig. 7.22)
- Glucose blocks this induction.

Haem breakdown

About 80–85% of haem that is broken down comes from old erythrocytes; the rest comes from cytochrome turnover (Fig. 7.23).

Location/site

Kupffer cells and macrophages of the reticuloendothelial system (mainly liver, spleen and bone marrow).

Pathway

The two steps in the pathway are (steps refer to Fig. 7.24):

1. Cleavage of the porphyrin ring to form biliverdin. Haem oxygenase found in microsomes splits the porphyrin ring by breaking one of the methenyl bridges between two pyrrole rings. This produces biliverdin,

Fig. 7.23 Haem breakdown.

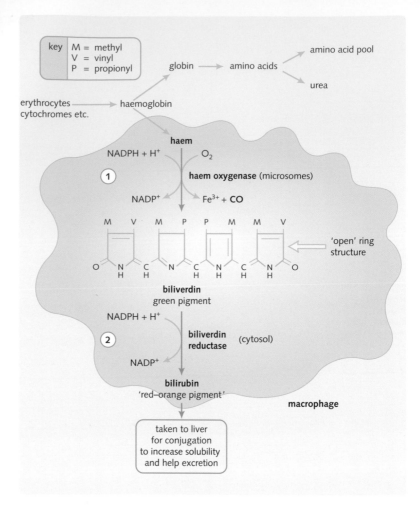

biliverdin
green pigment

bilirubin
'red–orange pigment'

taken to liver
for conjugation
to increase solubility
and help excretion

Fe^{3+} and carbon monoxide (this is the only reaction in vivo that produces carbon monoxide)

2. Reduction of biliverdin to bilirubin occurs in the cytosol.

Bilirubin metabolism

Bilirubin is non-polar and lipophilic and is only sparingly soluble in aqueous solutions. Within the blood, it is bound to albumin and very little remains free in solution. Bilirubin bound to albumin is taken up by the liver. Bilirubin is conjugated within the hepatic endoplasmic reticulum by a UDP glucuronyl transferase to produce a water-soluble bilirubin diglucuronide (Fig 7.24).

The conjugated bilirubin moves into the bile canaliculi of the liver and is then stored in the gall bladder. When stimulated by eating, bile (including the conjugated bilirubin) is secreted into the small intestine. Within the large intestine, bilirubin is further metabolized by bacteria present in the gut into urobilinogen. Some of this is absorbed from the intestine and enters the blood. Much of this in turn is taken up by the liver from the portal vein, but a small proportion enters the general circulation, is filtered through the glomerulus, and enters urine (giving its characteristic yellow colour).

Clinical Note

The liver has a large capacity to conjugate bilirubin and can normally cope with moderately elevated levels. However, in patients with haemolytic anaemia, such as during a sickle cell crisis, there is a very large increase in haem breakdown, resulting in high bilirubin levels, which exceed the conjugating capacity of the liver. This results in elevated plasma levels of unconjugated bilirubin, causing jaundice. In jaundice, the deposition of bilirubin leads to a yellow colouring of the skin, mucosal membranes and the sclerae of eyes (Fig.12.10 describes this clinical sign in the clinical assessment)

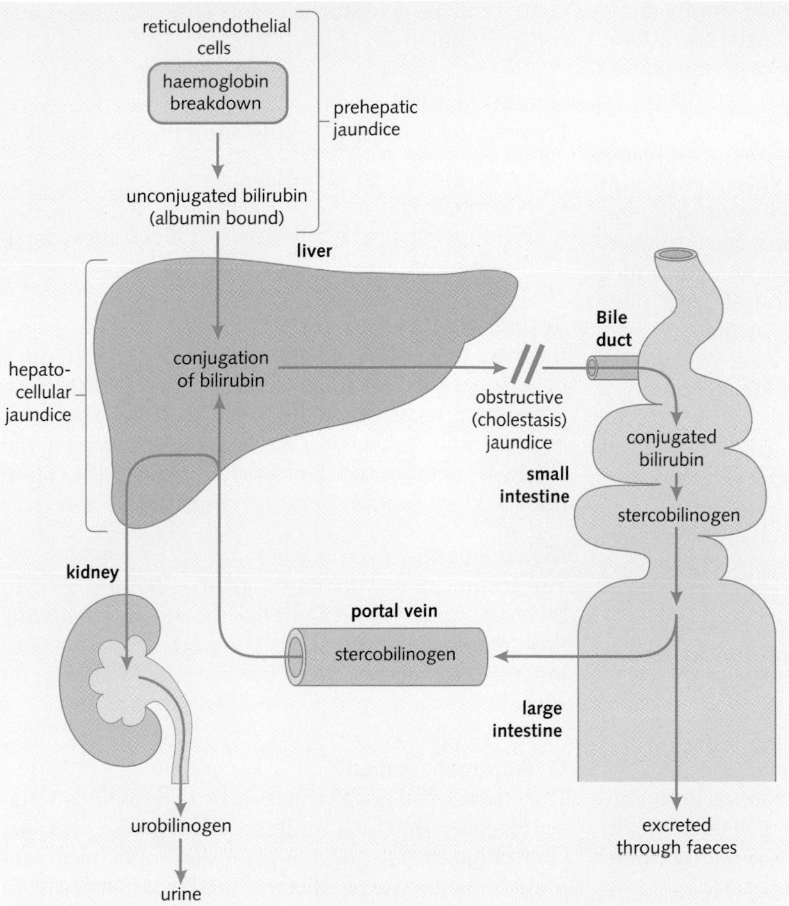

Fig. 7.24 Bilirubin metabolism.

	(1) **prehepatic jaundice**	(2) **hepatocellular jaundice**	(3) **obstructive jaundice**
causes	haemolysis antimalarial drugs (G6PDH deficiency)	viral hepatitis antibiotic drugs paracetamol overdose	gallstones pancreatic cancer antibiotics (flucloxacillin)
key features	↑ unconjugated bilirubin	↑ ALT ↑ AST	↑ conjugated bilirubin no unconjugated bilirubin (pale stools + dark urine) ↑ alkaline phosphates ↑ gGT

HINTS AND TIPS

Haem breakdown occurs at sites of minor trauma underneath the skin. The changing colours of a bruise represent the different pigments produced.

The porphyrias

This is a group of rare, inherited disorders in which there is a partial deficiency of one of the enzymes of haem synthesis. This results in the inhibition of haem synthesis and thus the formation of excessive quantities of either porphyrin precursors, for example δ-aminolevulinic acid (ALA) or porphobilinogen (PBG), or porphyrins themselves, depending upon which enzyme is deficient.

Clinical Note

PBG is readily measured in urine, and usually is crucial in the diagnosis of porphyrias.

The key, rate-limiting enzyme of haem synthesis is ALA synthase which is normally inhibited by haem (see Fig. 7.22). In porphyrias, the absence of haem releases the inhibition (and the control) of ALA synthase, resulting in the increased formation of intermediates preceding the defective enzyme in each porphyria.

When porphyrin precursors (ALA and PBG) are produced in excess, they cause mainly neuropsychiatric symptoms and abdominal pain. When porphyrins themselves are produced in excess, they cause skin photosensitivity (i.e., the skin burns and itches on exposure to light). This is because porphyrins absorb light, which excites them and induces the formation of oxygen free radicals. These can attack membranes, particularly lysosomal membranes, leading to the release of enzymes which damage underlying layers of skin, rendering it susceptible to the light.

Porphyrias are diagnosed on the basis of symptoms and the pattern of porphyrins and their precursors present in the blood and urine.

Porphyrias are classified as either hepatic or erythropoeitic and also as acute or chronic (Fig. 7.25). They are all rare; the most common in the UK is acute intermittent porphyria which is discussed below. The features of other types of porphyrias are summarized in Fig. 7.25.

Acute intermittent porphyria

Acute intermittent porphyria is an autosomal dominant disease with prevalence in the UK of 1:100 000. The defect is a deficiency of uroporphyrinogen I synthase. Characteristically, acute attacks are separated by long periods of remission. The attacks are precipitated by various factors, including alcohol, barbiturates, oral contraceptives, anaesthetic agents (e.g. halothane) and certain antibiotics.

Clinical features
Presentation is usually in early adult life and includes:

- Acute abdominal symptoms
- Neuropathy
- Neuropsychiatric symptoms (e.g. depression, anxiety and psychosis).

Results of laboratory tests
Increased levels of PBG and ALA can be found in the urine of these patients. The urine darkens to a port-wine colour on exposure to air, due to the presence of PBG. The classic bedside test for excess PBG is to add Ehrlich's reagent (an aldehyde) to urine, which causes it to go pink. The colour persists when excess chloroform is added.

Management
The treatment is with fluids, pain relief and a high-carbohydrate diet, which inhibits the pathway. Avoiding precipitants is important. It is important to ask about inherited disorders when pre-assessing patients for surgery.

Overall management
The effects of all porphyrias can be decreased by intravenous haemin which inhibits ALA synthase, the rate-controlling enzyme, regaining the control of haem synthesis. An increased dietary intake of antioxidant vitamins A, C and E also helps to protect against free radical damage. Intravenous haematin can be given.

Fig. 7.25 The porphyrias: summary.

Porphyria	Enzyme defect	Photosensitivity	Neurological symptoms	Biochemistry	
Acute intermittent (hepatic)	Uroporphyrinogen I synthase	No	Yes	Urine:	↑ δ-aminolevulinic acid (ALA) and porphobilinogen (PBG)
Congenital erythropoietic	Uroporphyrinogen III cosynthase	Yes	No	Red cells: Urine:	↑ UROgen I ↑ UROgen I and COPROgen I
Cutaneous (hepatic)	Uroporphyrinogen decarboxylase	Yes	No	Urine: Faeces:	↑ UROgen I and III ↑ COPROgen
Hereditary coproporphyria (hepatic)	Coproporphyrinogen III oxidase	Yes	Yes	Urine:	↑ PBG and COPROgen III
Variegate (hepatic)	Protoporphyrinogen IX oxidase	Yes	Yes	Urine: Faeces:	↑ PBG and ALA ↑ PROTOgen IX, COPROgen III
Erythropoietic	Ferrochelatase	Yes	No	Red cells:	↑ Protoporphyrin

Clinical Note

Porphyrias are very rare. You will seldom see or be asked about them. Fig. 7.25 summarizes all you need to know.

Lead poisoning

The human body contains about 120 mg of lead. Excessive ingestion or inhalation can result from contaminated food, water or air. In the UK, the common sources were old lead piping and petrol. Lead inhibits three key enzymes of haem synthesis, resulting in the accumulation of intermediates:

- ALA dehydrase: this leads to the accumulation of ALA, which can be measured in urine
- Coproporphyrinogen III oxidase: this leads to the accumulation of coproporphyrinogen III
- Ferrochelatase: this leads to the accumulation of protoporphyrin IX in erythrocytes.

Overall, this results in the inhibition of haem synthesis and microcytic anaemia. Lead also binds to bone. The main clinical features and diagnostic criteria are discussed in Fig. 7.26.

Fig. 7.26 Clinical features and diagnosis of lead poisoning.

Clinical features	Diagnosis
Acute exposure: • Severe weakness, vomiting, abdominal pain, anorexia and constipation	Blood lead levels >3 mg/L indicate significant exposure Urine: ↑ δ-aminolevulinic acid levels
Chronic exposure: • Causes staining of teeth and bones, myopathy, peripheral neuropathy, renal damage and sideroblastic anaemia • Eventually leads to encephalopathy and seizures • May cause mental retardation in children	Red cell: ↑ porphyrin levels and fluorescence Blood film: anaemia with basophil stippling; red cells may contain small, blue deposits

Treatment

Treatment is with lead chelators such as desferrioxamine mesilate, sodium calcium edetate or penicillamine. They all bind lead, forming a complex, which can be excreted in the urine.

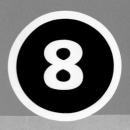
THE STATES OF GLUCOSE HOMEOSTASIS

Glucose homeostasis can be conveniently discussed by looking at three basic states: the fed, fasted (post-absorptive) and starved state (Fig. 8.1). The starved state can be further subdivided into early and late, since different metabolic fuels are used depending on the length of starvation (Fig. 8.2).

It is important to realize that glucose homeostasis is a dynamic process. There are no well-defined boundaries between the different states; instead, there is some degree of overlap between them.

The fed state

This is the period 0–4 hours after a meal and is summarized in Fig. 8.3. During the fed state (numbers refer to Fig. 8.3):

1. An increase in plasma glucose results in the release of insulin from the β cells in the pancreas. The availability of substrate and the increase in insulin stimulates

Fig. 8.1 Three states of glucose homeostasis.

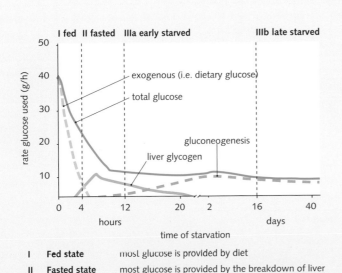

I	**Fed state**	most glucose is provided by diet
II	**Fasted state (post-absorptive)**	most glucose is provided by the breakdown of liver glycogen stores; increasing amounts are provided by gluconeogenesis
III	**Starved state**	most glucose comes from gluconeogenesis; the breakdown of protein and fat provides amino acids and glycerol, substrates for gluconeogenesis

Fig. 8.2 Three states of glucose homeostasis.

State	Time course	Major fuels used	Hormonal control
I Fed	0–4 h following a meal	Most tissues use glucose	↑ insulin results in: ↑ glucose uptake by peripheral tissues ↑ glycogen, TG, and protein synthesis
II Fasted (post-absorptive)	4–12 h after a meal	Brain: glucose muscle and liver: fatty acids	↑ glucagon and NA stimulate breakdown of liver glycogen and TG ↓ insulin
IIIa Early starvation	12 h → 16 days without food	Brain: glucose and some ketone bodies liver: fatty acids muscle: mainly fatty acids and some ketone bodies	↑ glucagon and NA → ↑ TG hydrolysis and ketogenesis ↑ cortisol → breakdown of muscle protein, releasing amino acids for gluconeogenesis
IIIb Prolonged starvation	> 16 days without food	Brain: uses more ketone bodies and less glucose to preserve body protein. Muscle: only fatty acids	↑ glucagon and NA

NA, norepinephrine; TG, triacylglycerol.

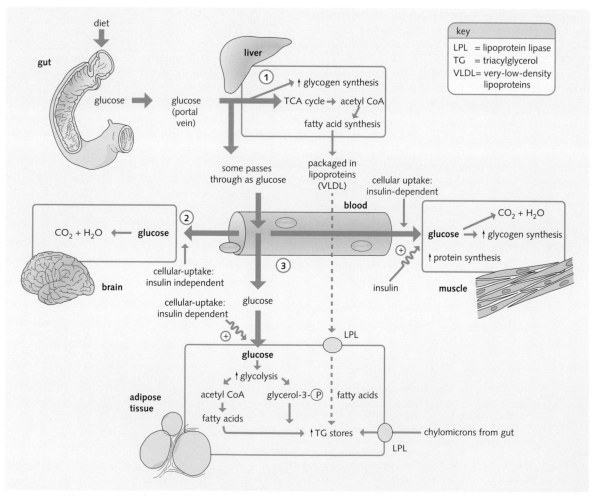

Fig. 8.3 Summary of fuel metabolism in the fed state (numbers 1–3 refer to the text).

glycogen, triacylglycerol (triglyceride), and protein synthesis by tissues; this is an anabolic state

2. Glucose is the sole fuel for the brain; its uptake there is insulin-independent

3. Muscle and adipose tissue also use glucose; however here its uptake is insulin dependent.

An increase in glucose and insulin activates glucokinase in the liver. Glucokinase, unlike hexokinase, is not inhibited by glucose-6-phosphate, enabling the liver to respond to the high blood glucose levels that occur after a meal. Glucokinase phosphorylates glucose, enabling its further metabolism, including glycogen synthesis (see Chapter 4).

Hexokinase, present in most cells, is also active when the concentration of glucose in the blood is low.

The fasted state

This is the period 4–12 hours after a meal, also called the post-absorptive state (Fig. 8.4). During the fasted state (numbers refer to Fig. 8.4):

1. The breakdown of liver glycogen stores provides glucose for oxidation by the brain. These stores are sufficient to last only between 12 and 24 hours

2. The hydrolysis of triacylglycerols from stores releases fatty acids, which are used preferentially as a fuel by muscle and liver

3. Muscle can also use its own glycogen as a fuel.

All these processes are activated by the increase in the ratio of glucagon to insulin. This activates (by phosphorylation) glycogen phosphorylase and hormone-sensitive lipase, leading respectively to glycogen breakdown and lipolysis.

The starved state

Early starved state

Once the liver glycogen begins to be depleted, an alternative substrate is required to provide glucose (Fig. 8.5). In short-term starvation (numbers refer to Fig. 8.5):

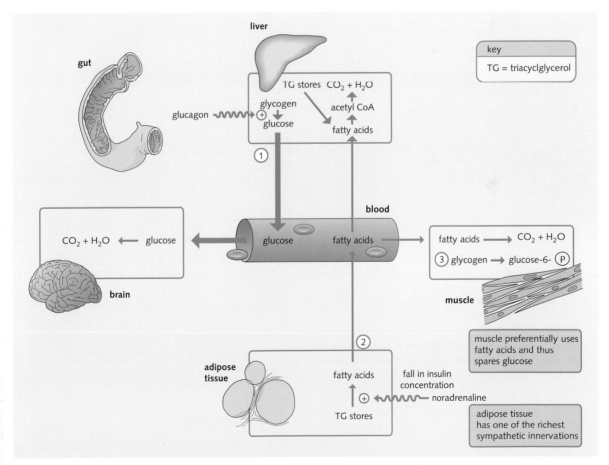

Fig. 8.4 Summary of fuel metabolism in the fasted state; 4–12 hours after a meal. A high glucagon to insulin ratio activates the breakdown of liver glycogen, which provides glucose for the brain. Both the fall in insulin concentration and the increase in norepinephrine promote hydrolysis of triacylglycerol stores, releasing fatty acids which can be used as a fuel by muscle and liver. Muscle uses its own glycogen as fuel (numbers refer to text above).

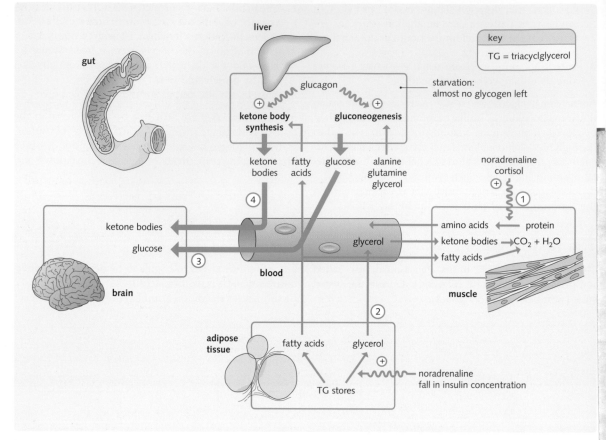

Fig. 8.5 Summary of fuel metabolism in early starvation. Norepinephrine and cortisol activate the breakdown of muscle protein to release amino acids, particularly alanine and glutamine. Norepinephrine also activates hydrolysis of triacylglycerols to release glycerol. Glycerol, alanine and glutamine are taken to the liver, where they enter gluconeogenesis and are oxidized to glucose. Glucose is used mainly by the brain. Fatty acids released from hydrolysis of triacylglycerols can be taken to the liver and used to generate ketone bodies, which can be used by brain and other tissues (numbers refer to text below).

1. Glucagon and later cortisol activate protein breakdown in muscle, which releases amino acids (particularly alanine and glutamine)
2. Hydrolysis of triacylglycerol stores (adipose tissue) releases glycerol. Both the amino acids and glycerol are used by the liver for gluconeogenesis
3. The glucose produced is used by the brain
4. The fatty acids released from triacylglycerols are also used by the liver to make ketone bodies which can be used as an alternative fuel by peripheral tissues as well as the brain.

> **Clinical Note**
>
> A comparison of the fed and the fasted state is a commonly examined 'metabolic' question, because it requires overall knowledge of protein, fat and carbohydrate metabolism and its regulation. The way to answer this for each state is to think about time-course, hormonal influences, main active pathways, substrate availability and any special tissue requirements.

Late starved state

This is the period of starvation of longer than 16 days. In prolonged starvation the breakdown of muscle protein slows down. This is because there is less need for glucose to be supplied via gluconeogenesis, because the brain adapts to using more ketone bodies. This is further helped by muscle using, almost exclusively, fatty acids as fuel.

Gluconeogenesis

Gluconeogenesis is the major source of glucose once glycogen stores are depleted. The main role of gluconeogenesis is the maintenance of blood glucose and the provision of glucose for the brain and erythrocytes during fasting. An increased glucagon:insulin ratio activates gluconeogenesis and causes the reciprocal inhibition of glycolysis (see Chapter 4). In muscle, cortisol activates protein breakdown, releasing, in particular, alanine and glutamine (alanine is one of the main substrates for gluconeogenesis).

Ketogenesis

Ketone body synthesis begins during the first few days of starvation and increases as the brain adapts to using ketone bodies as its major fuel, therefore reducing the need for glucose. Once significant ketone body synthesis occurs, a decrease in the level of gluconeogenesis from amino acids is seen. This results in a reduction in muscle proteolysis, therefore sparing protein.

After 2–3 weeks of starvation, muscle reduces its use of ketone bodies and uses fatty acids almost exclusively; this leads to an increase in ketone bodies available for the brain.

Both ketogenesis and gluconeogenesis are balanced to ensure efficient use of metabolic fuels during starvation. Gluconeogenesis activates ketogenesis by depleting oxaloacetate, which ensures that the concentration of acetyl CoA exceeds the oxidative capacity of the TCA cycle; acetyl CoA can therefore be used for ketone body synthesis.

HORMONAL CONTROL OF GLUCOSE HOMEOSTASIS

Insulin is an anabolic hormone that increases the glucose uptake and synthesis of glycogen, triacylglycerol and protein. Glucagon, norepinephrine, epinephrine and cortisol are catabolic hormones. The main effects of glucagon are summarized in Fig. 8.6. Norepinephrine and epinephrine (stress, or fight-and-flight hormones) have some similar effects to glucagon where they:

- Increase glycogen breakdown (in muscle only)
- Increase lipolysis in adipose tissue
- Stimulate protein breakdown.

Fig. 8.6 Summary of the main effects of insulin and glucagon.

Pathway	Insulin: anabolic	Glucagon: catabolic
Carbohydrate metabolism		
Glycogen	Increases glycogen synthesis in muscle and liver	Increases glycogen breakdown in liver only (NA and epinephrine increase breakdown in muscle) decreases glycogen synthesis
Glycolysis/ gluconeogenesis	Increases glycolysis Inhibits gluconeogenesis	Increases gluconeogenesis inhibits glycolysis
Glucose uptake	Increases uptake by peripheral tissues, not liver	No effect
Pentose phosphate pathway	Increases PPP, producing NADPH for lipogenesis	
Lipid metabolism		
Lipolysis and β oxidation	Inhibits	Activates
Ketone body synthesis	Inhibits	Activates
Lipogenesis	Activates	Inhibits
Protein metabolism		
Uptake of amino acids by tissues	Increases uptake by most tissues	Increases uptake by the liver for gluconeogenesis
Protein synthesis	Increases rate by most tissues	Decreases
Protein breakdown	Decreases	Stimulates breakdown
(NA, norepinephrine; PPP, pentose phosphate pathway).		

GLUCOSE HOMEOSTASIS IN EXERCISE

Sprinters

Sprinting is an anaerobic activity.

- In the muscle during intense activity, there is only time for anaerobic glycolysis, resulting in the build-up of lactate
- Lactate diffuses out of muscle and is taken to the liver where it is oxidized to pyruvate, which can then be converted back to glucose via gluconeogenesis
- The formed glucose diffuses out of the liver and returns to the muscle to be further used as fuel.

This series of reactions, which 'shifts the metabolic burden from the muscle to the liver', is known as the Cori cycle (Fig. 8.7). (Compare it with the glucose–alanine cycle.)

Long-distance running

Long-distance running is aerobic.

The body does not store enough glycogen to provide the energy necessary to run long distances. If the respiratory quotient (RQ: the ratio of the amount of O_2 consumed to the amount of CO_2 released) is measured during a run, initially it is about 1.0, indicating that

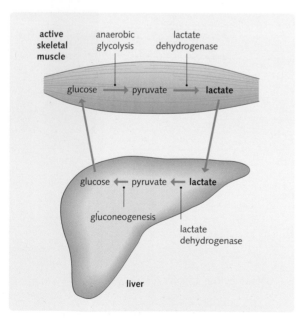

active skeletal muscle   anaerobic glycolysis   lactate dehydrogenase

glucose → pyruvate → lactate

glucose ← pyruvate ← lactate

gluconeogenesis

lactate dehydrogenase

liver

Fig. 8.7 The Cori cycle distributes the metabolic burden between the muscle and the liver. Lactate, which builds up in muscle during intense activity, is taken to the liver to be converted back to glucose via gluconeogenesis. This replenishes fuel for the muscle and prevents lactic acidosis.

mainly carbohydrate is being used. However, the RQ falls during running to a value of about 0.77 after about 1 hour, indicating that mainly fats are being oxidized.

The type and amount of substrate used varies with the intensity and duration of exercise, in a similar way to starvation. As glycogen stores are depleted, an increase in glucagon, norepinephrine and epinephrine stimulates lipolysis, releasing fatty acids for muscle to use to conserve glucose. An increase in these hormones, along with an increase in cortisol, leads to stimulation of gluconeogenesis and protein degradation in muscle. These changes are similar to those of the fasting state; the difference is that the level of ketone bodies in the blood is low. It is not clear whether this is because they are not being synthesized or if they are being oxidized as soon as they are formed.

Mechanism of action of insulin

Insulin is an anabolic hormone, and the understanding of its actions has recently greatly improved. It promotes the synthesis and storage of carbohydrates, lipids and proteins and inhibits their degradation and release back into the circulation; these actions involve multiple signaling pathways.

Basically, the binding of insulin to its tyrosine kinase receptor on the outside surface of the cells induces the receptor to undergo autophosphorylation at several tyrosine kinase residues located inside the cell. This autophosphorylation facilitates binding and phosphorylation of cytosolic substrate proteins, such as insulin receptor substrate-1 (IRS-1) and Cbl proteins. Upon phosphorylation, these proteins interact with other signaling molecules through their SH2 (Src-homology-2) domains, which then activate several diverse pathways.

Such pathways include activation of PI_3 kinase and TC10 (a small GTP binding protein). PI-3 kinase activates protein kinase B (PKB) and PKB in turn phosphorylates a range of target enzymes. The net result of these diverse pathways is regulation of glucose, lipid and protein metabolism as well as cell growth and differentiation (Fig. 8.8).

DIABETES MELLITUS

Classification

Diabetes mellitus is a syndrome caused by the lack, or diminished effectiveness, of insulin. It results in a raised blood glucose known as hyperglycaemia and can lead to the development of diverse vascular complications over long periods of time. There are two main types of diabetes:

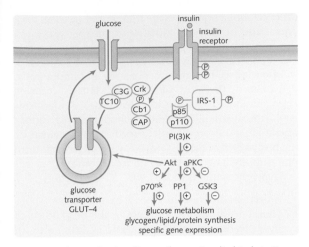

Fig. 8.8 The insulin signaling pathway. Insulin binds to its receptor, resulting in autophosphorylation. This then phosphorylates the protein Cbl which is in complex with the adaptor protein CAP. Cbl/CAP complex then interacts with the adaptor protein Crk which is constitutively associated with C3G, a GTP/GDP exchange protein. C3G activates TC10, which themselves promote GLUT4 translocation to the plasma membrane. Autophosphorylation of the insulin receptor also phosphorylates insulin receptor substrate 1 (IRS-1). IRS-1 attracts p85, which binds to p110, which then activates phophatidylinositol-3 kinase (PI-3 kinase). PI-3 kinase activates protein kinase B (PKB; Akt) which act on further pathways, resulting in glucose, lipid and protein metabolism, and specific gene expression. Akt also promotes GLUT-4 translocation to plasma membrane, resulting in increased glucose uptake.

- Type 1: formerly known as insulin-dependent diabetes mellitus (IDDM) in which there is an absolute failure of the pancreas to produce insulin
- Type 2: formerly known as non-insulin-dependent diabetes mellitus (NIDDM) in which there is a failure of the tissues to respond normally to insulin, together with a compensatory rise in plasma insulin concentration at early stages. As the disease progresses, insulin secretion deteriorates.

Type 1 diabetes mellitus

Type 1 was often referred to as juvenile-onset diabetes because it typically presents in childhood or puberty. It accounts for only 10–20% of the total number of people with diabetes and has an incidence rate of about 1 in 3000.

The aetiology of the disease is a complete deficiency of insulin that can only be corrected by life-long insulin treatment. There are three theories as to its cause:

- Auto-immune destruction of the β cells in the islets of Langerhans in the pancreas by islet cell auto-antibodies, resulting in insulin deficiency
- Genetic factors. The evidence for a genetic cause is that, firstly, there is a 50% concordance between

identical twins, which implies a mixture of both genetic and environmental factors. Secondly, there is a positive family history in approximately 10% of patients. Thirdly, more than 90% of patients with Type 1 diabetes carry HLA DR3 and DR4 antigens, compared with 40% of the general population
- A viral cause, for example mumps or Coxsackie B, has also been considered. However, it is likely that viral infections provide the stimulus for auto-immune destruction rather than actually initiating diabetes.

Therefore, the cause is probably a mixture of all three – auto-immune destruction of the β cells in genetically susceptible patients, which may be precipitated by a viral infection.

The presentation of the disease is usually of rapid onset, weeks or days, with the characteristic symptoms of polyuria, polydipsia and weight loss.

Type 2 diabetes mellitus

This was also known as maturity-onset diabetes, because it typically presents after the age of 35 years. The incidence is more common, and it accounts for 80–90% of the total number of people with diabetes.

> **Clinical Note**
>
> Insulin resistance (metabolic) syndrome is a new concept, which helps to identify individuals with risk factors for cardiovascular disease and type 2 diabetes (obesity, abnormal glucose tolerance). Defining criteria vary, but according to the International Diabetes Federation (2006) there needs to be:
>
> Central obesity (defined as waist circumference with ethnicity specific values, but if BMI is >30 kg/m², central obesity can be assumed)
> AND
> Any two of the following:
> - Raised triglycerides: >1.7 mmol/L
> - Reduced HDL cholesterol: <1.03 mmol/L in males, <1.29 mmol/L in females
> - Raised blood pressure: systolic BP >130 or diastolic BP >85 mmHg
> - Raised fasting plasma glucose (FPG) > (5.6 mmol/L).
> Note: If FPG >5.6 mmol/L, an oral glucose tolerance test is strongly recommended (but is not necessary to define the syndrome).
> Source: http://www.idf.org/webdata/docs/ MetSyndrome_FINAL.pdf

Type 2 diabetes is caused by:

- Impaired insulin secretion from the β cells; they fail to secrete enough insulin to correct the blood glucose level.
- Insulin resistance in the tissues; cells failing to respond adequately to insulin.

Genetic factors are very important; there is almost 100% concordance between identical twins and about 30% of patients have a first-degree relative with Type 2 diabetes. There is no auto-immune or viral involvement.

The presentation is of an insidious onset and more than 80% of patients are obese.

Other types of diabetes

There are a number of other types of diabetes, which usually occur secondary to a predisposing factor, for example:

- Gestational diabetes; onset of diabetes during pregnancy
- Secondary diabetes: this may be the result of damage to the pancreas itself, for example, in chronic pancreatitis or haemochromatosis, where iron may deposit in the pancreas (see Chapter 11). Diabetes may also occur secondary to the excessive secretion of catabolic hormones, resulting in hyperglycaemia and insulin resistance. For example, in acromegaly, where there is over-secretion of growth hormone, or in Cushing's syndrome, where there are high levels of glucocorticoids such as cortisol; also in poorly monitored long-term steroid therapy.

These other types of diabetes are covered in more detail in textbooks of endocrinology and clinical medicine.

Metabolic effects of diabetes mellitus

Type 1 diabetes mellitus

Insulin normally facilitates the uptake of glucose by peripheral tissues. In its absence, glucose remains in the blood, resulting in a decreased tissue availability of glucose, but a high plasma concentration of glucose. The phrase 'starvation in the midst of plenty' is frequently used to describe this. As there is a low concentration of insulin, the metabolic effects of glucagon and the

other catabolic hormones are unopposed (see Fig. 8.6). This results in the predominance of catabolic processes; the breakdown of carbohydrate, protein and fat (see Fig. 8.9). This aggravates hyperglycaemia, and leads to ketoacidosis, hypertriglyceridaemia and importantly, dehydration (because of osmotic diuresis, causing large amounts of glucose to enter urine). Ketoacidosis is life-threatening. In addition, because cells cannot obtain glucose from the diet they have to obtain it by the breakdown of body stores or by synthesizing it from non-carbohydrate precursors (gluconeogenesis).

Hyperglycaemia is caused by:

- A decreased uptake of glucose by the tissues
- Glucagon-stimulated increase in the breakdown of liver glycogen and gluconeogenesis, leading to an increased hepatic output of glucose.

Ketoacidosis is caused by:

- An increase in triacylglycerol hydrolysis in adipose tissue that releases fatty acids
- An increase in ketone body synthesis in liver.

The release of fatty acids is much greater than in starvation; therefore, the rate of formation of ketone bodies is much greater than the rate of use, leading to ketonaemia (see Chapter 5).

Hypertriglyceridaemia is an increase in the concentration of triacylglycerols in plasma. (Note that in clinical medicine triacylglycerols are usually referred to as triglycerides.) Some of the fatty acids released from triacylglycerols are packaged in the liver into very-low-density lipoproteins (VLDLs). Dietary triacylglycerols are assembled into chylomicrons. In the absence of insulin, the activity of lipoprotein lipase decreases, and the VLDLs and chylomicrons remain in the plasma, and are responsible for hypertriglyceridaemia (see Fig. 8.9).

Type 2 diabetes mellitus

The metabolic effects are essentially the same as for Type 1 but usually they are milder because insulin is present. However:

- The amount of insulin secreted from the pancreas may be insufficient to cope with the blood glucose level
- Target tissues or organs fail to respond correctly to insulin (they show insulin resistance).

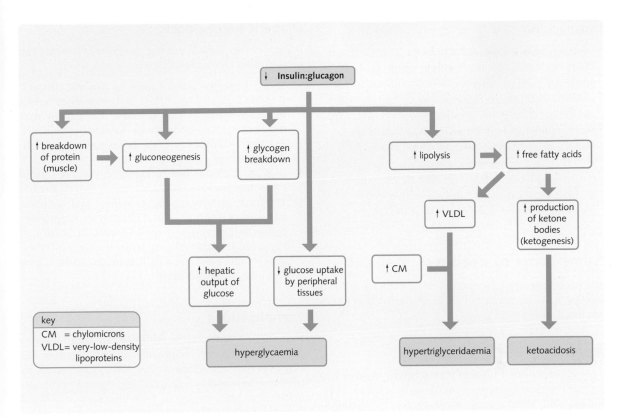

Fig. 8.9   Effect of an increased glucagon to insulin ratio in diabetes.

Fig. 8.10 Important differences between Type 1 diabetes and starvation.		
Feature	**Type 1 diabetes mellitus**	**Starvation**
Insulin	Absent or very low due to disruption of synthesis	Insulin produced but present at low level
Blood glucose	Hyperglycaemia	Normal blood glucose concentration maintained
Ketone body formation	Large increase in production of ketone bodies where rate of formation exceeds rate of use; can lead to life-threatening ketoacidosis	Increased concentration, but usually rate of formation equals rate of use

In Type 2 diabetes, insulin resistance may be due to a number of defects. For example, an abnormal insulin receptor or a defect in a glucose transporter. Insulin resistance in the liver results in uncontrolled glucose production and its decreased uptake by the peripheral tissues. Both phenomena contribute to hyperglycaemia. Hyperglycaemia in turn further stimulates insulin secretion by the pancreas. Type 2 diabetes is typically associated with older age of onset than Type 1 diabetes and, most importantly, with obesity.

Obesity is associated with an increase in the number and/or size of adipocytes. These cells overproduce hormones and cytokines, collectively known as adipokines, such as leptin and tumour necrosis factor-alpha, (TNF-α) which induce cellular resistance to insulin by interfering with the phosphorylation of the insulin receptor and IRS-1. Adipocytes also decrease synthesis of hormones such as adiponectin, which normally enhance insulin responsiveness. As a result, there is insulin resistance in muscle and liver. Initially, the pancreas maintains glycaemic control by overproducing insulin but prolonged overproduction of insulin eventually results in failure of the β-cells, leading to Type 2 diabetes. However, there is still hope for improvement since insulin resistance has been shown to be reversible with weight loss and increased exercise.

Symptoms of diabetes mellitus

The presentation of the symptoms of diabetes mellitus may be acute or emergency or insidious in onset (types are listed in Fig. 8.11).

Acute

Young people often present with a brief 2–4 week history of the classical symptoms, namely polyuria, polydipsia, and weight loss, accompanied by tiredness. These patients usually have Type 1 diabetes.

Subacute

The onset of symptoms is usually over months to years. Patients may still present with the classic symptoms although, quite often, tiredness is the prominent symptom, particularly Type 2 diabetes.

Asymptomatic

Glycosuria or raised blood glucose may be detected during a routine medical examination.

Diabetic ketoacidosis

If the early symptoms are not recognized, patients can present with ketoacidosis (see Fig. 8.12), where:

- Severe hyperglycaemia causes an osmotic diuresis. The consequent loss of fluid and electrolytes results in dehydration. If this is severe, the patient may be confused and be in shock. Remember to consider this diagnosis in patients presenting with abdominal pain
- Increased production of ketone bodies results in metabolic acidosis and characteristic ketotic breath. The acidosis typically causes nausea and vomiting and further loss of fluid and electrolytes. Respiratory compensation results in hyperventilation (Kussmaul breathing). Diabetic ketoacidosis is a medical emergency: failure to treat a patient in ketoacidosis may result in coma and death.

Complications

Patients may also present with diabetic complications such as retinopathy, neuropathy or nephropathy. For example, they may present after visits to the opticians (diabetic retinopathy), or with tingling and numbness in the leg, or with leg or foot ulcers or impotence (neuropathy).
The diagnosis of diabetes is discussed fully in Chapter 8.

Clinical features

Type 1 diabetes mellitus
The clinical features and diagnosis of Type 1 diabetes are listed in Fig. 8.13. The treatment consists of:

- Insulin. There are three main types of insulin: short-acting, intermediate-acting and long-acting. The duration of action of insulin is increased by forming a complex with a protamine salt and/or varying the size of the crystals

Fig. 8.11 Types of diabetes mellitus.	
Type	**Notes.**
Diabetes mellitus: Type 1, insulin-dependent diabetes mellitus Type 2, non-insulin-dependent diabetes mellitus	Overall incidence, approximately 2% in Western world Patients are usually younger than 25 years Patients are usually older than 25 years and can often be overweight
Impaired glucose tolerance	Affects about 5% of population; these patients are more likely to develop diabetes when they are older
Secondary diabetes	Either due to pancreatic damage, e.g. chronic pancreatitis, haemochromatosis or Wilson's disease, or due to endocrine disease, e.g. acromegaly, Cushing's disease
Note that a new category of impaired fasting glucose (>6 mmol/L) has been recently recognized	

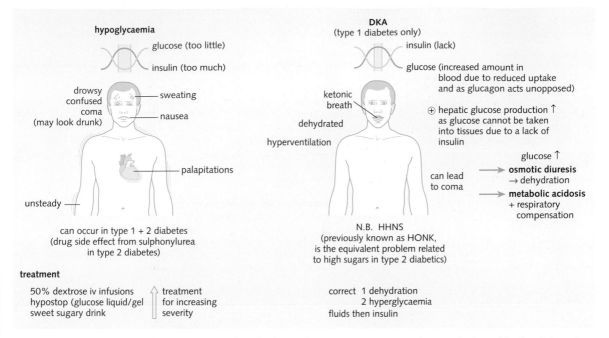

Fig. 8.12 Diabetic ketoacidosis. In the absence of insulin, hyperglycaemia causes osmotic diuresis. The loss of fluid and electrolytes results in dehydration. Increased ketogenesis causes metabolic acidosis. Respiratory compensation results in hyperventilation. Both dehydration and hyperglycaemia must be corrected in parallel with insulin treatment.

Fig. 8.13 Clinical features and diagnosis of Type 1 (insulin-dependent) diabetes mellitus.

Main clinical features	Diagnostic criteria
Classically: • acute onset of symptoms (2–4 weeks) polyuria, poly-dipsia, accompanied by weight loss, abdominal pain and tiredness • ketoacidosis: may present in diabetic coma	Presence of symptoms Raised random blood glucose, > 11.1 mmol/L Fasting blood glucose: venous plasma ≥7.0 mmol/L (oral glucose tolerance test is not necessary – reserved for borderline cases; glycosuria is not diagnostic due to variation in renal threshold for glucose)

- Diet. Ensuring the correct content and timing of meals. The diet should be high in fibre and unrefined carbohydrate, low in saturated fat and refined carbohydrate
- Education. It is crucial that patients understand their disease, and the short- and long-term benefits of treatment.

There are a number of methods for monitoring the control of diabetes and these are covered in detail in Chapter 12. They include:

- Measuring blood glucose levels, using reagent strips based on the glucose oxidase reaction, or portable glucose meters
- Monitoring the level of glycated haemoglobin (HbA$_{1c}$). This provides a measure of the average blood glucose control over the past 4–6 weeks

- The detection of ketones in urine (and blood), important for the detection of developing ketoacidosis
- Detection and monitoring of chronic complications.

Type 2 diabetes mellitus

Clinical Note

Type 2 diabetes is increasing in prevalence and not only can lead to specific long-term complications but also has an impact on cardiovascular risk. This should be considered and appropriately managed in patients identified as being 'at risk'.

Fig. 8.14 Diagnosis, management and treatment of Type 2 diabetes (non-insulin dependent diabetes, NIDDM). (References: http://guidance.nice.org.uk/CG66/Guidance/pdf/English)

Clinical features	Management
• Insidious onset: tiredness, polyuria, thirst, weight loss • Patients usually older and typically obese • May be asymptomatic – detection of ↑ blood glucose on routine check-up **Diagnosis**: as for Type 1 – symptoms usually less severe	**First line: Diet and lifestyle** **Second line: Oral hypoglycaemic drugs**: 4 main classes (in the usual order of use, with addition for further medications as needed for optimal control): 1) Biguanides, e.g. metformin: ↑ glucose uptake by peripheral tissues and ↓ glucose production by liver. Key point: metformin aids weight loss 2) Sulphonylureas, e.g. glibenclamide: ↑ insulin secretion by islet cells (inhibits ATP-sensitive K$^+$ channels in β cell membranes). Key point: due to this mechanism of action, this class of oral hypoglycaemics have a risk of hypoglycaemia 3) Thiazolidinediones, ↑ insulin sensitivity 4) Acarbose inhibits intestinal enzyme, glucosidase and therefore, delays the digestion of starch Metformin is usually the first choice, except in cases where the patient is not overweight or a rapid response to therapy is required because of hyperglycaemic symptoms, in which case sulphonylureas are initiated. **Third line: Insulin (used if oral therapy fails)**

The diagnosis, management and treatment of Type 2 diabetes are covered in Fig. 8.14.

Complications of diabetes

These develop slowly when diabetes is poorly controlled.

Acute complications (fig 8.15)

Hypoglycaemia

The aim of treatment of Type 1 diabetes with insulin is to maintain a normal blood glucose level, which decreases the long-term effects of diabetes. However, too much insulin or too infrequent 'top ups' of glucose (i.e. insufficient intake of carbohydrate) lead to a low blood glucose (hypoglycaemia). Hypoglycaemia causes unpleasant autonomic symptoms, such as sweating, nausea and palpitations, and more severe neuroglycopenic symptoms as a result of a decrease in glucose supply to the brain: drowsiness, unsteadiness, confusion and coma (these patients may look drunk). This is a very serious condition and must be treated without delay with an intravenous 50% dextrose infusion. Mild hypoglycaemia can be treated with sugar or sweet drinks.

Diabetic ketoacidosis (DKA)

In the absence of insulin, effects of glucagon are unopposed. Decreased uptake of glucose by tissues, coupled with an increased hepatic glucose production, leads to hyperglycaemia. This causes an osmotic diuresis, and the resulting loss of fluid and electrolytes causes dehydration. An increase in lipolysis leads to increased ketogenesis and a metabolic acidosis (ketones will be detected on urinalysis). Respiratory compensation results in hyperventilation.

Hyperosmolar hyperglycemic non-ketotic syndrome (HHNS) is a diabetic emergency which occurs rarely, mostly in elderly Type 2 diabetic patients. It is also due to hyperglycaemia. It is defined by a serum glucose that is usually higher than 33 mmol/l (600 mg/dl), and a resulting serum osmolarity that is greater than 350 mOsm. An osmotic diuresis will result in polyuria and severe volume depletion, which causes a hemoconcentration that further increases blood glucose level and osmolarity.

The main differences to a DKA are:

- Patient group
  - HHNS usually occurs in Type 2 diabetics, DKA usually in Type 1
  - HHNS usually affects older patients.
- Ketosis; absent in HHNS. (The presence of some insulin inhibits lipolysis so these acidic by-products may not form, unlike in DKA)
- Onset; HHNS can be insidious and develop over weeks, and in about a third of cases it is the first manifestation of type 2 diabetes. (Note that HHNS is very rare.)

Similarities include:

- Precipitating factors; both HHNS and DKA are usually precipitated by an illness/infection/acute illness (myocardial infarction)
- Dehydration; which is the principal problem in both

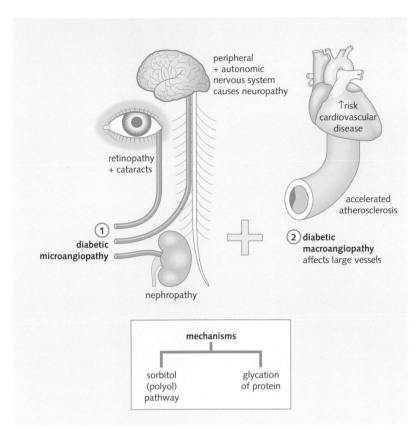

Fig. 8.15 Long-term complications of diabetes.

Clinical Note

Management of DKA and HHNS

Rehydration is the first priority, followed by management of electrolyte imbalances (potassium) and by control of blood glucose with an insulin infusion (sliding scale). Rehydration can be aggressive in young patients with ketoacidosis, but, care needs to be taken in elderly patients with HHNS who could have cardiovascular problems.

Sources

http://www.dh.gov.uk/en/Publicationsandstatistics/
    Publications/PublicationsPolicyAndGuidance/
    Browsable/DH_4902982
http://www.diabetes.org.uk/Guide-to-diabetes/
    Complications/Hyperosmolar_Hyperglycaemic_
    State_HHS/

- Both are life threatening; DKA continues to be a prominent cause of death, particularly in young diabetics. Cerebral oedema (swelling of the brain) is a serious complication of DKA and carries a high risk of permanent neurological damage and death. Equally, reported death rates from HHNS are very high (58%).

Be aware of warning signs: dry mouth, confusion, weakness, and visual losses. And knowledgeable about the emergency management of DKA and HHNS (Fig. 8.13).

Chronic complications

In the long term the major cause of death in Type 1 diabetes are chronic complications, particularly diabetic retinopathy, nephropathy and neuropathy. In type 2 diabetes, heart disease, peripheral vascular disease and stroke are the major causes of death.

Good control of diabetes (i.e. when the blood glucose is maintained close to normal) decreases the frequency and progression of microangiopathy (but apparently not macroangiopathy) (Fig. 8.14).

Fig. 8.16 Comparison of Type 1 and Type 2 diabetes mellitus.

	Type 1	Type 2
Usual age of onset	Young < 35 years (mean approx. 12 years)	> 35 years
Auto-immune factors	Yes	No
Genetic factors	Risk associated with certain HLA types	Yes – polygenic inheritance
Concordance identical twins	50%	Almost 100%
Symptoms	Polyuria, polydipsia, weight loss	Similar but usually less severe presentation
Signs	Wasting, dehydration, loss of consciousness	Obesity
Ketosis	Prone; leading to DKA	Rare; but HHNS can develop
Obesity	Infrequent	Frequent

The WHO criteria for diagnosis of diabetes are as follows: fasting venous plasma glucose equal or above 7 mmol/L. A glucose level of 6–7 mmol/L is defined as impaired fasting glucose (IFG). If the patient has no diabetic symptoms, diagnosis should not be based on a single glucose value.

HINTS AND TIPS

'Compare Type 1 diabetes mellitus with Type 2'. This is a commonly asked exam question; Fig. 8.16 should help.

Digestion, malnutrition and obesity

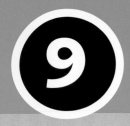

BASIC PRINCIPLES OF HUMAN NUTRITION

Definitions

Nutrients

Nutrients are essential dietary factors, such as vitamins, minerals, essential amino acids and essential fatty acids that cannot be synthesized by the body, and can only be obtained from the food we eat.

Macronutrients are present in our diets in large amounts, and make up the bulk of our diets. They can be found in carbohydrates, fat, protein and water.

Micronutrients are present in our diet, but in very small amounts. These are vitamins, minerals and trace elements. They do not provide energy, however they are still needed in adequate amounts to ensure that all our body cells function properly. Despite their presence in minute amounts their importance is paramount.

Staple foods

Staple foods are the principal sources of energy in the diet. They are specific to a particular country; for example, in parts of Africa and Asia cereals provide more than 70% of the energy in the diet. As countries become more prosperous, the percentage of energy derived from a single staple food declines. In the UK, flour and flour products provide only about 25% of food energy.

Digestion in the gastrointestinal tract

Figure 9.1 shows the anatomy of the intestinal tract and summarizes the main steps in the digestion of carbohydrates, proteins and fats.

Digestion of carbohydrates

Digestion of carbohydrates begins in the mouth and stomach. Saliva contains an enzyme, α-amylase, which hydrolyzes starch into maltose and other small polymers of glucose. Digestion continues in the stomach for about an hour before the activity of salivary amylase is blocked by gastric acid.

Pancreatic secretions, similar to saliva, contain large quantities of α-amylase. It is identical to the α-amylase in saliva, therefore virtually all the starches are digested by the time they enter the duodenum. Disaccharides and small glucose polymers are hydrolyzed into monosaccharides by intestinal epithelial enzymes.

- Lactose → galactose + glucose
- Sucrose → fructose + glucose
- Maltose and other small glucose polymers → glucose.

Digestion of proteins

Protein digestion begins in the stomach. The enzyme pepsin breaks down collagen to allow other enzymes to penetrate meats and digest cellular proteins. Most protein digestion occurs through the actions of pancreatic proteolytic enzymes.

- Trypsin and chymotrypsin break down protein molecules into small polypeptides
- Carboxypolypeptidase cleaves amino acids from the carboxyl ends of the polypeptides
- Proelastase gives rise to elastase, which then digests the elastin fibres that hold meat together.

The last stage of digestion of proteins is carried out in the intestinal lumen by enterocytes, which contain

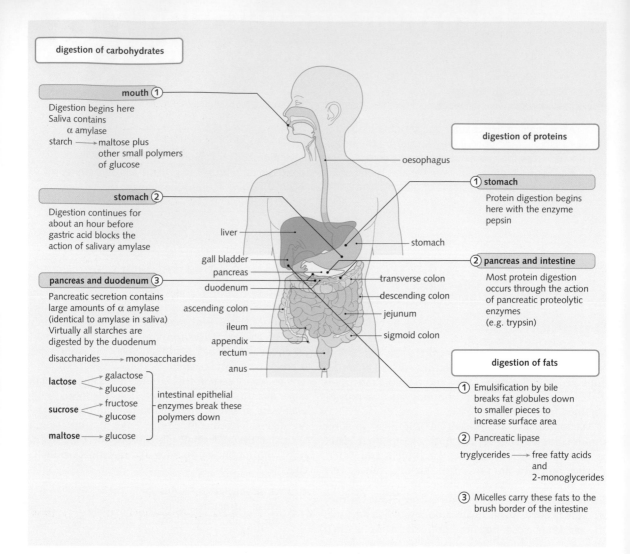

Fig. 9.1 The gastrointestinal tract.

multiple peptidases that break down remaining tripeptides and dipeptides into amino acids, which then enter the blood.

Digestion of fats

Fat digestion begins with the emulsification by bile acids and lecithin, where fat globules are broken into smaller pieces to increase their surface area. Pancreatic lipase breaks down triglycerides into free fatty acids and 2-monoglycerides which are carried to the brush border of the intestinal epithelial cells by micelles. Micelles are composed of a central fat globule (containing monoglycerides and free fatty acids) with molecules of bile salt projecting outward covering the surface of the micelle.

Methods of estimating an individual's dietary intake

There are three main methods for estimating an individual's dietary intake:

- Dietary recall. Ask the patient what he or she has eaten. This is the least accurate because it relies on the patient's recall and willingness to cooperate
- Food diary. This is slightly more accurate
- Complete chemical analysis. This is the most expensive but the most accurate method.

Dietary reference values

The definitions in Fig. 9.2 are in keeping with the dietary reference values (DRVs) for food energy and nutrients for the UK.

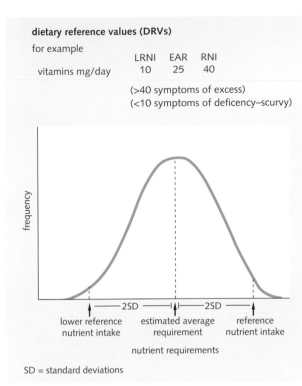

Estimated average requirement (EAR)
This is the average requirement of a group of people for energy or a nutrient. About 50% of the population will need less than the EAR and 50% will need more.

Reference nutrient intake (RNI)
This is the amount of nutrient that is enough or more than enough for about 97% of people in the group (EAR + 2SD)

Lower reference nutrient intake (LRNI)
This is the amount of nutrient that is sufficient for only a few people in a group with low needs (EAR − 2SD)

Adequate intake
This is the amount of nutrient enough for almost everyone, but not so much as to cause undesirable effects. This term is applied for nutrients for which there is not enough information known to estimate EAR, RNI or LRNI (e.g. vitamin E).

For instance, the DRVs for vitamin C are: LRNI, 10 mg/day; EAR, 25 mg/day; RNI, 40 mg/day. Therefore below the LRNI, symptoms of vitamin C deficiency (scurvy) are seen and above the RNI, symptoms of excess may be seen.

Fig. 9.2 Dietary reference values for food energy and nutrients.

ENERGY BALANCE

Food energy

The total energy content of food is the amount of energy released when food is completely burnt in air to CO_2 and H_2O, that is, the heat of combustion (Fig. 9.3). The total energy is equal to the sum of the digestible energy and the non-digestible energy (Fig. 9.4). From Fig. 9.3 it can be seen that protein has a higher total energy content than carbohydrate. However, protein is not as efficiently oxidized (it forms urea and requires ATP for this; see Chapter 6) and only about 4 kcal/g are available as metabolizable energy. Carbohydrate is oxidized completely to CO_2 and H_2O and all the energy produced is available for use; the metabolizable energy is also 4 kcal/g.

Body composition

An average 72-kg man is composed of:

- 15% fat
- 85% lean body mass (LBM).

Lean body mass (LBM) is made up of (these are approximate values):

- 72% water
- 20% protein
- 8% bone mineral.

Generally, women have a higher fat content (about 25% fat) than men. Fat content tends to increase with age. An average 72-kg man can survive on his energy stores for about 50–60 days provided he is given water. This is mostly due to fat reserves; glycogen stores last only

Fig. 9.3 Major sources of energy in the diet.

Energy source	Total kcal	Energy/g kJ
Fat: essential for absorption of fat-soluble vitamins (A, D, E and K)	9.2	38.6
Carbohydrate: as either starch, sugar or non-starch polysaccharide (NSP), i.e. fibre	4.0	16.8
Protein:	5.4	22.7
Alcohol: 'empty calories'	7.0	29.4

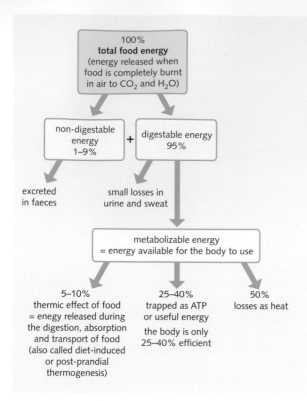

• Non-digestible energy is the energy in food that we cannot break down and is lost in faeces (e.g. cellulose)
• Digestible energy is the total energy minus energy that is lost in faeces.

Metabolizable energy is the energy available to the body for use; it has three fates:

• 50% is lost as heat
• 5–10% of energy is released during the digestion, absorption and transport of food. This is known as either the thermic effect of food, diet-induced thermogenesis (DIT), or post-prandial thermogenesis (they all mean the same thing)
• Only about 25–40% of the energy is trapped as ATP; that is, the body is only 25–40% efficient.

Fig. 9.4   Food energy utilization.

12–24 hours. Fig. 9.5 summarizes the methods available to measure body composition. However, most of the methods, with the exception of anthropometry, are rarely used in clinical practice.

Energy requirements

Energy is used by the body for three main processes (Fig. 9.6).

Basal metabolic rate

The basal metabolic rate (BMR) is the energy used to carry out normal body functions (such as breathing); it is the energy expended doing nothing. The units of BMR are kJ/hour/kg of body weight. To calculate the BMR:

• The patient must be at rest, lying down but not asleep
• The temperature of the environment must be moderate and constant
• The patient must be assessed about 12 hours after the last meal or any exercise.

The BMR is usually measured first thing in the morning. It is proportional to LBM, therefore, men have a higher BMR than women. Women have a greater percentage

Fig. 9.5 Measurement of body composition.	
Measurement	**Method**
Body density	Weigh in air to give fat content (density = 0.9 mg/mL); weigh in water to give lean body mass (density = 1.1 mg/mL)
Body water	The patient is injected with a known volume of tritiated water Its concentration at equilibrium is measured This is representative of lean body mass
Total body potassium	$^4 K^+$ is injected and its distribution assessed This is a measure of lean body mass as there is no potassium in fat
Body fat	The uptake of a fat-soluble gas, e.g. xenon or cyclopropane is measured Biopsy to measure concentration
Anthropometry	Measure: • weight and height • mid-arm circumference (biceps and triceps) • skin-fold thickness (subscapular and suprailiac) compare with normograms for weight and height

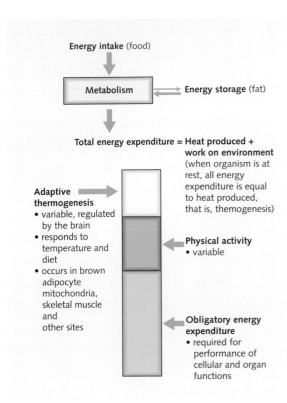

Fig. 9.6 Energy intake – food.

of fat which is less metabolically active. The BMR usually accounts for 50–70% of the total energy expended.

Thermic effect of food

This is the energy required for the digestion and absorption of food and accounts for 5–10% of the energy expenditure.

Physical activity

The amount of energy consumed depends on the duration and intensity of exercise. The physical activity ratio (PAR) can be measured for situations where activity is expressed as a multiple of the BMR (i.e. BMR = 1).

Activity	PAR = metabolic rate during exercise ÷ BMR
Lying	1.0
Sitting	1.2
Standing	1.7
Football	7.0

The physical activity level (PAL) can also be calculated. This is equal to the total energy expenditure in 1 day divided by the BMR.

Other factors can also affect energy requirements. For example:

- Environmental temperature changes. This is a very small effect unless the temperature is either extremely high or low
- Pregnancy and lactation. For the first 6 months of pregnancy no extra energy is necessary, but for the last 3 months, an extra 800 kJ (200 kcal) are needed each day. During lactation, an extra 2000 kJ (500 kcal) are required each day
- Growth. The energy requirement in the first year of life is double that of adulthood
- Age. The BMR decreases after the age of about 20 years.

How do we measure energy requirements?

Indirect calorimetry

The measurement of O_2 consumption allows indirect measurement of the metabolic rate. This is because 1 litre of O_2 consumed at rest is equal to 20 kJ of energy expenditure.

Indirect mass spectrophotometry

The incorporation of doubly labelled water ($^2H_2{}^{18}O$) into body fluids and its loss in the urine can be measured. H is incorporated only into H_2O but O is incorporated into both H_2O and CO_2. The difference between them is equal to the CO_2 produced.

Regulation of food intake

A number of systems are thought to participate in the regulation of food intake (Fig. 9.7).

Overall control is by the hypothalamus. Hormones and signals from the stomach, pancreas, and adipose tissue interact to control the balance of hunger/satiety and energy expenditure, through the mechanisms described in the figure.

Key hormones/signals:

- Ghrelin is secreted by the stomach and stimulates NPY/AgRP-expressing neurons, increasing appetite
- Cholecystokinin (CCK) is known to decrease appetite. CCK slows gastric emptying, maintaining gastric distension, which is thought to be an important satiety signal
- Pancreatic signals include insulin, which regulates food intake, promotes satiety by stimulating the uptake of glucose by peripheral tissues. Therefore, levels of glucose and glucagon regulate intake. Originally it was thought that low plasma glucose levels had a direct stimulatory effect on the hunger centre. Now it is believed that it is the increased availability of glucose to tissues that produces satiety (the glucostat hypothesis)

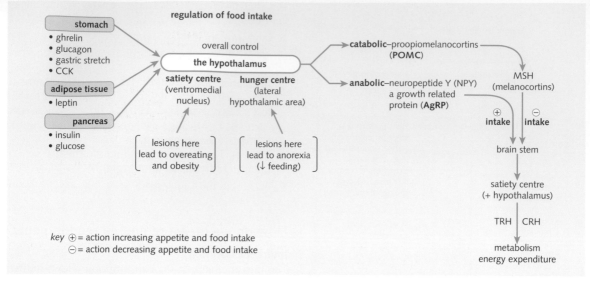

Fig. 9.7 Regulation of food intake.

- Adipose tissue is an active endocrine organ producing adipokines such as leptin.
  - Leptin has a key role in decreasing appetite and increasing thermogenesis, and leptin levels are proportional to body fat content. Animal studies on leptin found deficient cases to be hyperphagic and obese.

Obesity

If energy intake is equal to energy expenditure, there is no change in body mass. Obesity develops when there is an imbalance; and energy intake is greater than expenditure.

Definition

Obesity can be categorized in terms of the body mass index (BMI) (Fig. 9.8). The cut-off values for classifications are in the table below, but consideration of ethnic group should be noted, as cut-offs for obesity in China are BMI > 28 and in Japan > 25 (lower thresholds due to the negative consequences of a higher BMI).

$$BMI \ (kg/m^2) = weight/(height)^2$$

Obesity is rising to epidemic proportions in men, women and children, especially in countries with Western influences. This problem is beginning to replace infectious diseases and under nutrition as the most significant contributor to ill health worldwide, as it is associated with an increased risk of various clinical disorders. In developing countries, it is estimated that more than 115 million people suffer from weight-related problems.

Fig 9.8 Categories for BMI.

BMI	Classification
< 18.5	Underweight
18.5–24.9	Ideal weight
25.0–29.9	Overweight
>30	Obesity
BMI in obese patients	**Sub-classifications of obesity:**
30–34.9	Class 1 Moderate
35–39.9	Class 2 Severe
≥40	Class 3 Morbid

Aetiology

Fig. 9.9 discusses some of the proposed theories for obesity. Twin studies suggest a genetic background. However, genetic factors are greatly influenced by environmental and socio-economic factors. Poor education, high alcohol intake, and less energy expenditure, increase the incidence of obesity. This may also be related to the type of food consumed, which is largely governed by financial status. The most obvious cause of obesity is an excessive intake of calories accompanied by a decrease in energy expenditure. The reasons for overeating are usually complex and may be psychological in origin, related to stress or a life event. Only rarely are there metabolic causes.

Fig. 9.9 Causes of obesity.

Cause	Evidence	Comments
Excessive intake of calories	Psychological factors, stress or social reasons	Most common cause
Genetic	Identical twins are not always the same weight Adopted children resemble their new family weightwise	Likely genetic predisposition but also modified by environmental factors (diet, social-economic status) Recent evidence suggests that there is a 'gene' for obesity
Socio-economic	In the West, low socio-economic class → obesity In the East, high socio-economic class → obesity	Survey in Finland and Scotland showed obesity is associated with: • low education • high alcohol intake • giving up smoking • getting married
Endocrine	Adrenal hyperfunction (Cushing's syndrome), hypothyroidism, and Type 2 diabetes mellitus are all associated with obesity	Most obese people do not have endocrine problems
Energy expenditure	Diet-induced thermogenesis (DIT) is greater in lean people (N.B. basal metabolic rate is not lower in obese people!)	Maybe obese people are better at conserving energy

---

HINTS AND TIPS

The main cause of obesity is usually an excessive intake of calories accompanied by a decrease in energy expenditure.

Clinical consequences

Obesity is associated with an increased risk of:

- Type 2 diabetes. Obesity results in persistently high insulin levels, leading to a down-regulation of insulin receptors and thus insulin resistance in the tissues
- Coronary heart disease. There is an increase in morbidity and mortality caused by coronary heart disease in obese individuals. It may be that other risk factors are more likely to be present in obese patients

- Hypertension
- Respiratory problems
- Stroke
- Osteoarthritis and back pain
- Gout.

HINTS AND TIPS

Morbidity is the incidence or prevalence of disease in a population. Mortality is the number of deaths from disease in a population.

Prevention and treatment

Treatment of obesity is generally unsatisfactory. Possibilities include:

- Reduction of energy intake. The main treatment of an obese patient is an appropriate diet, with plenty of support and encouragement from a doctor. Lots of different weight-reducing diets have been formulated; most do not work, particularly in the long term. For example, on a low-carbohydrate diet, where bread, potatoes, cakes and any starch-containing foods are cut out of the diet, initially, weight loss is fast (0.5 kg/day) but most of the loss is water. Protein is also broken down to maintain the blood glucose, but is replaced as soon as the diet is stopped. The loss of fat is the same as for a normal mixed diet. However, low-carbohydrate diets improve glucose tolerance
- Other diets such as low-fat diets and low-cholesterol diets are also used to help treat obesity. Recent trials, utilizing diets low in saturated fat and supplemented with polyunsaturated fatty acids, mainly from omega-3 fatty acids (three helpings of oily fish per week, fish oil capsules and alpha-linoleic acid margarine), have been shown to be beneficial in helping patients to lose weight
- Most weight-reducing diets allow an intake of 1000 kcal/day. This must be a balanced intake of protein, carbohydrate and fat (i.e. a mixed diet). Why is it that 80–100% of obese people regain lost weight? During starvation, the metabolic rate falls by

15–30%. Therefore, after dieting, to remain at a lower weight, a lower energy intake must be maintained otherwise the weight will be put straight back on. The only way to lose weight is a prolonged moderation of intake and then a permanent change in eating habits to maintain the weight loss

- Increase energy expenditure in a way appropriate to age and health
- Drug therapy should only be considered after dietary, exercise and behavioural approaches have been started and evaluated for patients who have not reached their target weight loss or have reached a plateau on dietary, activity and behavioural changes alone. Any medications should be reviewed regularly. There is only one key medication you need to know about: *Orlistat*, which is a pancreatic lipase inhibitor which is licensed for use together with a mildly hypocaloric diet in those with a BMI of greater than $30\,kg/m^2$. Part of its effect may be related to the reduction of fat intake necessary to avoid severe gastrointestinal effects such as steatorrhoea. It should only be continued beyond 3 months if the patient has lost at least 5% of their initial body weight since starting the drug treatment. Appetite suppressants such as phentermine (a catecholaminergic drug with minor sympathomimetic and stimulant effects) are not presently used. Sibutramine has recently been suspended and is no longer used. Currently, research is being done on unraveling the links between obesity and adipokine secretion to investigate leptin and other adipokines for use in the diagnosis and treatment of obesity
- Surgery. Examples include: jaw wiring, gastric plication (stapling the walls of the stomach together to form a smaller stomach), bypass of the small intestine, and gastric distension.

Clinical Note

Bariatric surgery (surgery to aid weight loss) is a last resort – considered only for patients with:

- Morbid obesity (BMI $\geq 40\,kg/m^2$ OR $35–40\,kg/m^2$) AND other significant disease (diabetes, high blood pressure) that may be improved if they lose weight. In addition to meeting all of the following criteria:
- ≥ 18 years
- Receiving treatment in a specialist obesity clinic (providing full assessments, counseling and support pre and post-surgery)
- Unable to maintain weight loss despite trying all other appropriate non-surgical treatments
- No medical or psychological contraindications for this type of surgery
- Understand the need for long term follow-up.

PROTEINS AND NUTRITION

Definitions

Reference proteins

Reference proteins contain all the amino acids in the exact proportions needed for protein synthesis. Albumin (found in egg white) and casein (milk) are closest to the ideal. Other proteins are compared with these reference proteins.

Limiting amino acids

A limiting amino acid is the essential amino acid present in a protein in the lowest amount relative to its requirement for protein synthesis. Examples of protein-containing foods and their limiting amino acids are:

- Wheat, limited by lysine
- Meat and fish, limited by methionine and cysteine
- Maize, limited by tryptophan.

Combining different protein-containing foods, such as meat and the pulses, ensures an adequate intake of all the amino acids, that is, protein complementation (e.g. eating baked beans on toast). This is particularly important in vegetarian diets.

Protein quality

The quality of any protein can be assessed using a rating system based on a number of variables.

Chemical score

The chemical score is the ratio of the amount of limiting amino acid to its requirement, expressed as percentage points. For example, if the amount of limiting amino acid in a test protein is 2% and the amount of limiting amino acid in the reference protein is 5%; the chemical score is 40%.

Biological value

The biological value is the proportion of the absorbed protein which is retained by the body for protein synthesis.

Net protein utilization

The net protein utilization (NPU) is the proportion of dietary protein which is retained by the body for protein synthesis. For example:

Diet	NPU
Mixed Western diet	70% (70% dietary protein is retained for protein synthesis)
Meat-based diet	75%
Cereal-based diet	50-60%
Egg-based diet	100%

Net dietary protein as a percentage of energy

Net dietary protein as a percentage of energy (NDPE%) is the proportion of total dietary energy provided by fully 'usable' protein. This method provides a way of comparing different diets. For example:

- Cereal-based diets provide 5–6%
- Western diets provide 10–12%
- In India, the diet provides 10%.

Children require an NDPE% of greater than 8%, that is, at least 8% of their diet must come from usable protein. Adults require an NDPE% of greater than 5%. In areas where the staple food is starch (e.g. yam, cassava), the diet provides only low levels of protein. It would be physically impossible to consume the amount of food necessary to satisfy the protein requirement, especially for children, and this leads to protein deficiency states. Cereal-based diets are adequate for adults but not children.

Protein requirement

Diet should provide the essential amino acids and enough amino acid nitrogen to synthesize the non-essential amino acids. These are required for:

- Maintenance of tissue proteins in adults
- Formation of body proteins during periods of growth, pregnancy, lactation, infection, and after major trauma or illness such as cancer.

The recommended protein requirement for an adult in the UK is 0.8 g/kg/day of protein and should not be greater than 1.5 g/kg/day.

The RNI for protein is 55 g/day for men and 44 g/day for women.

Protein–energy deficiency states

Protein–energy malnutrition (PEM) arises when the body's need for protein or energy, or both, is not met by the diet. It is most commonly seen in developing countries. However, in the industrialized world, it can be present in the elderly or chronically ill patients.

Causes of PEM

These can be one or a combination of the following:

- Decreased dietary intake
- Malabsorption
- Increased requirement; for example, in preterm infants, infection (septic state increases catabolism), major trauma or surgery
- Psychological; for example, depression or anorexia nervosa.

HINTS AND TIPS

The bulk of excess protein is oxidized via gluconeogenesis to glycogen or fat and stored by the body. Therefore, protein is not a slimming food. One famous diet consists of a protein-sparing modified fast (PSMF) which is hydrolyzed gelatine and collagen, thus it is cheap. However, during the hydrolysis process a lot of electrolytes are lost, including potassium, which may lead to serious problems.

In developing countries, PEM manifests as two conditions in children:

- Marasmus: lack of protein and energy (i.e. starvation)
- Kwashiorkor: lack of protein only – energy supply is adequate.

Incidence

In developing countries, 20–75% of children below 5 years of age have some form of malnutrition. Five million children die every year because of malnutrition.

Aetiology and mechanisms of pathogenesis

Marasmus

Marasmus is the childhood form of starvation (Figs 9.10 and 9.11). Both protein and energy are limited, leading to a low concentration of insulin but increased levels of glucagon and cortisol, that is, a starved state (see Chapter 8). As no fuel is available for the body, muscle protein and fat are broken down to provide energy, which leads to wasting. Muscle protein is broken down to amino acids which are used for the synthesis of albumin by the liver; therefore, this prevents oedema.

Kwashiorkor

Translated this means the 'disease the first child gets when the second child is born'. In kwashiorkor severe protein deficiency occurs but energy is maintained (Figs 9.12 and 9.13). It usually occurs when a young child is weaned from breastfeeding because of the arrival of a new baby. The first child is fed a low-protein, high-starch diet instead. Kwashiorkor often develops after an acute infection, such as measles or gastroenteritis, when the demand for protein is increased.

As energy is not limiting, there is a high insulin to glucagon, and insulin to cortisol ratio. Amino acids are taken up by muscle for protein synthesis. This diverts amino acids from the liver, so fewer are available for albumin synthesis: the resulting low albumin levels reduce the plasma oncotic pressure, causing oedema. The oedema causes a deceptively fat appearance and

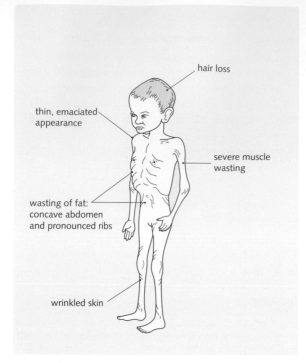

Fig. 9.10   Marasmus.

hair loss

thin, emaciated
appearance

severe muscle
wasting

wasting of fat:
concave abdomen
and pronounced ribs

wrinkled skin

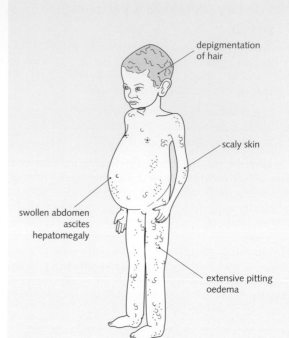

Fig. 9.12   Kwashiorkor.

depigmentation
of hair

scaly skin

swollen abdomen
ascites
hepatomegaly

extensive pitting
oedema

Fig. 9.11 The clinical features of marasmus.

Very thin, wasted appearance
Obvious muscle wasting and loss of body fat
<60% normal body weight
Age: usually <18 months
No oedema
Wrinkled skin, hair loss and apathy
Plasma albumin is usually **normal**
Diarrhoea and infection may be present
Electrolyte disturbances: low potassium and sodium
common
Anaemia

Fig. 9.13 The features of kwashiorkor.

Oedema: 'hides' severe wasting of underlying tissues
Age: usually 2–4 years
Scaly skin: 'flaky point' rash with hyperkeratosis
Depigmentation of hair
Distended abdomen caused by ascites and enlarged
fatty liver
Hypothermia and bradycardia
Apathy
Anaemia: due to folate, iron or copper metabolism
disturbances
Low plasma albumin
Usually diarrhoea and/or infection
Low potassium, sodium, glucose, and other electrolyte
disturbances

children are known as water or 'sugar' babies. It is possible there may also be some degree of energy loss in kwashiorkor and therefore other factors may contribute to, or cause, the oedema. For example:

- Excessive generation of free radicals causing membrane damage and oedema
- Infection diverts protein synthesis from albumin to the synthesis of immunoglobulins and acute-phase proteins (e.g. C-reactive protein).

A comparison of kwashiorkor and marasmus is given in Fig. 9.14.

Management and treatment of PEM

It is important to restore fluid and electrolyte balance first. Following this:

- Any infection, hypothermia or hypoglycaemia present can be treated
- Carefully re-feed initially, just enough to maintain a steady state to satisfy the normal daily requirement. Milk is often given with flour or maize, slowly and regularly. There is a risk of refeeding syndrome, which results within the first few days of starting to feed after a period of starvation/prolonged undernutrition. The availability of glucose causes surges in insulin levels, which moves phosphate, potassium, and other electroltytes into cells, reducing levels in the blood. These low levels, especially hypophosphataemia, can result

130

Fig. 9.14 A comparison of marasmus and kwashiorkor.

Feature	Marasmus	Kwashiorkor
Deficiency	Protein and energy	Protein only
Age	Usually <18 months	Older: 1–5 years
Oedema	Absent Severe wasting of body protein and fat	Present Oedema hides wasting of body protein
Body weight	< 60% normal	60–80% normal
Cause	Severe malnutrition	Malnutrition infection
Features	Wrinkled skin Hair loss Thin and emaciated	Scaly skin and dermatitis Sparse, depigmented hair Distended abdomen Hepatomegaly

in seizures, arrhythmias and can even have life-threatening consequences
- Eventually, high-energy foods are given to restore weight and also any necessary vitamin and mineral supplements.

Prognosis

Mortality rates for children with severe malnutrition are about 50%. The rate is so high because adequate treatment is usually not available.

Consequences of prolonged PEM

Malnourished children are less active and more apathetic; these behavioural abnormalities are usually reversed by re-feeding. However, severe, prolonged malnutrition causes much reduced brain growth and permanent damage to both physical and mental development. Immunity is impaired, leading to delayed wound healing; protein loss from muscle may eventually include the diaphragm, leading to death. The physiological effects of severe prolonged malnutrition are listed in Fig. 9.15.

Prevention

Prevention of childhood malnutrition is a World Health Organization priority. The main targets are to provide:

- Food supplements and additional vitamins to 'at-risk' groups
- Family planning
- Immunization programmes.

However, drought, famine and war in affected countries often make these targets impossible to achieve.

In Western countries, a degree of PEM may be seen in hospitalized patients with the following conditions:

- Anorexia
- Trauma, severe infection, major surgery, or burns
- Cancer.

That is, anything that causes a negative nitrogen balance (see Chapter 6).

> **HINTS AND TIPS**
>
> Malnutrition in adults in developing countries has symptoms similar to those seen in children but the results are not as devastating. This is because adults are already physically and mentally mature and are therefore more resilient.

Parenteral and enteral nutrition

Nutritional support is provided for all patients who are severely malnourished or are unable to eat because of physical illness. Whenever possible, enteral nutrition is used, that is, delivery of nutrients via the gastrointestinal tract, including eating and drinking normally, or a nasogastric (NG) tube or gastrostomy; a tube placed directly in the stomach. Enteral nutrition is more natural, cheaper and far less hazardous in terms of the effects on fluid and electrolyte balance than parenteral nutrition. Enteral nutrition is always given in preference if the gastrointestinal tract is functional. Parenteral nutrition may be indicated in the following situations:

- Intestinal failure; either as the result of surgery (gut resection) or because of a fistula or gastrointestinal tract obstruction by tumour.
- Unconscious patients with a very high energy requirement; that is, those in hypercatabolic state, for example severe trauma or burns patients.

Administration

Administration is usually via a central venous catheter into the superior vena cava, or sometimes into a

Fig. 9.15 The physiological effects of severe prolonged malnutrition.

Effect	Consequence
Decreased brain development	Permanent damage to both physical and mental development
Defective immune system	Decreased cell-mediated response, immunoglobulin production is maintained: this can have harmful effects as it depletes production of other proteins
Loss of protein	Firstly from muscle, then viscera → death
Electrolyte losses	May effect Na^+/K^+ pump and the maintenance of ion gradients across cells
Low haemoglobin	Anaemia
Low serum albumin (only kwashiorkor)	→ oedema
Impaired gastrointestinal function	Bacterial overgrowth and malabsorption
Fatty liver	Fat accumulates since its transport requires apolipoproteins that are deficient (not seen in marasmus)

peripheral vein. It involves the intravenous infusion of a mixture of high-concentration glucose, fat emulsion, amino acids, vitamins, electrolytes and trace elements.

Monitoring the patient

The most frequent complication of total parenteral nutrition (TPN) is infection of the delivery line; therefore, a meticulous aseptic technique is essential. Also, these patients require careful daily clinical monitoring to avoid complications:

- Fluid balance. The patient requires a daily fluid balance chart
- Plasma electrolytes (sodium, potassium, chloride, bicarbonate, urea, and creatinine) and glucose are measured at least once a day to prevent the development of refeeding syndrome
- Regular haematological measurements (full blood count and so on) are necessary, as is the monitoring of iron, vitamin B_{12} or folate deficiencies

- In a patient with stable renal function, 24 h urinary urea excretion provide an index of the body's protein status. This is not used as a routine test
- Liver function tests are checked about three times a week
- Vitamins and trace elements are periodically checked.

Clinical Note

Refeeding syndrome is usually within 4 days of starting artificial refeeding (enteral or parenteral) in patients who are severely malnourished and it encompasses potentially fatal metabolic disturbances (a fall in serum phosphate, potassium, magnesium, glucose, and thiamine), which can cause confusion, coma, convulsions, and even death.

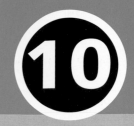
VITAMINS

Definition

Vitamin: A complex organic substance required in the diet in small amounts, the absence of which leads to a deficiency disease.

Vitamins can be divided into two main groups, fat-soluble and water-soluble.

Fat-soluble vitamins

Vitamins A, D, E and K. These are:
- Stored in the liver
- Not absorbed or excreted easily
- Can be toxic in excess (particularly A and D) (Fig. 10.1).

Water-soluble vitamins

The B-group vitamins and vitamin C. These are:
- Not stored extensively
- Required regularly in the diet
- Generally non-toxic in excess (within reason).

All B vitamins are coenzymes in metabolic pathways.

FAT-SOLUBLE VITAMINS

Vitamin A (retinol)

RNI

Sources: 700 mg/day for men; 600 mg/day for women.

Animal sources are butter, whole milk, egg yolk, liver and fish liver oils; they contain retinol.

Plant sources are most green, yellow or orange vegetables; they contain β-carotene, the precursor of retinol.

Absorption and transport of vitamin A

Retinol is absorbed in the intestinal mucosa and esterified to long-chain fatty acids, forming retinyl esters.

These are packaged in chylomicrons and transported to the liver for storage. When required, retinol is released and transported, bound to retinol-binding protein. Retinol can be oxidized to other active forms, namely retinoic acid and retinal. β-carotene is absorbed in the intestine and converted into retinal.

Functions

There are three active forms of vitamin A:

- Retinoic acid. This acts as a typical steroid hormone. It binds to chromatin to increase the synthesis of proteins controlling cell growth and differentiation of epithelial cells. Therefore, it increases epithelial cell turnover
- Retinal. 11-cis retinal binds to opsin to form rhodopsin, the visual pigment of the rod cells in the retina, involved in vision and particularly night vision (Fig. 10.2)
- β-carotene is an antioxidant. The role of antioxidants in the prevention of heart disease and lung cancer is being studied intensively, but has not yet produced any conclusive results.

Deficiency

Incidence

Vitamin A deficiency is rarely seen in developed countries because liver stores are sufficient to last 3–4 years. It is commonly found in children in developing countries such as India and parts of South-East Asia, where about 500 000 children each year are blinded as a result of vitamin A deficiency.

Causes

Vitamin A deficiency may be caused by a decreased dietary intake; usually only seen in very severe malnutrition. It may also occur secondary to fat malabsorption.

Clinical features

In the eye, the symptoms are progressive:

- Initially, deficiency causes impaired dark adaptation and night blindness. This is reversible

Fig. 10.1 Vitamins with significant toxicity.

Vitamin	Toxicity
Vitamin A	Hypervitaminosis A Dermatitis, mucous membrane defects and hair loss Hepatomegaly, thinning and fracture of the long bones Increased intracranial pressure Toxicity is very unlikely with normal sources, be wary when prescribing high doses of retinoic acid for severe acne sufferers
D	The most toxic of all vitamins. As it is fat soluble, it is stored in the body. Normally, this is well tolerated but in high doses over a period of time, hypervitaminosis D may occur. This presents with nausea, vomiting and muscle weakness. Very high levels of vitamin D result in greatly increased rates of calcium absorption and bone resorption, causing hypercalcaemia and calcium deposition in tissues, particularly the arteries, heart, liver, kidneys and pancreas. This is known as metastatic calcification and may interfere with the correct functioning of the organs, possibly causing renal stones, calcification of other arteries and heart failure
E	The least toxic of all the fat-soluble vitamins
B1	Rare; headaches, insomnia and dermatitis
Niacin	High intake disturbs liver function, carbohydrate tolerance and urate metabolism. (>200 mg/day) causes vasodilatation and flushing
Pyridoxine B6	Rare; an excess can result in sensory neuropathy. It can be used in treatment of premenstrual tension
C	Kidney stones, diarrhoea and systemic conditioning (requirements increasing as the body adapts to metabolizing more)

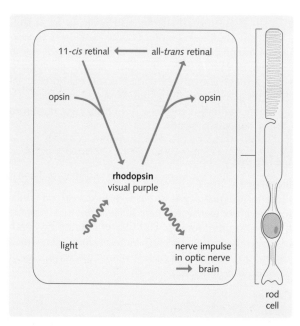

Fig. 10.2 Role of vitamin A in vision. 11-*cis* retinal binds to opsin, converting it to rhodopsin, the visual pigment of the rod cells in the retina involved in vision and dark adaptation to light. Low light intensity (scotopic vision) activates a series of photochemical reactions that bleach rhodopsin, converting it to all-*trans* retinal, which triggers a nerve impulse in the optic nerve to the brain.

- Severe prolonged deficiency results in xerophthalmia: a dryness of the cornea and conjunctiva due to progressive epithelial keratinization. Bitot's spots may be seen, which are white plaques of keratinized epithelial cells on the conjunctiva
- If untreated, keratomalacia develops, causing corneal ulceration and the formation of opaque scar tissue (cataracts); this causes irreversible blindness.

In the skin, decreased epithelial cell turnover produces:

- Thickening and dryness of skin due to hyperkeratosis
- Impaired mucosal function.

Diagnosis and treatment

Diagnosis and treatment are usually on the basis of the above clinical features. The following can also be measured:

- The plasma concentration of vitamin A and retinol binding protein
- The response to replacement therapy.

Urgent treatment with vitamin A (as retinol palmitate) orally or intramuscularly prevents blindness. If the deficiency is severe and has already caused keratomalacia, eyesight cannot be restored. It is interesting to note that vitamin A is also used successfully to treat a number of skin problems, including acne (Fig. 10.3).

Fig. 10.3 Uses of vitamin A in the treatment of skin disorders.

Condition	Treatment
Moderate acne	Topical retinoic acid (all *trans* retinoic acid)
Severe disfiguring acne Psoriasis	Isotretinoin (13-*cis* retinoic acid) orally Acitretin (Both are contraindicated in pregnancy as they are teratogenic)

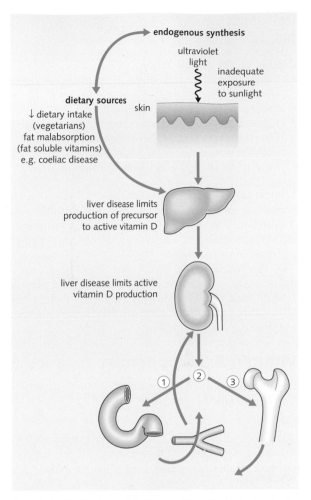

Fig. 10.4 Synthesis, metabolism and functions of vitamin D. The active form has three main effects:
1. Increases uptake of Ca^{2+} (and inorganic phosphate) from the intestine
2. Increases reabsorption of calcium from the kidney
3. Increases resorption of bone (when necessary) so that calcium is released.
The causes of deficiency are also highlighted in blue at the levels of synthesis affected.

Teratogenicity

Pregnant women must not take more than 3.3 mg/day because vitamin A causes congenital defects. Therefore, they must avoid vitamin A supplements or eating liver because it contains about 13–40 mg of vitamin A per 100 g. Isotretinoin treatment for acne is absolutely contraindicated in pregnancy.

Vitamin D₃ (cholecalciferol)

RNI
There is no RNI for vitamin D because it is synthesized by the body.

Sources
The sources of vitamin D include:

- Diet: in fish liver oils as cholecalciferol
- Endogenous synthesis: most vitamin D is made by the body.

Vitamin D is a derivative of cholesterol and is therefore not present in plants; vegetarians must make their own.

Synthesis
Vitamin D is manufactured in the skin by the action of sunlight of wavelength 290–310 nm. No radiation of this length is available between October and March in the UK; therefore, the body relies on stores made during summer.

Cholecalciferol undergoes two hydroxylation reactions, the first in the liver and the second in the kidney, to form the active form, 1,25-dihydroxycholecalciferol (Fig. 10.4). Vitamin D is mostly stored as 25-hydroxycholecalciferol in the liver.

Functions
The main role of vitamin D is in calcium homeostasis, which it controls in three ways (Fig. 10.4):

- Increases uptake of calcium (and inorganic phosphate) from the intestine (main role)
- Increases the reabsorption of calcium from the kidney

- Increases resorption of bone (when necessary) so that calcium is released.

Therefore, vitamin D increases the plasma concentration of calcium ions.

Mechanism of action
The active form, 1,25-dihydroxycholecalciferol, is a steroid hormone. In intestinal cells it binds to a cytosolic receptor. The resulting complex enters the nucleus and binds to chromatin at a specific site (enhancer region or response element) to increase the synthesis of a calcium-binding protein, cal-bindin, resulting in increased calcium reabsorption in the intestine.

Deficiency

The causes of deficiency are outlined in Fig. 10.4.

Groups at risk of deficiency

- Children and women of Asian origin in sunlight-poor areas
- Elderly and housebound individuals
- Babies breastfed in winter because light of the correct wavelength for production of vitamin D is not available for mothers
- Vegans (vitamin D is not present in plants).

Clinical features and pathogenesis

Vitamin D deficiency disrupts bone mineralization. In children, this causes rickets; in adults, it causes osteomalacia. These disorders are covered later in this chapter with calcium deficiency.

A disruption of calcium homeostasis also causes hypocalcaemia and hypophosphataemia (low plasma calcium and phosphate). This may cause symptoms of neuromuscular irritability, numbness, parasthesiae, tetany and, possibly seizures.

Vitamin E (tocopherol)

Vitamin E consists of eight naturally occurring tocopherols; α-tocopherol is the most active.

RNI

None. A diet high in polyunsaturated fatty acids (PUFA) requires a high vitamin E intake.

Sources

Vegetable oils, especially wheatgerm oil, nuts and green vegetables.

Absorption and transport

Tocopherol is found 'dissolved' in dietary fat and is absorbed with it. It is transported in the blood by lipoproteins, initially in chylomicrons which deliver dietary vitamin E to the tissues. Vitamin E is transported from the liver with very-low-density lipoproteins (VLDL) and is stored in adipose tissue. Therefore, a defect in lipoprotein and fat metabolism may lead to a deficiency of vitamin E.

Functions and deficiency

The functions and clinical manifestations of a deficiency of vitamin E are listed in Fig. 10.5.

Deficiency

Incidence

In humans, vitamin E deficiency is very rare and is only seen in:

- Premature infants, causing haemolytic anaemia of the newborn. Vitamin E crosses the placenta in the

Fig. 10.5 Vitamin E: function and effects of deficiency. PUFA, polyunsaturated fatty acid; LDL, low-density lipoprotein

Functions	Deficiency
Naturally occurring antioxidant which prevents oxidation of cell components by free radicals, e.g. PUFA present in cell membranes	Very rare except in premature infants in whom it can cause haemolytic anaemia of newborn

last trimester of pregnancy; therefore, premature infants have very small vitamin E stores. Their erythrocyte membranes are fragile and are susceptible to free radical damage, leading to lysis of erythrocytes. Vitamin E supplements are given to pregnant mothers to prevent this

- Children and adults, secondary to severe fat malabsorption. For example, biliary atresia, cholestatic liver disease or a lipoprotein deficiency (e.g. abetalipoproteinaemia).

Clinical features

Vitamin E deficiency causes muscle weakness, peripheral neuropathy, ataxia and nystagmus. In children with abetalipoproteinaemia, vitamin E therapy can prevent the occurrence of severe spino-cerebellar degeneration and gross ataxia.

Vitamin K

RNI

None.

Sources

The sources of vitamin K include:

- Diet: especially green vegetables, egg yolk, liver and cereals
- It is made mostly by the normal bacterial flora of jejunum and ileum
- Human milk contains only a small amount.

Functions and deficiency

The functions and clinical manifestations of a deficiency of vitamin K are listed in Fig. 10.6.

Deficiency

A true deficiency is rare because most of the body's vitamin K is synthesized by bacteria in the gut.

Fig. 10.6 Functions and deficiency of vitamin K.

Functions	Deficiency
Vitamin K is a coenzyme for the carboxylation of glutamate residues of blood clotting factors II, VII, IX and X Carboxylation activates clotting factors and thus clotting cascade Anticoagulants warfarin and dicoumarol inhibit vitamin K	True deficiency is rare because bacteria in the gut usually produce enough Long-term antibiotic therapy leads to ↓ bacteria and ↓ vitamin K, resulting in poor blood clotting and bleeding disorders May result in haemorrhagic disease of the newborn

Causes

The main causes of vitamin K deficiency are:

- A decreased level of bacteria in the gut (e.g. due to long-term antibiotic therapy)
- A decrease in dietary intake
- Newborn babies have sterile guts and cannot make vitamin K initially
- Oral anticoagulant drugs (e.g. warfarin) are vitamin K antagonists

Mechanism

A deficiency of vitamin K results in low levels of the vitamin K-dependent clotting factors II, VII, IX and X and inhibition of the clotting cascade. Patients will have an increased tendency to bleed and bruise.

Diagnosis and treatment

The diagnosis and treatment of vitamin K deficiency is covered in Fig. 10.7.

Deficiency in newborn babies

Newborn babies have sterile gut and have no bacteria to make vitamin K. The newborn infant has virtually no hepatic stores of vitamin K and it is present in only low concentrations in human milk. Vitamin K deficiency causes haemorrhagic disease of the newborn (HDNB).

Fig. 10.7 Diagnosis and treatment of vitamin K deficiency.

Diagnosis	Treatment
Clinical features: bruising and bleeding, e.g. haematuria or bleeding from the GI tract Increased prothrombin time (PTT) Increased activated partial thromboplastin time (APTT) less marked than PTT	Vitamin K supplements

HINTS AND TIPS

HDNB is a coagulation disturbance, resulting from vitamin K deficiency and consequently impaired hepatic production of factors II, VII, IX and X. Premature infants, infants exposed to perinatal asphyxia and breastfed babies are most at risk of developing HDNB. It classically presents in the fourth day of life with gastrointestinal bleeding. Usually, the bleeding is minor but can also result in major haemorrhage and death. Therefore, every newborn baby in the UK is given prophylactic intramuscular or oral vitamin K.

WATER-SOLUBLE VITAMINS

Vitamin B_1 (thiamine)

RNI

1.0 mg/day for men; 0.8 mg/day for women.

Sources

Wholegrain cereals, liver, pork, yeast, dairy products and legumes.

Active form

Thiamine pyrophosphate (TPP), which is formed by the transfer of a pyrophosphate group from ATP to thiamine.

Functions

The functions of thiamine are listed in Fig. 10.8, with its mechanism of action described in Fig. 10.9.

Deficiency diseases

A deficiency of thiamine causes:

- Beriberi. This occurs in two forms: wet beriberi, which results in oedema, cardiovascular symptoms and heart failure, and dry beriberi, which causes muscle wasting and peripheral neuropathy
- Wernicke's encephalopathy which is associated with alcoholism
- Korsakoff' s psychosis.

Beriberi

Incidence

Beriberi (Fig. 10.10) is now seen only in the poorest areas of South-East Asia where the staple food is

Fig. 10.8 Thiamine: functions and effects of deficiency.

Functions	Deficiency
Thiamine pyrophosphate is cofactor for **four key enzymes:** • pyruvate dehydrogenase • α-ketoglutarate dehydrogenase (TCA cycle) • branched-chain amino acid α-ketoacid dehydrogenase • transketolase (pentose phosphate pathway)	Decreased activity of pyruvate dehydrogenase and α-ketoglutarate dehydrogenase causes: • accumulation of pyruvate and lactate • decreased acetyl CoA and ATP formation and decreased acetylcholine and central nervous system activity Decreased activity of pentose phosphate pathway results in low levels of NADPH necessary for fatty acid synthesis; therefore this leads to a decrease in synthesis of myelin, which may cause peripheral neuropathy

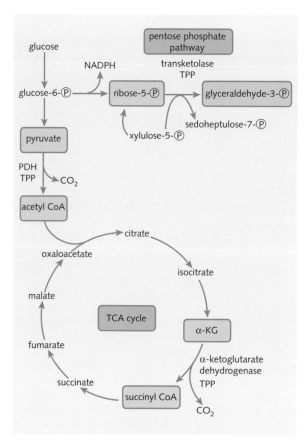

Fig. 10.9   Mechanism of action of thiamine. Thiamine pyrophosphate (TPP), the active form of thiamine, acts as coenzyme for pyruvate dehydrogenase and α-ketoglutarate dehydrogenase reactions in the TCA cycle and for transketolase in the pentose phosphate pathway.

Fig. 10.10 Types of beriberi.

	Clinical features	Signs
Wet beriberi	Oedema: spreads to involve the whole body → ascites and pleural effusions Congestive heart failure	Raised JVP Tachycardia and tachypnoea
Infantile beriberi	A form of wet beriberi that occurs in breastfed babies whose mothers are thiamine-deficient	Acute onset: anorexia and oedema that can involve the larynx → aphonia Tachycardia and tachypnoea develop → death
Dry beriberi	Gradual, symmetrical, ascending peripheral neuropathy resulting in progressive paralysis	Initially, stiffness of legs → weakness, numbness, and 'pins and needles' ascends to involve trunk, arms and eventually brain

polished rice, that is, the husk that contains most of the vitamins, including thiamine, has been removed.

Diagnosis

Diagnosis is by measurement of the transketolase activity in erythrocytes, before and after the addition of TPP. A greater than 30% increase in activity with TPP indicates a deficiency. Thiamine can now also be measured directly in plasma.

Treatment

Initially, treatment is with intramuscular injections of thiamine for approximately 3 days (varies according to severity) followed by daily, oral supplements of thiamine. For wet beriberi, treatment results in a dramatic decrease in oedema and a quick improvement of symptoms. For dry beriberi, there is a slower improvement.

Fig. 10.11 Clinical features of Wernicke's encephalopathy and Korsakoffs psychosis.

Clinical features	Causes
Wernickes' encephalopathy: • acute confusional state • ataxia; cerebellar signs • ophthalmoplegia and nystagmus • peripheral neuropathy **Diagnosis:** made on clinical grounds; condition is reversible with immediate thiamine therapy If untreated it may develop into **Korsakoffs psychosis:** a severe irreversible syndrome characterized by loss of short-term memory	Alcohol Ischaemic damage to brainstem Major cause of dementia in developed countries Progression from untreated Wernicke's encephalopathy

Wernicke-Korsakoff syndrome

Incidence
As thiamine is present in most foods, a dietary deficiency is rare in developed countries. The deficiency manifests itself as Wernicke's encephalopathy (Fig. 10.11). In the UK, a low thiamine intake is seen in:

- Chronic alcoholics: alcohol inhibits the uptake of thiamine
- The elderly
- People with diseases of the upper gastrointestinal tract (e.g. gastric cancer).

Toxicity
Toxicity is rare but an excess causes headaches, insomnia and dermatitis.

Vitamin B$_2$ (riboflavin)

RNI
1.3 mg/day for men; 1.1 mg/day for women.

Sources
Milk, eggs, liver. Riboflavin is readily destroyed by ultraviolet light.

Active forms
Riboflavin occurs in two active forms:

- Flavin mononucleotide (FMN)
- Flavin adenine dinucleotide (FAD).

Fig. 10.12 Riboflavin: functions and effects of deficiency.

Functions	Deficiency
FAD and FMN are coenzymes for a number of oxidases and dehydrogenases They can accept two hydrogens to form FADH$_2$ and FMNH$_2$ respectively and take part in redox reactions, e.g. electron transport chain or act as antioxidants	Rare except in elderly or alcoholic individuals Symptoms of deficiency: • angular stomatitis (inflammation at sides of mouth) • cheilosis (fissures at corners of the mouth) • cataracts • glossitis (inflamed tongue)

Functions and deficiency
The functions and clinical manifestations of a deficiency of riboflavin are listed in Fig. 10.12. Riboflavin is not toxic in excess.

Niacin or nicotinic acid

RNI
17 mg/day for men; 13 mg/day for women.

Sources
Wholegrain cereals, meat, fish and the amino acid tryptophan.

Synthesis of niacin from tryptophan
The synthesis of niacin from trytophan is a very inefficient process: as much as 60 mg of tryptophan is needed to make 1 mg of niacin. Synthesis requires thiamine, riboflavin and pyridoxine as cofactors, and only occurs after the needs of protein synthesis are met. This means, in theory, that niacin deficiency can be treated with a high-protein diet, but lots would be needed!

Active forms
NAD+ and NADP+.

Functions and deficiency
The functions and clinical manifestations of a deficiency of niacin are listed in Fig. 10.13.

Fig. 10.13 Niacin: functions and effects of deficiency.

Functions	Deficiency
NAD$^+$ and NADP$^+$ are coenzymes for many dehydrogenases in redox reactions NAD is required for repair of UV light-damaged DNA in areas of exposed skin (nothing to do with redox state) Nicotinic acid is used for treatment of certain dyslipidaemias because it inhibits lipolysis, leading to decreased VLDL synthesis (see Chapter 5)	Pellagra Symptoms, the **3Ds:** **d**ermatitis **d**iarrhoea **d**ementia leading to death

Pellagra: a disease of the skin, gastrointestinal tract and central nervous system

Incidence

Pellagra is rare and is found in areas where maize is the staple food. It is now seen only in certain parts of Africa. Maize contains niacin in a biologically unavailable form, niacytin. Niacin can only be removed from the maize by alkali treatment (Mexicans soak maize in lime juice to release the niacin). Pellagra (Fig. 10.14) can also occur in conditions in which large amounts of tryptophan are metabolized; for example, carcinoid syndrome, which is very rare.

Causes

The causes of pellagra are:

- Dietary deficiency of niacin
- Protein deficiency (as niacin is made from tryptophan)
- Vitamin B_6 and pyridoxal phosphate deficiency (pyridoxal phosphate is a cofactor for niacin synthesis from tryptophan)
- Hartnup's disease: a failure to absorb tryptophan from the diet (Fig. 6.6).
- Isoniazid treatment for tuberculosis inhibits vitamin B_6, causing a decrease in tryptophan synthesis.

Diagnosis

Diagnosis is by the measurement of niacin or its metabolites (N-methylnicotinamide or 2-pyridone) in the urine.

Treatment

As niacin can be formed from tryptophan, treatment involves:

- High-dose niacin supplements
- A high-protein diet.

Mild cases are reversible, dementia usually is not, and may lead to death.

Toxicity

A high intake upsets liver function, carbohydrate tolerance and urate metabolism. More than 200 mg/day will cause vasodilatation and flushing.

Vitamin B_6

Vitamin B_6 exists in three forms: pyridoxine, pyridoxal and pyridoxamine.

RNI

1.4 mg/day for men; 1.2 mg/day for women.

Sources

Whole grains (wheat or corn), meat, fish and poultry.

Active form

All three forms can be converted to the coenzyme pyridoxal phosphate (PLP).

Functions and deficiency

The functions and clinical manifestations of a deficiency of vitamin B_6 are listed in Fig. 10.15.

Pyridoxine deficiency

Causes

Dietary deficiency is extremely rare but may be seen in:

- Newborn babies fed formula milk
- Elderly people and alcoholics
- Women taking oral contraceptives
- Patients on isoniazid therapy for treatment of tuberculosis.

Fig. 10.14 Clinical features and symptoms of pellagra.

Clinical features	Symptoms
3Ds: Dermatitis; deficiency of NAD, inhibits DNA repair of sun-damaged skin	Photosensitive symmetrical skin rash occurs when skin is exposed to sunlight: • skin may crack and ulcerate • on neck, extent depends on area of skin exposed
Diarrhoea	May also see glossitis and angular stomatitis
Dementia	Dementia occurs in chronic disease and is usually irreversible; may develop tremor and encephalopathy

Fig. 10.15 Vitamin B_6: functions and effects of deficiency.

Functions	Deficiency
• Pyridoxal phosphate is a co-enzyme for many enzymes	→ primary deficiency is very rare
• In amino acid metabolism: aminotransferases and serine dehydratase	→ abnormal amino acid metabolism
• In haem synthesis, ALA synthase (catalyses rate-limiting step)	→ hypochromic, microcytic anaemia
• Glycogen phosphorylase	
• Conversion of tryptophan to niacin	→ secondary pellagra
• Indirect role in serotonin and norepinephrine synthesis as they are derived from aminoacids	→ convulsions and depression

The drug isoniazid binds to pyridoxal phosphate to form an inactive hydrazone derivative, which is rapidly excreted, causing the deficiency.

Clinical features
The main features include:

- Hypochromic, microcytic anaemia
- Secondary pellagra
- Convulsions and depression.

Treatment
Vitamin B_6 supplements are given to all patients on isoniazid therapy

Toxicity
Toxicity is rare. Vitamin B_6 is actually used in the treatment of premenstrual tension (PMT). An excess is, however, associated with the development of a sensory neuropathy.

Pantothenic acid

Sources
Most foods, especially eggs, liver and yeast.

Active form
Component of coenzyme A.

Functions and deficiency
The functions and manifestations of a deficiency of pantothenic acid are listed in Fig. 10.16. Panthothenic acid is not toxic in excess.

Biotin

Sources
Most foods, especially egg yolk, offal, yeast and nuts. A significant amount is synthesized by bacteria in the intestine.

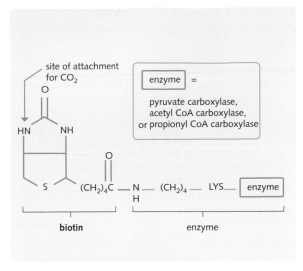

Fig. 10.17 Biotin is a coenzyme for carboxylation reactions. It binds to a lysine residue in carboxylase enzyme molecules.

Active form
As a coenzyme for carboxylation reactions, biotin binds to a lysine residue in carboxylase enzymes (Fig. 10.17).

Functions and deficiency
The functions and clinical manifestations of a deficiency of biotin are listed in Fig. 10.18.

Vitamin B_{12} (cobalamin)

RNI
1.5 mg/day.

Sources
Only animal sources: liver, meat, dairy foods; vegans are at risk of deficiency.

Fig. 10.16 Functions and effects of deficiency of pantothenic acid.

Functions	Deficiency
As coenzyme A, it is involved in the transfer of acyl groups, e.g. acetyl CoA, succinyl CoA, fatty acyl CoA	Very rare; causes 'burning foot syndrome'
It is also a component of fatty acid synthase: acyl carrier protein (see Chapter 4)	N.B. a deficiency in rats causes depigmentation of fur, i.e. it turns grey. Not toxic in excess

Fig. 10.18 Biotin: functions and deficiency.

Functions	Deficiency
It is an activated carrier of CO_2	Very rare on a normal diet, may cause dermatitis
It is a coenzyme for: • pyruvate carboxylase in gluconeogenesis (see Chapter 5) • acetyl CoA carboxylase in fatty acid synthesis (see Chapter 4) • propionyl CoA carboxylase in β oxidation of odd-numbered fatty acids (see Fig. 10.20) • branched-chain amino acid metabolism	Can be induced by: • eating lots of raw egg whites, rich in a glycoprotein, avidin, that binds to biotin in the intestine preventing its absorption • long-term antibiotic therapy, which kills intestinal bacteria

Active forms

Two active forms: deoxyadenosylcobalamin and methyl-cobalamin.

Absorption and transport

The absorption and transport of vitamin B_{12} occurs in several steps (numbers refer to Fig. 10.19):

1. Vitamin B_{12}, released from food in the stomach, becomes bound to a glycoprotein carrier, intrinsic factor (IF), produced by gastric parietal cells
2. The complex of B_{12} and intrinsic factor binds to receptors on the mucosal cells of the terminal ileum
3. B_{12} is absorbed and transported to tissues, attached to transcobalamin II. About 2–3 mg of B_{12} are stored by the body, mainly in the liver; this is relatively large compared with its daily requirement.

Functions

Vitamin B_{12} is a carrier of methyl groups. It is the coenzyme for two enzymes:

- Methylmalonyl CoA mutase, as deoxyadenosylcobalamin, to assist in the breakdown of odd-numbered fatty acids (Fig. 10.20)

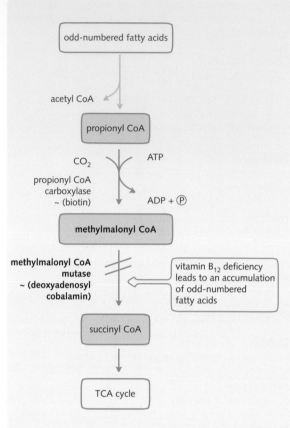

Fig. 10.20   β Oxidation of odd-numbered fatty acids. B_{12} is a carrier of methyl groups. It is the coenzyme for methylmalonyl CoA mutase, assisting in the breakdown of odd-numbered fatty acids.

- Homocysteine methyltransferase, as methylcobalamin, to assist in the synthesis of methionine. This reaction also reverses the methylfolate trap, regenerating tetrahydrofolate (THF) from methyl-THF (discussed below with folate).

Deficiency and toxicity

A significant amount of vitamin B_{12} is stored; it takes about 2 years for symptoms of deficiency to develop. Deficiency can cause two main problems:

- The accumulation of abnormal odd-numbered fatty acids, which may be incorporated into the cell membranes of nerves, resulting in neurological symptoms, inadequate myelin synthesis and nerve degeneration
- Secondary 'artificial' folate deficiency since folate is 'trapped' as methyl THF. This causes a decrease in nucleotide synthesis, resulting in megaloblastic anaemia (see Chapter 7).

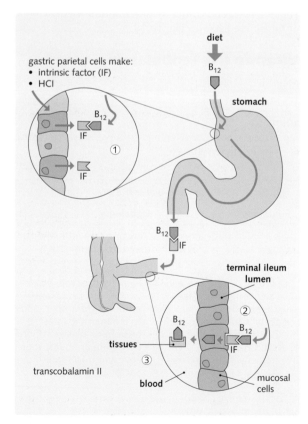

Fig. 10.19   The absorption and transport of vitamin B_{12} (numbers refer to the text).

Subacute combined degeneration of the spinal cord is the metabolic disorder due to vitamin B_{12} and even folate deficiency. It is characterized by a symmetrical loss of posterior columns, causing an ataxic gait, asymmetrical upper motor neurone signs in the lower limbs, but absent reflexes, peripheral sensory neuropathy, optic atrophy and dementia. It is treated with intramuscular injections of hydroxycobalamin.

The most common cause of vitamin B_{12} deficiency is pernicious anaemia, an auto-immune condition where antibodies are made by the body to intrinsic factor.

Causes of deficiency

Reduced intake, for example, by vegans because vitamin B_{12} is only found in animal-derived foods. Reduced absorption caused by:

- A lack of intrinsic factor (e.g. pernicious anaemia)
- Diseases of the terminal ileum which is the site of B_{12} absorption (e.g. Crohn's disease or tuberculosis)
- Bypass of the B_{12} absorption site (e.g. fistulae or surgical resection of gut)
- Blind-loop syndrome: parasites compete for B_{12}.

Body stores (mainly in the liver) are large relative to the daily requirement, therefore a reduced intake alone takes about 2–3 years to cause a deficiency.

Pernicious anaemia

Pernicious anaemia is the commonest cause of vitamin B_{12} deficiency.

Incidence

It is more common in older women and is often associated with fair-haired and blue-eyed individuals, and also the presence of other auto-immune disorders (e.g. thyroid disease and Addison's disease).

Pathogenesis

Pernicious anaemia is an auto-immune disorder where antibodies are made to either:

- Gastric parietal cells, causing atrophy or wasting of the cells, thus preventing the production of intrinsic factor and stomach acid (Fig. 10.21A)
- Intrinsic factor itself (Fig. 10.21B); antibodies bind to the intrinsic factor, preventing it from either binding to vitamin B_{12} (blocking antibodies) or binding to the receptors in the terminal ileum (binding antibodies). A lack of intrinsic factor leads to a decreased uptake of vitamin B_{12}. The clinical features of pernicious anaemia are discussed in Fig. 10.22.

Diagnosis

Diagnosis is performed by analysis of the blood film and bone marrow specimens and by the Schilling test, which measures the absorption of vitamin B_{12}:

- Radioactive vitamin B_{12} is given orally
- A 24 hr urine collection is performed to measure the percentage of the dose of radioactive vitamin B_{12} excreted in the urine
- If the subject is vitamin B_{12} deficient, less than 10% will be excreted because the vitamin B_{12} is being used to replenish depleted stores
- If the result is abnormal, the test is repeated with the addition of intrinsic factor
- If excretion is now normal, the diagnosis is pernicious anaemia.

Treatment

The treatment of vitamin B_{12} deficiency is intramuscular injections of hydroxycobalamin for life. Initially, these are more frequent to fill the stores. Pernicious anaemia carries a slightly increased risk of carcinoma of the stomach.

The toxicity of vitamin B_{12} is low.

Folate

RNI

200 mg/day

Sources

Green vegetables, liver and wholegrain cereals.

Active form

5,6,7,8-THF, which is involved in the transfer of one-carbon units.

Absorption and storage

Folate is absorbed in the duodenum and jejunum. About 10 mg of folate is stored, mainly in the liver.

The role of folate and vitamin B_{12}

All one-carbon THF units are interconvertible except N^5-methyl THF; the THF cannot be released from it and is trapped, forming the 'methyl-folate trap'.

The only way to re-form THF is via vitamin B_{12}-dependent synthesis of methionine: the methionine salvage pathway (Fig. 10.23).

Functions and deficiency

The functions and clinical manifestations of a deficiency of folate are listed in Fig. 10.24.

Folate deficiency

The stores of folate are small relative to the daily requirements, therefore a deficiency state can develop in a few months, particularly if it is associated with a period of rapid growth.

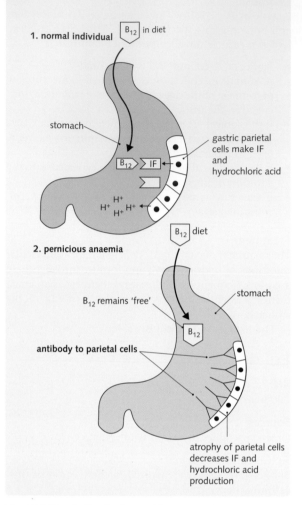

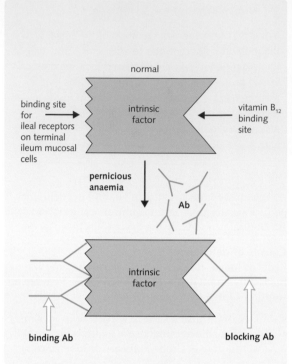

Fig. 10.21B Antibodies to intrinsic factor. Intrinsic factor contains two binding sites; one for vitamin B_{12} and a second one for ileal receptors in the terminal ileum, its site of absorption. In pernicious anaemia, antibodies produced may bind to either or both of these sites.

Fig. 10.21A Antibodies in pernicious anaemia.
1. In normal individuals, vitamin B_{12} released from food in the stomach becomes bound to intrinsic factor (IF) produced by gastric parietal cells
2. In individuals with pernicious anaemia, antibodies to the gastric parietal cells cause wasting of the cells and therefore prevent production of intrinsic factos by them. Vitamin B_{12} is not absorbed, resulting in B_{12} deficiency.

Causes
- Decreased intake: a poor diet is the most common cause (e.g. in slimmers, elderly people and alcoholics)
- Increased requirement: during periods of rapid cell growth, such as:
  - Pregnancy, infancy or adolescence
  - Cancer, inflammatory states or recovery from illness
  - Haemolytic anaemias
- Malabsorption: in coeliac disease or after gut resection
- Drugs:
  - Anticonvulsants impair absorption (e.g. phenytoin and phenobarbitone)
  - Dihydrofolate reductase inhibitors (e.g. methotrexate)
  - Antimalarial drugs (e.g. pyrimethamine)
- Secondary to B_{12} deficiency: vitamin B_{12} is essential to maintain an adequate supply of the active form of folate, that is 5,6,7,8-tetrahydrofolate. It regenerates THF from N^5-methyl-THF in the methionine salvage pathway (Fig. 7.3). Even if there are adequate amounts of folate in the diet, in the absence of vitamin B_{12}, folate deficiency arises.

Clinical features and diagnosis of folate deficiency
The clinical features and diagnosis of folate deficiency are covered in Fig. 10.25.

Treatment
The treatment of folate deficiency is daily oral folate supplementation.

Folate deficiency in pregnancy
The development of the neural tube in the fetus is dependent on the presence of folic acid. Pregnant women should take prophylactic folate supplements to reduce the risk of neural tube defects such as spina bifida or anencephaly. The critical time is the first few weeks after

Fig. 10.22 Clinical features and mechanism of pernicious anaemia.

Clinical features	Mechanism
Megaloblastic anaemia: blood film: macrocytes (MCV > 100 fL) bone marrow: megaloblasts (developing red cells where nuclei mature more slowly than the cytoplasm)	B_{12} deficiency causes secondary folate deficiency, which leads to decreased production of DNA and defective cell division
Neurological abnormalities: peripheral neuropathy affecting sensory neurons of posterior and lateral columns of spinal cord; leads to subacute combined degeneration of spinal cord	Pathogenesis of CNS damage unknown impairment of CNS amino acid and fatty acid metabolism has been implicated
Lemon yellow colour	Combination of jaundice from red cell lysis and pallor because of anaemia
Glossitis, diarrhoea, and weight loss	
Gastric atrophy and achlorhydria (↓ hydrochloric acid production)	Antibodies to gastric parietal cells

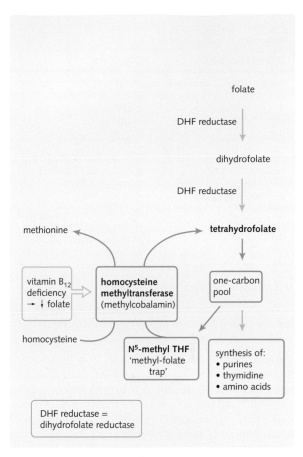

Fig. 10.23 Folate and vitamin B_{12}. The only way to re-form tetrahydrofolate is via vitamin B_{12}-dependent synthesis of methionine: the methionine salvage pathway.

conception: women should therefore start supplements before conception to cover this period. A woman who has already had a baby with a neural tube defect has about a 1:20 risk of a second affected baby; the use of folate supplements has been shown to reduce this risk.

A comparison of folate and vitamin B_{12} deficiencies

A comparison of folate and vitamin B_{12} deficiencies is given in Fig. 10.26. A deficiency of either can cause a macrocytic, megaloblastic anaemia. Patients suspected of having either deficiency, must always be investigated for both folate and B_{12} deficiency since the administration of folic acid corrects the anaemia but masks a B_{12} deficiency. Therefore, folate should never be given alone in treatment of pernicious anaemia and other B_{12} deficiency states because it may precipitate an irreversible peripheral neuropathy.

Fig. 10.24 Folate: function and deficiency

Functions	Deficiency
Synthesis of: • amino acids, e.g. glycine and methionine • purines, AMP, and GMP (see Chapter 7) • thymidine (see Chapter 7)	**Megaloblastic anaemia:** • decrease in purines and pyrimidines leads to a decrease in nucleic acid synthesis and cell division • shows up mostly in cells that are rapidly dividing, e.g. bone marrow and gut • large, immature red blood cells are present

Vitamin C (ascorbate)

RNI
40 mg/day.

Sources
Citrus fruits, tomatoes, berries and green vegetables.

Active form
Ascorbate.

Functions and deficiency
The functions and clinical manifestations of a deficiency of ascorbate are listed in Fig. 10.27.

Fig. 10.25 Clinical features and diagnosis of folate deficiency.

Clinical features	Diagnosis
Megaloblastic anaemia: this is identical to vitamin B_{12} deficiency (see Fig. 10.22)	Blood film: macrocytes (MCV > 100 fL) megaloblasts in bone marrow
Growth failure	Low serum folate
N.B. peripheral neuropathy and neurological symptoms do not occur in folate deficiency	Red cell folate is a better test of folate stores normal = 135–750 mg/mL
	Must always consider and eliminate vitamin B_{12} deficiency and malignancy

Vitamin C deficiency: scurvy

In the past, this used to be common among sailors who spent weeks at sea without any fresh fruit or vegetables.

Causes

Scurvy is caused by a poor dietary intake of fresh fruit and vegetables. In the UK, it is seen in elderly people, alcoholics and smokers. Smokers require twice the normal intake of vitamin C (80 mg/day). Humans have about 6 months' store of vitamin C.

Clinical features

The clinical features of scurvy are described in Fig. 10.28.

Fig. 10.26 A comparison of vitamin B_{12} and folate deficiency; main differences.

Characteristics	Vitamin B_{12}	Folate
Most common cause	Pernicious anaemia	↓ dietary intake
Onset	Slow, 2–3 years	Develops over weeks
Neurological symptoms	Frequent + severe	Never
Drug-related	No: vitamin B_{12} deficiency usually causes secondary folate deficiency	Yes: anticonvulsants, diydrofolate reductase inhibitors
		Folate deficiency occurs frequently on its own because of ↓ intake or ↑demand

Fig. 10.27 Ascorbate: function and deficiency.

Functions	Deficiency
Co-enzyme in hydroxylation reactions: • proline and lysine hydroxylases in collagen synthesis • dopamine β-hydroxylase in epinephrine and nor-epinephrine synthesis Powerful reducing agent: • reduces dietary Fe^{3+} to Fe^{2+} in the gut, allowing its absorption (therefore, deficiency can lead to anaemia) Antioxidant and free-radical 'scavenger' • inactivates free oxygen radicals which damage lipid membranes, proteins and DNA • also protects other antioxidant vitamins A and E	**Scurvy:** most symptoms are due to a decrease in collagen synthesis, leading to poor connective tissue formation and wound healing

Fig. 10.28 Clinical features of scurvy.

Clinical features	Diagnosis
• Swollen, sore, spongy gums with bleeding; loose teeth	Hypochromic, microcytic anaemia caused by secondary iron deficiency.
• Spontaneous bruising and petechial haemorrhages	Low plasma ascorbate level (not very accurate)
• Anaemia	The measurement of ascorbate concentration in white blood cells provides an assessment of tissue stores
• Poor wound healing	
• Swollen joints and muscle pain	

Treatment

The treatment of vitamin C deficiency is 1 g daily of ascorbate and lots of fresh fruit and vegetables in the diet.

The megadose hypothesis

Some researchers believe that large doses of vitamin C cure many illnesses, such as the common cold and certain immune-mediated diseases, and even help in cancer prevention and promote fertility. The benefits of large doses are unresolved and under review. It is thought that 1–4 g/day of vitamin C can decrease the severity of symptoms of cold but not decrease the incidence. Vitamin C is an antioxidant and it is thought that, along with vitamins

A and E, it might decrease the incidence of coronary heart disease and certain cancers by scavenging free radicals, preventing oxidative damage to cells and their components. This has not been confirmed.

Toxicity

A high intake of vitamin C may lead to the formation of kidney stones, diarrhoea and also cause systemic conditioning, that is, requirements increase as the body adapts to metabolizing more.

HINTS AND TIPS

The role of ascorbate in hydroxylation reactions: Hydroxylase enzymes contain iron, which exists in two oxidation states: Fe^{3+} which is inactive, and Fe^{2+} which is reduced and active. Ascorbate is necessary to maintain iron in its reduced and active state (Fe^{2+}).

HINTS AND TIPS

The best way to learn this sort of information is to take a large piece of paper and for each vitamin list only the main points mentioned above. Examiners love to ask about deficiency diseases.

Symptoms of vitamin deficiencies

Fat-soluble vitamins: A, D, E and K

The symptoms and signs of each individual vitamin deficiency are covered in Chapter 11 and therefore will only be covered briefly here (Fig. 10.29). General causes of deficiency are:

Fig. 10.29 Differential diagnosis of fat-soluble vitamin deficiency diseases.

Vitamin deficiency	Differential diagnosis
Vitamin A: night blindness and keratomalacia	Other causes of degenerative eye changes, e.g. infection such as syphilis, gonorrhoea, chlamydia in neonates (rare)
Vitamin D: rickets or osteomalacia	• Ca^{2+} deficiency • renal disease – causing ↓ activity of 1-α hydroxylase • liver disease: causing ↓ acitivity of 25-α hydroxylase
Vitamin K: increased bleeding produces clotting problems (in newborn babies, causes haemorrhagic disease of the newborn)	• inherited coagulation disorders, e.g. haemophilia, von Willebrand's disease • anticoagulant therapy: warfarin/dicoumarol • antibiotic therapy which destroys vitamin K-producing bacteria in gut
Vitamin E: very rare	

- Decreased intake, which may be due either to generalized malnutrition, mainly seen in developing countries; or to poor diet, commonly seen in the elderly and in the housebound in developed countries, or it may occur in people on a vegan diet
- Fat malabsorption; for example, due to liver and biliary tract disease or obstruction preventing bile salts from facilitating absorption

Water-soluble vitamins (B and C)

The symptoms of a deficiency of vitamins B and C are listed in Fig. 10.30.

Fig. 10.30 Symptoms of water-soluble vitamin deficiencies.

Vitamin deficiency	Main symptoms
Vitamin B_1-thiamine: Wet beriberi	Oedema, tachycardia, shortness of breath and other signs of heart failure
Dry beriberi	Ascending peripheral neuropathy: initially weakness and numbness of legs that ascends to involve trunk, arms and eventually brain
Wernicke–Korsakoff syndrome	Confusion, ataxia, ophthalmoplegia and peripheral neuropathy
Niacin: pellagra	3 Ds: dermatitis, dementia and diarrhoea
Vitamin B_6: secondary pellagra	Very rare
Vitamin B_{12}: megaloblastic, macrocytic anaemia	See 'symptoms of anaemia' in Chapter 12
Folate: megaloblastic, macrocytic anemia	See 'symptoms of anaemia' in Chapter 12
Vitamin C: scurvy	Failure of wound healing hypochromic, microcytic anaemia Swollen, sore, spongy gums with bleeding

Nutrition: Minerals and trace elements

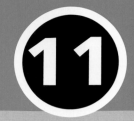

11

Objectives

After reading this chapter you will be able to:
- Describe the main causes and clinical features of mineral deficiencies along with the treatments available

CLASSIFICATION OF MINERALS

There are 103 known elements. Living organisms are composed mainly of 11 of these. Namely carbon, hydrogen, oxygen, nitrogen and the seven major minerals:

- Calcium, phosphorus and magnesium, which are used mainly in bone
- Sodium, potassium and chloride, which are the main electrolytes present in the intracellular and extracellular fluid
- Sulphur, which is used mainly in amino acids.

The RNI is greater than 100 mg/day for each of these (the exception is sulphur for which no RNI has been published).

In addition, there are at least 12 other elements that are required in the diet in smaller quantities. These are known as the essential trace elements, for which the RNI is less than 100 mg/day: iron, zinc, copper, cobalt, iodine, chromium, manganese, molybdenum, selenium, vanadium, nickel and silicon.

CALCIUM

Calcium is the most abundant mineral in the human body. There is about 1.2 kg of calcium in the average 70-kg adult, of which 99% is in bone.

RNI
The RNI of calcium is 700 mg/day; it is higher during periods of growth, pregnancy, lactation and after the menopause.

Sources
Milk and milk products; a lot of foods are fortified with calcium, for example, bread.

Absorption
Absorption of calcium from the diet is variable depending on the following factors:

- Lactose and basic amino acids increase absorption because they form complexes with calcium

- Fibre decreases absorption, therefore, vegans need a lot more calcium.

Active forms
The ionized form, Ca^{2+}.

Main functions
The main functions of calcium are listed in Fig. 11.1.

Regulation of calcium
Calcium levels are controlled by three hormones which also regulate plasma phosphate levels:

- Parathyroid hormone, which increases plasma calcium but decreases levels of inorganic phosphate
- Vitamin D, which increases both plasma calcium and inorganic phosphate levels
- Calcitonin, which decreases both plasma calcium and inorganic phosphate levels.

Calcium deficiency

In children, calcium deficiency causes rickets (derived from the old English word 'wrickken' meaning to twist).

Fig. 11.1 Main functions of calcium.	
Function	**Examples**
Structural role	Bone and teeth Calcium is present as calcium phosphate (hydroxyapatite) crystals
Muscle contraction	Calcium binds to troponin C
Nerve impulse transmission	Calcium is released in response to hormones and neurotransmitters
Blood clotting	Coenzyme for coagulation factors
Ion transport and cell signalling	Intracellular second messenger

In adults, calcium deficiency causes osteomalacia. They both may occur:

- From dietary deficiency of calcium, particularly in developing countries
- Secondary to vitamin D deficiency. Vitamin D is necessary for the intestinal absorption of calcium and phosphate (Fig. 11.2)
- From malabsorption (e.g. coeliac disease).

Pathogenesis

Both rickets and osteomalacia are the result of inadequate mineralization of bone, resulting in a reduction in its normal strength, leading to soft, easily deformed bones. The difference is that they occur at different stages of bone development. In rickets the production of undermineralized bone results in a failure of adequate growth, whereas in osteomalacia, demineralization of existing bones leads to an increased risk of fractures.

- Rickets. The characteristics of rickets are shown in Figs 11.3 and 11.4. Treatment is with calcium supplements and education on a balanced diet. Vitamin D supplements may also be required

Fig. 11.2 Synthesis, metabolism and functions of vitamin D. Active form, 1,25-dihydroxycholecalciferol has three main effects which increase the plasma calcium concentration:
1. Increases uptake of Ca^{2+} (and inorganic phosphate) from the intestine
2. Increases reabsorption of calcium from the kidney
3. Increases resorption of bone (when necessary) so that calcium is released.

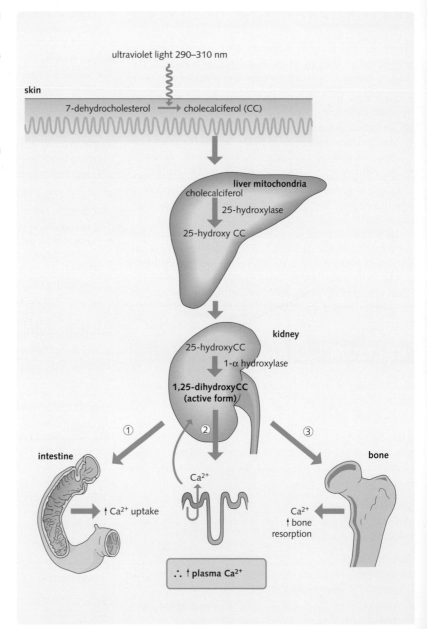

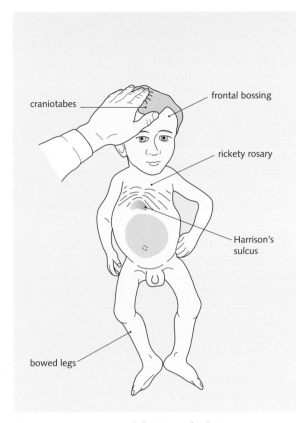

Fig. 11.3 Characteristic deformities of rickets.

Fig. 11.4 The clinical features and diagnosis of rickets.

Clinical features	Diagnosis
Bowed legs: short stature and failure to thrive	↓ serum calcium and phosphorus
Craniotabes: skull bones easily indented by finger pressure	↑ alkaline phosphatase: secreted by osteoblasts to compensate and ↑ bone formation
Rickety rosary: expansion or swelling at costochondral junctions	X-rays show defective mineralization of pelvis, long bones and ribs
Harrison sulcus: indrawing of softened ribs along attachment of diaphragm → 'hollowing'	N.B. low calcium results in ↓ neuromuscular transmission; therefore infant may present with seizures
Expansion of metaphyses especially at wrist	
Delayed dentition	

Fig. 11.5 Clinical features of osteomalacia.

Clinical features	Diagnosis
Spontaneous, incomplete (subclinical) fractures, often in long bones or pelvis	Low serum calcium
Bone pain	Bone biopsy shows increase in non-mineralized bone matrix
Weakness of proximal muscles causing a proximal myopathy with a characteristic waddling gait	X-rays show defective mineralization of long bones and pelvis

- Osteomalacia. This is seen particularly in elderly people and is usually secondary to vitamin D deficiency. The characteristics of osteomalacia are shown in Fig. 11.5
- Osteoporosis. This is the progressive reduction of total bone mass, usually due to the effects of oestrogen deficiency, post-menopause. It is prevented by the use of hormone replacement therapy but calcium is also thought to have a role in its prevention. Adequate calcium nutrition when young helps to achieve a peak bone mass and this decreases the effects of loss and osteoporosis in later life. Calcium supplements both before and after menopause, usually with vitamin D, are recommended.

Calcium overload: hypercalcaemia

Causes
Major causes of hypercalcaemia are primary hyperparathyroidism and malignant disease and have nothing to do with nutrition, and are therefore, beyond the scope of this book. Very rarely, hypercalcaemia is associated with the excessive ingestion of milk and antacids for the control of indigestion. This decreases the renal excretion of calcium: milk–alkali syndrome.

Clinical features
Calcium ions are normally found in cells and deposited calcium salts are present in bones and teeth. In overload, calcium salts are deposited in normal tissues, leading to tissue metastatic calcification and impaired function. This may cause renal stones, arrhythmias, heart failure and calcification of the arteries. Muscle weakness, tiredness, anorexia, constipation and a sluggish, nervous response may also be seen.

PHOSPHORUS

RNI
550 mg/day

Sources

Most foods; a dietary deficiency has not been described.

Functions

Phosphorus works in conjunction with vitamin D and calcium:

- It has a structural role in bones and teeth
- It is required for the production of ATP and other phosphorylated metabolic intermediates. Therefore, it is fundamental to the maintenance of function of cells in the body.

Deficiency and toxicity

The clinical manifestations of a deficiency and excess of phosphorus are listed in Fig. 11.6.

MAGNESIUM

RNI

270 mg/day.

Sources

Most foods, especially green vegetables.

Functions

The functions of magnesium are:

- Structural role in bones and teeth
- Cofactor for more than 300 enzymes in the body, that is, those enzymes that catalyse ATP-dependent reactions. Magnesium binds to ATP, forming a magnesium–ATP complex which is the substrate for enzymes such as kinases
- Interacts with calcium to affect the permeability of excitable membranes and neuromuscular transmission.

Deficiency

Seen in alcoholics; patients with liver cirrhosis; following diuretic therapy; and in renal and intestinal disease. The symptoms are:

- Muscle weakness
- Secondary calcium deficiency
- Confusion, hallucinations, convulsions and other neurological symptoms
- Can also lead to hypokalaemia.

Excess

Extremely rare.

SODIUM, POTASSIUM AND CHLORIDE

Sodium, potassium and chloride function together to regulate the osmolality of intracellular and extracellular fluids. Sodium is the most important one in this respect. Importantly, both high and low potassium concentration in plasma can cause severe cardiac problems. The characteristics of sodium and potassium are listed in Fig. 11.7.

Fluid and electrolyte balance management is an important aspect of medicine, and rarely well understood.

Key intravenous fluids you may prescribe for patients include 3 main classes:

- Crystalloids (0.9% Saline, 5% Dextrose (glucose)) and on rarer occasions Hartmann's
- Colloids (gelofusine, albumin)
- Blood and blood products.

The choice depends on whether you wish to replete the circulatory volume, top up electrolytes or maintain fluid balance. The fluids all have different compositions of electrolytes and should be used with caution in certain groups of patients. Key composition of commonly prescribed crystalloids:

It is important to note that Hartmann's solution is the most physiological of the solutions with a composition and osmolality most similar to plasma values (normal plasma Osm: 275–299 milli-osmoles per kilogram). Also note that 0.9% Saline is often referred to as 'normal saline'; please remember this is not a 'normal' fluid as the name implies, and as with all fluids, it should be only prescribed once existing electrolyte and fluid statuses are known.

SULPHUR

The dietary intake of the sulphur-containing amino acid methionine is essential for synthesis of cysteine (see Fig. 6.11); both can then be incorporated into proteins and enzymes.

Fig. 11.6 The effects of phosphorous deficiency and excess.

Deficiency	Excess
If severe (<0.3 mmol/L), will affect the function of all cells causing: • muscle weakness • in erythrocytes leads to a decrease information of 2,3-bisphosphoglycerate and therefore, reduces unloading of oxygen to tissues • rickets and osteomalacia	May combine with calcium to produce calcium phosphate and be deposited in tissues

Solution	pH	Na$^+$	Cl	K$^+$	Ca^{++}	Lactate	Glucose	Osmolality (Osm)
0.9% 'normal' saline	5.0	154	154	0	0	0	0	308
Hartmann's solution/ compound sodium lactate	6.5	30	109	4	3	28	0	275
% Dextrose	4.0	0	0	0	0	0	50 g/L	252

Fig. 11.7 The characteristics of sodium and potassium.

	Sodium	Potassium
RNI Sources Functions	1.6 g/day Salt, most foods Principal cation of ECF: plasma concentration maintained between 135 and 145 mmol/L; necessary for: • control of ECF volume • Na$^+$/K$^+$-ATPase and uptake of solutes by cell • Na$^+$ gradient provides driving force for secondary active transport • neuromuscular transmission	3.5 g/day Most foods Principal cation of ICF: plasma concentration 3.5–5.0 mmol/L fundamental to: • Na$^+$/K$^+$-ATPase and uptake of molecules by cell • neuromuscular transmission • acid–base balance • cardiac muscle contraction
Deficiency	• disturbances common in hospitalized patients; causes of loss include: vomiting, diarrhoea, use of diuretics, Addison's disease, hyperglycaemia (causing an osmotic diuresis) or renal failure • sodium loss is usually accompanied by water loss, leading to decrease in plasma volume and signs of circulatory failure and collapse	• loss may be secondary to vomiting and the use of diuretics, diarrhoea, excess steroids, hyper-aldosteronism (e.g. Conn's syndrome), Cushing's syndrome or alkalosis • high chance of cardiac arrhythmias and neuromuscular weakness • remember, intravenous insulin treatment without supplementation of potassium leads to hypokalaemia
Excess	Role in hypertension: sodium overload linked to water overload can lead to oedema and to cardiac failure	• the most common cause of potassium retention and hyperkalaemia is renal failure • both severe hypokalaemia and hyperkalaemia are dangerous and require immediate treatment

Clinical Note

Hyperkalaemia is a medical emergency and requires immediate attention, especially when the potassium concentration is above 6 mmol/l or there are associated ECG changes. Refer to local and current guidelines when managing, focus on the protection of the cardiac membrane by giving calcium gluconate intravenously. This buys one time to treat the hyperkalaemia by giving infusion of both insulin and glucose to shift potassium ions into the cell, lowering the plasma potassium concentration.

Hypokalaemia (<2.5 mmol./L) is also a medical emergency that can result in cardiac arrythmias and muscle weakness. This should be managed with potassium replacement.

IRON

RNI

The daily loss of iron from the body is 0.5–1.0 mg/day and is due to:

- Gastrointestinal tract turnover, about 0.5 mg/day
- Desquamation of intestinal mucosal cells and biliary excretion, about 0.3 mg/day
- Sweat and desquamation of skin cells, about 0.1 mg/day
- Urinary losses, about 0.1 mg/day.

Small daily losses are accounted for by the absorption of dietary iron in the duodenum. The demand for iron increases during growth, pregnancy and menstruation (1 ml of blood loss is equal to 0.5 mg of iron). The daily iron requirements are:

- Adult male   1.0 mg
- Child   1.5 mg
- Menstruating woman   2.0 mg
- Pregnant woman   3.0 mg

Only 10% of dietary iron is absorbed, therefore, the amount ingested daily is equal to the daily requirement × 10. Therefore, the RNI = 10–20 mg/day.

Sources
Liver, meat, green vegetables and cereals. Dietary iron exists in two forms:

- Haem iron, which is derived from haemoglobin or myoglobin in meat and is rapidly absorbed
- Non-haem iron, which is present in vegetables and cereals and is absorbed slowly.

Absorption, transport and storage
A summary of the absorption, transport, and functions of iron is given in Fig. 11.8. Total body iron is about 3–5 g. About 60% is in haemoglobin and most of the rest is stored mainly as ferritin, which is a protein–iron complex. A small amount of iron is also stored as haemosiderin.

Figure 11.9. summarizes the functions of body iron.

Iron deficiency anaemia

Bioavailability
Haem iron, present in meat, is readily absorbed. Inorganic (non-haem) iron, present in vegetables and cereals, is mostly in the oxidized (Fe^{3+}) state and must

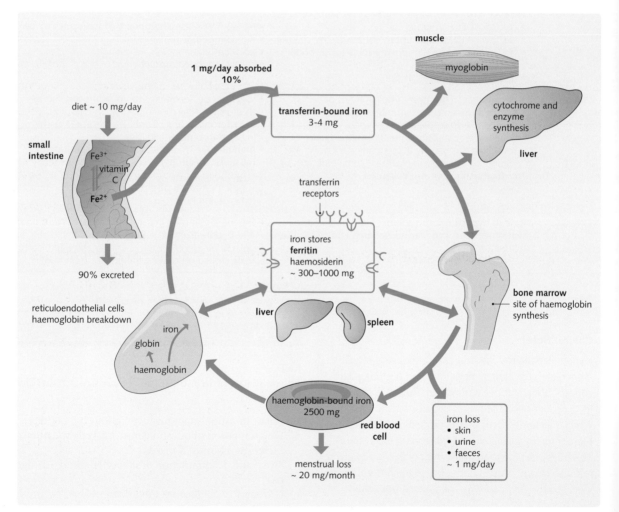

Fig. 11.8 A summary of the absorption, transport and functions of iron. Iron is transported in the blood bound to transferrin; each molecule of transferrin binds two Fe^{2+} ions. This transports iron from sites of absorption and haemoglobin breakdown to storage sites: mainly the reticuloendothelial cells (bone marrow, spleen), hepatocytes (liver) and muscle cells. These cells have transferrin receptors enabling iron to be taken up by receptor-mediated endocytosis. Iron is also transported to these sites for production of haemoglobin (bone marrow), myoglobin (muscle) or production of enzymes (liver).

Fig. 11.9 The distribution and function of total body iron.

Site	Function	Amount of iron (mg)	Percentage total body iron
Total body iron		3500–5000	100
Haemoglobin	Oxygen transport	2500	60–70
Ferritin (2/3) and haemosiderin (1/3)	Iron storage: mainly liver, spleen and bone marrow	1000	27
Myoglobin	Oxygen transporter in muscle	130	3.5
Uncharacterized iron-binding molecules	Storage	80	2.2
Cytochromes and other iron-containing enzymes	Electron transport chain Cytochrome P450 (drug metabolism) Catalase (H_2O_2 breakdown) peroxidase	8	0.2
Transferrin	Transports iron from intestines to tissues	3	0.08

be reduced for absorption. Factors affecting bioavailability include:

- Absorption is favoured in the ferrous (Fe^{2+}) as opposed to the ferric (Fe^{3+}) form
- Stomach hydrochloric acid and ascorbic acid both favour absorption by reducing iron to the ferrous form
- Increased erythropoietic activity (e.g. due to bleeding, haemolysis or high altitude) increases absorption
- Alcohol increases absorption. Phosphates and phytates (from plants) form insoluble complexes with iron and prevent absorption.

Causes of deficiency

Inadequate intake
This is probably the most common cause of iron deficiency, particularly in a vegan diet.

Increased requirement
This occurs in premature babies as iron is transferred to the fetus during the last trimester of pregnancy. It also occurs during infancy, adolescence and pregnancy, that is, during periods of increased growth.

Blood loss
1 mL of blood contains 0.5 mg of iron. Therefore, a small blood loss of 3–4 mL/day over a period of weeks to months can cause chronic iron deficiency. Losses can be from:

- The gut (e.g. due to peptic ulcer, hiatus hernia, cancer of the stomach or caecum and ulcerative colitis)

- Menstrual loss, if periods are particularly heavy.

Always look for causes of chronic blood loss in a person with iron deficiency anaemia.

Malabsorption
Due to high levels of phytates in the diet, secondary to vitamin C deficiency or after surgery (partial or total gastrectomy).

Often, there is more than one cause, for example, a poor quality diet and heavy periods in an adolescent.

Groups in the population at risk of deficiency
Infants, toddlers, adolescents, pregnant women, menstruating women and elderly people are all at risk of iron deficiency.

Highlight the importance to learning this concept of bioavailability for exams.

Clinical Note

Bioavailability is the efficiency (%) with which any dietary nutrient is used in the body. A number of factors can influence the absorption and use of nutrients. For example:

1. The chemical form of the nutrient
2. Antagonistic or facilitatory ligands
3. The breakdown of the nutrient
4. The pH and redox state
5. Anabolic requirements, endocrine influences, infection, and so on.

Clinical features and diagnosis of iron deficiency anaemia

The clinical features and diagnosis of iron deficiency anaemia are covered in Fig. 11.10.

Management and treatment

Finding the cause is essential. The treatment for iron deficiency anaemia is oral iron supplements (e.g. ferrous sulphate or gluconate). If malabsorption is suspected, use intramuscular or intravenous iron. Iron supplements should be given for long enough to correct the haemoglobin level; when this is normal, iron must then be continued for 3–6 months to replenish stores.

Prognosis

Pathological changes are reversed by adequate replacement therapy.

Iron overload

Iron overload leads to iron deposition in the tissues, which may interfere with their function (Fig. 11.11).

Causes

There are two principal causes of iron overload. There is an inherited form, called idiopathic primary haemochromatosis, which has a homozygote prevalence in the population of 0.5%. Iron overload may also be acquired, where it occurs secondary to an increased administration of iron. This is called transfusional iron overload.

Idiopathic primary haemochromatosis

Pathogenesis

Idiopathic primary haemochromatosis is an autosomal recessive disorder, characterized by the excessive absorption of iron in the small intestine. The gene defect is located on chromosome 6. Only homozygotes manifest clinical features; the accumulation of iron is gradual. It usually presents in the fifth decade when levels of iron are about 40–60 g compared with 3–5 g in a normal person. The disease is clinically manifested more commonly in men as women can compensate for the excess absorption by menstrual bleeding. The course of the disease depends on the amount of dietary iron and the presence of other dietary factors, such as vitamin C or alcohol.

Clinical consequences

Iron is deposited as insoluble haemosiderin, forming yellow granules in tissues (Fig. 11.12), which eventually interfere with tissue function. An increase in iron levels leads to an increase formation of free radicals, especially the hydroxyl radical. At normal iron levels, a reactive superoxide radical $O_2{}^\bullet$ is removed effectively by the enzyme superoxide dismutase, as shown in the reaction below:

$$2O_2{}^\bullet + 2H^+ \rightarrow H_2O_2 + O_2$$

However, in iron overload, Fe^{3+} reacts with the superoxide radical to form an extremely reactive hydroxyl radical, $OH^\bullet$. this hydroxyl radical is capable of damaging biological molecules, particularly lipids, leading to lipid peroxidation and membrane damage (especially of lysosomal membranes).

$$O_2{}_-{}^\bullet + Fe^{3+} \rightarrow Fe^{2+} + O_2$$

$$Fe^{2+} + H_2O_2 \rightarrow Fe^{3+} + OH^- + OH^\bullet$$

Fig. 11.10 Clinical features and diagnosis of iron deficiency anaemia.

Signs and symptoms	Diagnosis
↓ **Production of haemoglobin:** less oxygen reaches the tissues especially the brain and heart muscle causing pallor, tiredness, shortness of breath, giddines, palpitations symptoms usually occur when haemoglobin < 8 g/dL	**Blood tests:** • ↓ haemoglobin, serum ferritin and iron • FBC, blood film • ↑ total iron-binding capacity (TIBC) (due to increase in 'free' transferrin)
Epithelial abnormalities: angular stomatitis (cracked corners of mouth) glossitis (sore tongue) koilonychia (spoon-shaped nails)	**Gold standard** for diagnosis of iron deficiency is the absence of iron stores in the bone marrow **Blood film:** microcytic, hypochromic erythrocytes, i.e. small, pale erythrocytes where: • MCV (mean cellular volume) < 80 fL • MCH (mean cell Hb) < 27 pg **N.B.** normal haemoglobin concentration is 13–18 g/dL in men, 11.5–16 g/dL in women

Fig. 11.11 Sites of iron deposition in iron overload.

Tissue	Effect
Liver	Liver fibrosis and pigmentation resulting in cirrhosis and eventually liver failure; may progress to hepatocellular carcinoma (30%)
Pancreas	'Bronze diabetes': iron damages islet cells causing diabetes mellitus
Heart	Heart failure
Skin	Grey/bronze skin colour because of increased production of melanin
Testes	Impotence
Joints	Arthropathy

Zinc deficiency

Acrodermatitis enteropathica

Acrodermatitis enteropathica is an extremely rare, autosomal recessive disorder that leads to the malabsorption of zinc in the small intestine. It presents in infancy with a severe symmetrical, eczematous rash around orifices and on the hands and feet. Frequently, the lesions become severely infected with *Candida* or bacterial infections, leading to death. Infants may also develop growth retardation, hypogonadism and poor wound healing.

Treatment

The condition is completely cured by zinc therapy. Zinc deficiency is also a very rare complication of parenteral nutrition when insufficient supplementation is given.

Fig. 11.12 The role of zinc in the body.

Functions	Deficiency
Co-factor of over 100 enzymes, e.g.: • dehydrogenases, e.g. LDH • peptidases • carbonic anhydrase • enzymes of DNA and protein synthesis • superoxide dismutase Transcription factors contain 'zinc fingers' that enable them to bind DNA	Causes: growth retardation, hypogonadism, and delayed wound healing These effects are mainly a result of decreased activity of the enzymes of DNA synthesis

This results in the oxidation and destruction of cell membranes and tissues.

Treatment

The treatment for idiopathic primary haemochromatosis is regular venesection (i.e. removal of blood) to reduce the iron load. Plasma iron and ferritin levels are used to monitor the treatment. Once the excess iron is removed, the frequency of venesection is reduced.

Transfusional iron overload: transfusion siderosis

Causes

Repeated blood transfusions over a long period of time can cause iron overload. The ability of the reticuloendothelial cells (spleen, liver and bone marrow) to store iron is exceeded and iron is deposited at other sites. As with primary iron overload, iron is deposited mainly in the skin, heart, liver and pancreas. Patients with any condition requiring regular blood transfusions are regarded as high risk (e.g. thalassaemia major, aplastic anaemia).

Treatment

Chelation therapy with desferrioxamine is highly effective in chelating the iron, thus enabling its excretion.

ZINC

The daily zinc requirement is 2–3 mg/day but absorption is only about 30% effective. Therefore, the RNI is 10 mg/day. Zinc can be found in most foods. The total body zinc is 2–3 g. It is found in all tissues but high concentrations are present in the liver, kidney, bone, retina, muscle and prostate. The role of zinc in the body is described in Fig. 11.12.

COPPER

RNI
1.2 mg/day.

Sources
Liver is a very good source.

Copper metabolism

The total body copper is about 75–150 mg. High copper concentrations are found in the liver, brain, heart and kidneys. Dietary copper is absorbed in the stomach and duodenum and transported to the liver loosely bound to albumin; the absorption is about 30% effective. It is incorporated into caeruloplasmin, a glycoprotein synthesized by the liver, which transports copper to the tissues where it can be used for the synthesis of other copper-containing enzymes. Normally, it is excreted in the bile (daily loss is approximately 2–3 mg/day). In the blood, 80–90% of the copper present is bound to caeruloplasmin.

Function

Copper is required for the synthesis of a number of copper-containing enzymes (Fig. 11.13).

Copper deficiency: Menkes' kinky hair syndrome

Menkes' kinky hair syndrome is a rare, X-linked disease with an incidence of 1 in 50 000–100 000. It is caused by the defective absorption of copper from the intestine, leading to a decreased synthesis of copper-containing enzymes (Fig. 11.14).

Fig. 11.13 The role of copper and the effects of copper deficiency.

Affected enzyme	Functional role	Effect of deficiency
Caeruloplasmin	Promotes absorption of iron	Iron deficiency anaemia
Lysyl oxidase	Cross-links collagen and elastin	Weak-walled blood vessels
Tyrosinase	Melanin production	Failure of pigmentation
Dopamine β-hydroxylase	Catecholamine production	Neurological effects
Cytochrome c oxidase	Electron transport chain	Decreased ATP formation
Superoxide dismutase	Scavenges the superoxide radical and prevents lipid peroxidation and membrane damage	Tissue damage

Fig. 11.14 Clinical features of copper deficiency.

Clinical features	Explanation
Depigmentation of hair 'steely hair'	↓ tyrosinase and melanin production
Arterial degeneration	↓ lysyl oxidase resulting in defective collagen and elastin
Neuronal degeneration and mental retardation	↓ catecholamine neurotransmitters
Growth failure and anaemia	↓ caeruloplasmin

Fig. 11.15 Clinical features of copper overload.

Clinical effects of copper accumulation	Diagnosis
Liver: chronic hepatitis → cirrhosis	Low serum concentration of caeruloplasmin
Brain: severe, progressive neurological disability including tremor, mental deterioration and loss of co-ordination	↑ urinary copper Excess copper in liver biopsy
Eyes: characteristic yellow-brown Kayser-Fleischer rings around corneal limbus	

Treatment

Copper therapy has no significant effect. The life expectancy is less than 2 years.

Copper overload: Wilson's disease

Aetiology

Wilson's disease is a rare, autosomal recessive disorder (incidence of 1 in 100 000). The defect has been identified on chromosome 13 and results in failure of the liver to excrete copper in the bile. Copper incorporation into caeruloplasmin is also impaired. Copper accumulates and is deposited in the liver, basal ganglia of the brain, kidneys and the eyes, causing damage (Fig. 11.15).

Treatment

Wilson's disease is treated by daily chelation therapy with D-penicillamine. This is very effective at binding copper and eliminating it in the urine. However, the resulting liver and neurological damage is permanent.

IODINE

The human body contains about 15–20 mg of iodine, most of which is in the thyroid gland. It is essential for the synthesis of the thyroid hormones thyroxine and triiodothyronine.

Deficiency

Endemic goitre

Endemic goitre, a generalized enlargement of the thyroid gland, occurs in areas where the soil and water lack iodine, such that the daily intake is less than 70 mg (usually mountainous areas). In the UK, it used to be found in people in Derbyshire, causing the so-called Derbyshire neck. The problem has now been eliminated in most countries by the addition of iodine to table salt and its prevalence is mostly restricted to developing countries.

Pathogenesis of goitre

Normally iodine is used to make thyroxine and triiodothyronine. Increased levels of these hormones exert a negative feedback effect on the hypothalamus and

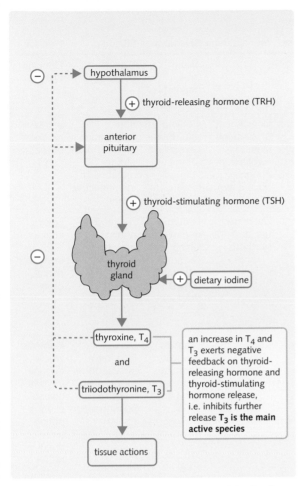

Fig. 11.16   The hypothalamic–pituitary–thyroid feedback system: normal status. In the presence of dietary iodine, thyroid hormones are produced which exert a negative feedback effect on hypothalamus and pituitary, inhibiting release of TRH and TSH.

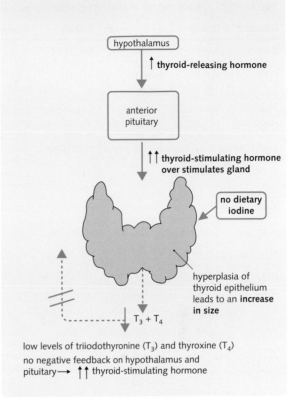

Fig.11.17   The hypothalamic–pituitary–thyroid feedback system: dietary iodine limiting. Decreased production of thyroid hormones releases negative feedback on hypothalamus and anterior pituitary.

anterior pituitary inhibiting further release of thyroid-releasing hormone and thyroid-stimulating hormone (Fig. 11.16), resulting in a decrease in their synthesis. However, low levels of iodine decrease thyroxine formation by the thyroid gland. This releases the negative feedback on the hypothalamic-pituitary axis, causing an uncontrolled increase in thyroid-stimulating hormone secretion. High levels of TSH overstimulate the thyroid gland, causing hyperplasia of the thyroid epithelium and generalized enlargement (Fig. 11.17). The addition of iodine to the diet should reverse this effect.

Cretinism

Pregnant mothers who are deficient in iodine may give birth to babies who are hypothyroid. Growth and mental development in these babies are severely impaired and may be irreversible. The diagnosis is made by the neonatal screening test, the Guthrie test, which is performed on all newborn babies and looks for raised thyroid-stimulating hormone levels. The same sample is used to screen for phenylketonuria. Treatment is lifelong oral replacement of thyroxine. Cretinism can be prevented by the iodination of salt in the maternal diet.

Clinical Note

Hypothyroidism has an insidious onset with vague, non-specific and diverse features. It usually presents with fatigue, weight gain and cold intolerance. It may also present with bradycardia, constipation, delayed puberty, growth and mental retardation, and dry, scaly, cold and thickened skin.

Fig. 11.18 The characteristics of some of the other trace elements.

Element	Iodine	Chromium	Cobalt	Manganese	Molybdenum	Selenium	Silicon	Fluoride
Source	Supplemented salt RNI = 140 µg	Meat, liver, yeast, whole grains	Foods of animal origin			Meat, green vegetables RNI = 60 µg	Green vegetables	Drinking water
Main function	Synthesis of thyroid hormones	Possibly improves glucose tolerance	Constituent of vitamin B_{12} as cobalamin	Cofactor for enzymes: decarboxylases, transferases, superoxide dismutase	Constituent of xanthine oxidase: involved in purine breakdown	Cofactor of glutathione peroxidase	Bone calcification, glycosamino-glycan metabolism in connective tissue	Increases hardness of teeth
Deficiency	Goitre in adults Cretinism in babies	Impaired glucose tolerance (reported very rarely in patients on parenteral nutrition)	As for vitamin B_{12} deficiency	Unknown	Decreased uric acid synthesis	Endemic in parts of China → cardio-myopathy (Keshan disease)	Decrease in normal growth	Low intake leads to increased dental caries
Excess	Toxic goitre Hyperthyroidism	Nonspecific: nausea, diarrhoea and irritability		Inhalation poisoning leading to psychotic symptoms and parkinsonism (rare)		Leads to hair loss, dermatitis, and irritability	Silicosis: long-term inhalation of silicon dust leads to pulmonary fibrosis	Fluorosis: where fluorine infiltrates enamel causing pitting and discolo-ration of teeth

Iodine overload

Excessive dietary iodine may cause the symptoms of hyperthyroidism, that is, an overactive thyroid.

OTHER TRACE ELEMENTS

The characteristics of some of the other trace elements not covered here are listed in Fig. 11.18.

HINTS AND TIPS

Know about iron deficiency and overload, calcium deficiency, and copper overload because they are commonly asked about.

SYMPTOMS OF MINERAL DEFICIENCIES

The symptoms and signs of each individual mineral deficiency are covered in this chapter. The symptoms of the more important mineral deficiency disorders are listed in Fig. 11.19. The differential diagnosis is biased towards metabolic causes.

Symptoms	Cause
Fig. 11.19 Symptoms of mineral deficiencies.	
Iron deficiency: anaemia (symptoms of anaemia have been covered earlier)	May be due to: ↓ blood loss: either acute or chronic ↓ dietary intake ↓ absorption caused by: intestinal malabsorption such as ulcerative colitis, Crohn's disease and coeliac disease, ↑ phosphates and phytates in diet or vitamin C deficiency ↑ requirement: periods of growth and pregnancy
Calcium (and phosphate) deficiency: • in children: rickets; present with soft, easily deformed bones, short stature and failure to thrive • in adults: osteomalacia ('brittle bones')	• ↓ dietary intake • secondary to vitamin D deficiency: vitamin D is necessary for intestinal absorption of calcium and phosphate • intestinal malabsorption • renal failure • hypothyroidism
Iodine deficiency: goitre can lead to symptoms of hypothyroidism: tiredness, weight gain, anorexia, cold intolerance, constipation	• auto-immune: Hashimoto's thyroiditis • after surgery for hyperthyroidism

Clinical assessment of metabolic and nutritional disorders

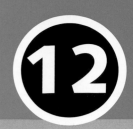

Objectives

After reading this chapter you should be able to:

- Describe the metabolic causes of the common presenting complaints
- Describe the symptoms of the major metabolic and nutritional disorders
- Work out a differential diagnosis for the major metabolic and nutritional disorders
- Take a good history and perform a general examination
- Summarize the main points of history taking and examination with an emphasis on eliciting signs and symptoms of metabolic disorders
- Understand the indications for and basic principles behind the routine investigations
- Understand how to interpret the results of routine investigations in order to make a thorough assessment of the patient's nutritional status

PRESENTATION OF METABOLIC AND NUTRITIONAL DISORDERS

COMMON PRESENTING COMPLAINTS

This section deals with some examples of common presenting complaints, and symptoms of metabolic disorders. For each complaint, the major metabolic causes are considered.

Remember, for each symptom there are also lots of non-metabolic causes, which might be more common but are beyond the scope of this book. For further discussions of these, refer to a general medicine textbook.

Fatigue

Fatigue is one of the most common general presenting complaints and patients may describe: 'tiredness', 'lack of energy' (one of the most common general symptoms), 'weakness' or 'exhaustion'.

It is important to obtain a clear history (when it started, its progression, precipitating and relieving factors, and any associated symptoms) to help detect the cause. Always clarify whether tiredness occurs on effort or rest. A good follow-up question to differentiate psychological from physical causes is 'What slows you down when you attempt doing anything strenuous?'. The main metabolic causes of fatigue are described in Fig. 12.1.

Weight loss

Weight loss is associated with many different conditions. Only the main metabolic causes are considered here.

Working definition
A loss of 5% or more of the usual body weight over a period of 6 months.

It is essential to take a clear and well-documented history from the patient and to attempt to quantify true weight loss over a specific time period and to establish changes in diet and exercise. The difficulty of doing this accurately is well recognized, unless the patient is continually weighed and monitored over a period of time. Indicators of weight loss include:

- Changes in clothing or belt size
- Verification from friends or relatives.

Other methods of nutritional assessment are covered in Chapter 11.

Involuntary weight loss is often a clue that the patient has a serious underlying disease such as cancer. Figure 12.2 lists the common metabolic causes of weight loss.

Symptoms of anaemia

Anaemia occurs when the blood haemoglobin level is below the normal range for the patient's age and sex. The normal haemoglobin range in males is 13.5–18.0 g/dL and in females is 11.5–16.0 g/dL.

The symptoms depend on the severity of the anaemia; a small reduction in haemoglobin is usually

Fig. 12.1 Main metabolic causes of fatigue.

Causes	Examples and notes
Anaemia	This may be secondary to: • iron/B_{12}/folate deficiency • haemolytic anaemia, e.g. G6PDH or pyruvate kinase deficiency (see Fig. 12.3 for other examples)
Hypothyroidism	This may be due to an iodine deficiency or an auto-immune disease, Hashimoto's thyroiditis
Diabetes mellitus	See types of diabetes (see Fig. 8.11)
Malnutrition: 1) Undernutrition 2) Overnutrition/ obesity	General vitamin deficiencies Protein–energy malnutrition (PEM): marasmus or kwashiorkor (see Chapter 9) Tiredness, glucose intolerance, risk of hypertension
Ca^{2+} or vitamin D deficiency	Osteomalacia (weak, easily deformed bones)
Glycogen storage disorders	e.g. McArdle's disease (see Chapter 4)

asymptomatic. Most symptoms are non-specific and result from a decreased oxygen supply to the tissues:

• Fatigue
• Headaches
• Fainting
• Breathlessness
• Importantly, anaemia could unearth coronary heart disease by precipitating angina (chest pain, brought on by exercise, relieved by rest)
• Similarly, peripheral vascular disease may become symptomatic (intermittent claudication: leg pain precipitated by walking and quickly relieved by rest)
• Palpitations.

As these symptoms are relatively non-specific, to find out the cause of the anaemia, a number of laboratory tests may be performed, including:

• Full blood count, which includes the measurements of haemoglobin concentration, the red cell count, and several calculated indices, such as the mean cell volume and the mean cell haemoglobin (see Fig. 12.20)

Fig. 12.2 Common metabolic causes of weight loss.

Main cause	Differential diagnosis
Decreased calorie intake	• Malnutrition: common in developing countries, and in the UK may be seen in the elderly • Cancer (due to anorexia) • Alcoholism • Anorexia nervosa • Depression
Increased loss or energy expenditure	• Hyperthyroidism • Poorly controlled diabetes • Cancer

HINTS AND TIPS

For iron deficiency anaemia, there are unique signs and symptoms which help in clinical diagnosis. They are: painless glossitis (smooth tongue), angular stomatitis (sores at corner of the mouth), koilonychia (spoon-shaped nails) and unusual dietary cravings such as pica (soil-eating).

HINTS AND TIPS

Mean cell volume (MCV) is a useful indicator of the type of anemia and possible causes (see Fig. 12.3).

• Blood film, which provides information on the morphology of cells
• Reticulocyte count
• Serum iron and total iron-binding capacity/ transferrin
• Serum ferritin
• Vitamin B_{12} and folate levels
• Schilling test. This is specific for pernicious anaemia.

These tests and their results are discussed fully in Chapter 11.

Causes of anaemia

There are many causes of anaemia, ranging from acute blood loss to hereditary haemolytic anaemias such as sickle cell anaemia. The main metabolic causes of anaemia are listed in Fig. 12.3.

Fig. 12.3 Metabolic causes of anaemia.

Cause	Notes
Microcytic anaemia (MCV < 75 fL)	
Iron deficiency	Decrease in haem and red blood cell production
Lead poisoning	Lead inhibits three enzymes of haem synthesis (see Chapter 7)
Vitamin C deficiency	Vitamin C is required for absorption of Fe^{2+}
Normocytic anaemia (MCV 76–100 fL)	
Haemolytic anaemia	Deficiency of erythrocyte enzymes such as pyruvate kinase or G6PDH (see Chapter 4)
Macrocytic anaemia (MCV > 100 fL)	
Pernicious anaemia	Auto-immune condition in which antibodies against intrinsic factors prevent B_{12} absorption in the terminal ileum, leading to B_{12} deficiency (see Chapter 10)
Folate/B_{12} deficiency	Folic acid and vitamin B_{12} required for DNA synthesis; results in megaloblastic anaemia (see Chapter 10)

Dehydration

This is commonly a problem in elderly patients and assessment of volume status, detailed clinical skills and investigation of prior events are required. Establishing the duration and form of fluid loss from diuresis, diarrhoea and vomiting, or bleeding can give an estimate of the amount and type of fluid that needs replacement. If accurate quantification of loss is needed; monitor inputs and outputs (from bowel, bladder, or surgical drains). Symptoms of volume depletion are usually secondary to decreased tissue perfusion.

Symptoms and signs
Usually non-specific. Lassitude, muscle cramps and dizziness. Signs are more important and include low skin turgor/tension, dry mucous membranes, acute weight loss, jugular venous pressure (JVP), sunken eyes, postural hypotension, increased heart rate and reduced urine output.

Dehydrated patients tend to have an increased plasma sodium concentration and elevated urea and creatinine concentration. In the so-called pre-renal uraemia (when a decrease of the glomerular filtration rate is due to volume depletion rather than to nephron destruction), plasma urea increase exceeds that of creatinine.

Fluid overload
This is an important state to recognize, especially in patients with heart failure or renal failure. It can be detected from symptoms such as shortness of breath, paroxysmal nocturnal dyspnoea (waking at night/when lying flat due to shortness of breath) and signs including: peripheral or sacral oedema (if sedentary; pitting), crepitations on auscultation of the chest, raised JVP and weight gain.

Fluid overload is often associated with hyponatraemia.

Clinical Note

Fluid status is an important aspect of the examination especially for cardiovascular, renal and surgical patients.

Symptoms of amino acid disorders

All amino acid disorders are rare. Most present in infancy as developmental delay, vomiting, failure to thrive, mental retardation and seizures. The symptoms are all non-specific, making the differential diagnosis complex. All neonates are now screened for phenylketonuria at a few days of age using the Guthrie test. The other amino acid disorders must be considered and eliminated when infants present with these symptoms without other adequate explanation; for example, in the absence of infection (Fig. 12.4). Their diagnosis depends on the measurement of metabolites in the blood and urine.

Fig. 12.4 Differential diagnosis of amino acid disorders in infants.

Phenylketonuria
Inborn errors of carbohydrate metabolism, e.g. galactosaemia, glycogen storage disorders
Neurological disorders, e.g. febrile convulsions, infantile spasms
Infections (common), e.g. gastroenteritis, urinary tract infection
Coeliac disease (1 in 2000 in the UK)
Acute abdomen

HISTORY TAKING

THINGS TO REMEMBER WHEN TAKING A HISTORY

'The history is usually the most important part of the consultation.'

Before you begin, as with any examination:

- Always introduce yourself, clarify the patient's identity and cross-check patient data with case notes
- Look around the bedside for clues such as monitors, treatments, supportive equipment (glasses, walking sticks and frames)
- Observe the patient initially from the end of the bed and afterwards assess in more detail
- Look at their overall state (physical and psychiatric): are they agitated/distressed/in pain or uncomfortable? This should take only a few seconds, and should precede your introductory history questions to ensure you address issues of pain/discomfort, and avoid asking obvious or unsuitable questions before proceeding with the history taking.

Structure of a history

This is a basic plan designed for you to copy and take with you when you first start clerking patients, which should be memorized and become automatic after several uses.

Personal information

- Name and sex
- Age/date of birth
- Occupation
- Ethnicity.

Presenting complaint (PC)

This should be a short statement of the symptoms the patient is complaining of, in his or her own words. For example, pain.

History of presenting complaint (HPC)

Try to get the patient to tell the story in his or her own words from when he or she thought it began. For most symptoms you will need to know:

- What is the time course/duration? When did the problem start or when did the patient first feel unwell?
- Was the onset rapid or slow?
- What is the nature of the complaint? And has it changed? If it is pain: what is its site, radiation and

so on; if it is vomiting: how often does it happen and how much is there? What's the colour? Is there any visible blood?

- Does the symptom show a pattern? Is it continuous, intermittent or continuous with acute exacerbations?
- Are there any precipitating or relieving factors? For example, is it related to meals or the type of food eaten, or to stress? Is it helped by painkillers or any other medication?

HINTS AND TIPS

For pain, a useful mnemonic to remember is SOCRATES:

Site
Onset
Character (e.g. sharp, dull, colicky)
Radiation
Associated symptoms (e.g. nausea, vomiting)
Timing
Exacerbation and relieving factors
Severity (e.g. on a scale of 1 to 10)

- Are there any other relevant or associated symptoms? For example, for chest pain, ask about palpitations, sweating and nausea
- Has it happened before? Ask about any previous treatment or investigations for the complaint.

Use simple terms as much as possible and avoid medical jargon.

Review of symptoms

Some of these symptoms may have already been covered in the history of the presenting complaint. You need to use your discretion about the extent of this enquiry. Good general systemic enquiry questions which can help detect thyroid/metabolic disorders, infections, malignancies, even lymphoma, include:

- Weight changes
- Appetite changes
- Fatigue
- Fever
- Lumps and bumps (lymph node enlargements)
- Everything else – ask the patient if there is anything else they would like to add that they have noticed?

Cardiovascular system, ask specifically about:

- Chest tightness and pain
- Palpitations

- Changes in exercise tolerance (quantify by stairs climbed or distance walked before onset of breathlessness)
- Remember: Dyspnoea is shortness of breath; orthopnoea is breathlessness when lying down flat (quantify in terms of number of pillows the patient must sleep on to prevent dyspnoea); paroxysmal nocturnal dyspnoea is waking up at night breathless
- Claudication (calf pain on walking). Ask how far can the patient walk without discomfort. Importantly, does it happen when walking on the flat or on inclines and stairs
- Leg pain at rest
- Ankle oedema

Respiratory system, ask specifically about
- Persistent cough – is it productive?
- Sputum: amount, colour
- Haemoptysis (coughing up blood)
- Shortness of breath
- Wheeze.

Gastrointestinal system, ask specifically about
- Change in appetite
- Change in weight
- Nausea or vomiting (haematemesis (vomit containing blood))
- Difficulty swallowing (dysphagia)
- Heartburn or indigestion
- Change in bowel habit: diarrhoea, constipation, frequency
- Change in nature of stools: consistency, colour, mucus, melaena (black tarry stools due to digested blood), and do they float in the toilet pan (steathorrhoea).

Urinary system, ask specifically about
- Frequency
- Urgency
- Nocturia
- Urine stream: hesitancy, dribbling
- Dysuria (pain on passing water)
- Haematuria
- Incontinence.

Skin, ask specifically about
- Rashes or sensitive skin
- Dermatitis
- Eczema/psoriasis
- Remember that the skin is frequently affected by substances encountered at work and at home.

Musculoskeletal system, ask specifically about
- Location: generalized aches and pains or discomfort affecting a specific muscle?
- Painful joints
- Stiffness
- Swelling
- Arthritis
- Diurnal variations in symptoms (i.e. with time of the day)
- Functional deficit (i.e. can they undo buttons?).

Nervous system, many questions so use a structure
Work from top to toe to remember symptoms.

- Headaches
- Fits, faints and funny turns. Dizziness
- Anxiety, depression or suicidal thoughts
- Changes in vision, hearing, speech or memory
- Changes in sleep pattern
- Pins and needles, paraesthesiae; especially ask about sensation in the peripheries/glove and stocking distribution
- Ataxia; lack of coordination of muscle movements
- Motor function of the limbs; power, tone, coordination, tremors/uncontrolled movements.

Menstruation and obstetric history
This should only be taken when relevant. For example, 'last menstrual period', should be checked when the presenting complaint is abdominal pain to consider ectopic pregnancy as a differential diagnosis.

Past medical history (PMHx)
Ask the patient about previous illnesses, hospital admissions, operations and investigations, with dates.

HINTS AND TIPS

You may find the mnemonic MTHREADS:

Myocardial infarction
Tuberculosis
Hypertension
Rheumatic fever
Epilepsy
Asthma
Disbetes
Stroke

You should always ask specifically about these conditions, as well as anaemia and jaundice.

Ask about the patient's nutritional history. A lot of metabolic and nutritional disorders present in infancy. When dealing with children, ask the parents specifically about problems during the pregnancy or birth, or when their child was a neonate; for example, problems with feeding, bowels or failure to thrive. Enquire about developmental milestones: smiling, sitting, walking and talking.

Drug history (DH)

Is the patient currently on any medication (either over-the-counter or prescription). Ask about the dosage. If relevant, ask about alternative therapies, herbal medicine and recreational drugs. Also remember to ask female patients if they are on the oral contraceptive pill, as many do not regard it as a drug.

Allergies

Is the patient allergic to any medicines or foods that they know of? Ask specifically about penicillin. If they say they are allergic, ask about what happened when they took the medicine or food.

Smoking

How many per day and how long ago did the patient start? If they say they have given up, you must also ask when – it might be just yesterday! A useful way of quantifying smoking is in pack years: 20 cigarettes smoked per day for 1 year equals 1 pack year.

HINTS AND TIPS

The CAGE questionnaire is a useful screening test for alcoholism, with two or more positive answers suggesting an alcohol problem. Have you ever:
Felt you should **C**ut down on your drinking?
Been **A**nnoyed at others' concerns about your drinking?
Felt **G**uilty about drinking?
Had alcohol as an **E**ye-opener in the morning?

Alcohol

How many drinks or units each week? An alcohol unit = 10 ml/8 g pure alcohol = 25 ml single measure of whisky or a third of a pint of beer or half a standard (175 ml) glass of red wine. The limits are 21 units for males and 14 units for females per week.

Family history (FH)

Ask about any known illnesses in first-degree relatives, in particular, diabetes and heart disease. Remember to ask specifically about premature heart disease ('Has there been any talk in the family about a lot of people having heart disease at a young age?' The accepted definition of premature disease is onset below age 55 in men and 65 in women). It may help to make a quick sketch of the family tree.

A number of inborn errors of metabolism are inherited as autosomal recessive disorders and have a high incidence amongst populations where marriages between first cousins are quite common, for example, Ashkenazi Jews. Be tactful when asking about a family history of malignancy.

Social history (SH)

Ask about marital status, number of children, and the type of accommodation. Ask about the patient's occupational history: current and previous jobs, exposure to chemicals or asbestos and any time off work due to illness. Ask about financial and personal worries and any risk-related behaviour, for example, taking illegal drugs or any risky homosexual or heterosexual contacts.

Summarize

This should be a brief recall of the main points. For example: Jonathan Brown, a 4-year-old boy referred by his general practitioner, presenting with a 6-week history of increasing thirst, polyuria and weight loss. His mother has insulin-dependent diabetes mellitus. On examination . . .

COMMUNICATION SKILLS

Medical schools now place great emphasis on communication skills and their importance in the practice of medicine. Examinations now feature some form of structured clinical examination, e.g. OSCEs.

Communication skills contribute heavily to the global score in clinical exams, so it is important to develop a rapport with the patient or actor, especially as in addition to giving you a good global score it will encourage them to divulge more information/clues. So make sure you practice communicating with your friends in clinical scenarios.

The importance of communication

How you communicate is absolutely essential. Good communication makes patients more comfortable and greatly facilitates the correct diagnosis. On the other hand, poor communication is the most common cause of patients' complaints.

Obstacles to communication

There are many factors that can make it difficult to talk with patients and colleagues. It is important to be aware of these and address the ones you can do something about, while making allowances for those you can't. For example:

- Noisy environment and lack of privacy – try to find a quiet room or cubicle in which to see your patient, if possible

- Pain – does the patient need analgesia now, rather than after the history?
- Other medical factors – breathlessness, hearing impairment and confusion (acute or chronic) can all make communication difficult. Patience and persistence are required in these situations
- Language and cultural barriers – if you encounter problems, try to take the history with a member of the family who can interpret. If this is not possible, it may be possible to obtain the help of an interpreter. In an acute situation, you may have to make do with smiles, drawings and gestures to establish the important points, such as the presence and site of pain
- Hostility – some people may feel (rightly or wrongly) aggrieved by some aspect of the treatment they had already received. It is vital that you do not take this personally or be drawn into a confrontation. Try to remain calm and civil, empathise with the patient and apologise if appropriate. If all else fails, politely explain that you don't feel anything is being achieved and come back later.

Verbal communication skills

It is important to put the patient at ease during a consultation, although this is often easier said than done, as people are often understandably concerned in the clinical situation. The following are important skills:

- ALWAYS begin by checking very carefully the patient's identity, explaining who you are, and gaining their consent to take a history
- Empathise with the patient: this means trying to understand their point of view, and is not the same as sympathy. It is perfectly good practice to use such phrases as 'I understand' or 'That must have been very frightening', etc. when a patient is relating the details of their history
- Use open questions to start, such as: 'What made you come to see a doctor today?' or 'Have you any other problems that have been worrying you?' Always ask the old doctor's question: 'How do you feel generally?'; you will be surprised how many things you will learn. It is a good idea to let the patient talk freely for the first minute or so, before you focus the history with closed questions such as: 'Does the pain catch you when you breathe in?'
- Avoid using 'leading' questions, which direct the patient as to what to say, e.g. compare 'Does the pain go anywhere?' an open-ended question with: 'Does the pain shoot down your left arm?' a leading question
- Use interjectors ('I see') to maintain the flow of conversation
- Check that you have understood what the patient has told you by repeating a summary back to him or her

- Avoid medical jargon
- Reflect the terminology your patient uses for symptoms and diagnoses as appropriate.

Non-verbal communication skills

A large proportion of our communication 'bandwidth' is non-verbal. This includes body posture, facial expression and gestures; we are conscious of some of these things, but most are subconscious. Non-verbal cues are very important in a clinical setting, both in achieving a rapport with patients and in gaining insight into their condition. The following points may be helpful during a consultation:

- Sit with the patient so that your eyes are on roughly the same level, preferably without a desk as a barrier between you. Maintain a comfortable distance, and try to face them while you are talking. It is also useful to make sure you have a comfortable position to write when you are taking a history; kneeling by the bedside is sometimes the best option
- Maintain good eye contact, even if the patient doesn't. However, try not to stare
- Use non-verbal cues to show you are listening, and encourage the patient: nodding, smiling and even appropriate laughter can help to put the patient at ease. Smiling is particularly important
- It is worth having practice sessions with friends before you go into an exam, as they can point out any nervous habits that you might be unaware of.

Objectives in the consultation

Have a mental checklist of objectives when you go into a consultation – especially when this is part of an exam. Once again, the key to this is practice, preferably on the wards, but you can also run through mock scenarios in a study group if you are short of time. You may also need to produce this kind of list in a short-answer exam paper or viva. For example:

- Introduce yourself and establish a rapport with the patient
- Find out why the patient has presented to you and the impact of the condition.

Are there any other concomitant health problems?

- Find out what the patient understands about the problem, and if they have their own theory as to what has caused it; ensure you explore their main concerns
- What are the patient's expectations of this consultation – what do they want from meeting with you today?
- Explore the problem with history and examination, and formulate a plan for further management, i.e. investigations and treatment

- Explain your findings and plan to the patient as clearly as possible
- Give the patient time to react to new information.

CALF (Check-Ask-Literature-Follow-up) is a good way to use the last few minutes of an OSCE station to your advantage to cover the last four points can be remembered with the mnemonic 'CALF'.

Clinical Note

When interviewing the patient, remember to ask about the patient's perspective; this can gain you extra points in exams. Determine, acknowledge and appropriately explore the patient's ICE; Ideas, Concerns and Expectations. Also ask how their problems are affecting their life, and encourage the patient to express their feelings.

PHYSICAL EXAMINATION

This section deals with the main signs on examination that are caused by an underlying metabolic disorder, which may be observed on examination. This is not a comprehensive guide to clinical assessment, so you should refer to a detailed clinical examination textbook for this. Some of the signs mentioned are relatively non-specific and may be related to other diseases, which may indeed be a lot more common than the metabolic cause. Others may be specific to, and in fact be diagnostic of, a metabolic disorder. Just remember, a lot of metabolic disorders are very rare and you may go through all your working life without seeing them.

General inspection

This section considers the main signs that are indicative of an underlying metabolic cause. These signs are often non-specific and, therefore, there may be other possible non-metabolic causes that must be considered and eliminated in the differential diagnosis. In any clinical examination it is important that you are seen to generally inspect the patient. Stand at the foot of the bed and observe the patient taking a breath in and out.

The main signs you need to look out for are: wasting, cachexia and obesity (Fig. 12.5), pallor, jaundice (see Fig. 12.10), respiratory distress (see Fig. 12.12) and tremors (Fig. 12.6).

Checklist of an examination:

1. Introduce yourself, gain informed consent, wash your hands

Fig. 12.5 Assessment of wasting and obesity underlying metabolic causes.

Physical examination	Symptoms and signs	Possible diagnosis
Wasting: mild-moderate generalized loss of muscle and weight	• When severe, patient has a thin emaciated appearance, almost skeletal, and it is referred to as cachexia • Skin is wrinkled and there may be hair loss	• Cachexia implies serious underlying cause, such as cancer or AIDS • In developing countries wasting probably due to malnutrition due to insufficient intake causing by marasmus • In children also consider malabsorption e.g. coeliac disease
Obesity: observe; can also: • Measure weight and height and calculate body mass index (BMI) • Compare with tables of ideal weight for height (mid-arm circumference and skin-fold thickness are rarely useful in practice)	• When severe it is obvious on inspection • BMI $> 30 \, kg/m^2$ is regarded as obese (see Chapter 9)	Usually energy input is greater than energy output Obesity is also seen in: • Cushing's syndrome • Hypothyroidism It may also be: • Drug-induced, e.g. corticosteroids • Consider the possibility of Type 2 diabetes mellitus

Fig. 12.6 Assessment of tremors, and their significance in metabolic disorder. Four common tremors are covered below.

Physical examination	Symptoms and signs	Possible diagnosis
Patient holds arms outstretched in front of them with hands flat Place a piece of paper on them	Look for fluttering of paper → tremor present	**Essential or physiological tremor:** Normal tremor associated with anxiety, ↑ caffeine and ↑ exercise Also seen in: hypoglycaemia, alcoholism, hyperthyroid (thyrotoxic) patients, and Wilson's disease
Ask patient to hold arms outstretched with wrists hyperextended	Observe flapping motion of hands	**Flapping tremor:** CO_2 retention caused by hyperventilation may be seen in people with diabetes or can be seen with hepatic encephalopathy in chronic liver disease
Observe hands at rest and with the patient distracted	Look for a 'pill rolling' 3 Hz/second tremor of the hands worse at rest	**Resting tremor:** Parkinsonism
Finger-nose test	Tremor arises on movement associated with cerebellar lesions	**Intention tremor:** seen in chronic alcoholics with Wernicke-Korsakoff syndrome

2. Position and expose the patient (at 45 degrees for cardiovascular and respiratory examinations with the chest exposed, and at 180 degrees with the abdomen exposed (xiphisternum to pelvis) for abdominal examinations)
3. Ask if they are in any pain and ensure they are comfortable
4. General observations; stand back and observe (appearance, level of consciousness, colour and distress) at rest
5. Examine starting at the hands, assessing the limbs, head and neck in turn
6. Move onto detailed examination (inspection, palpation, percussion, auscultation) of the relevant system; respiratory, cardiovascular, abdominal, neurological
7. Comment on extra parts of the examination that you would ideally also perform
8. Thank the patient and ensure they are comfortable.

Limbs

Examination of the limbs for underlying metabolic disorder can be conveniently divided into assessment of skin and joint problems associated with metabolic disorders (Fig. 12.7) and vascular supply (Fig. 12.8). Remember to check peripheral pulses.

Main metabolic problems to consider in examination of the limbs

Diabetic patients: Look specifically for ischaemic and neuropathic damage leading to ulceration and deformity of limbs (see Chapter 8).

Patients with peripheral vascular disease: Look for arterial ulceration and, in extreme disease, gangrene.

Hands

There are a number of signs on the hands and nails indicative of underlying metabolic disorder. They are often subtle (Fig. 12.9). Clubbing, which is a common exam question, may be indicative of liver cirrhosis due to a number of causes, some of which are listed in Fig. 12.9. However, it is most commonly caused by suppurative lung disease or infective endocarditis and therefore these must always be highest on your list of differential diagnoses. It may also be congenital.

Clinical Note

Examination of the limbs should include:
- Assessment of vascular supply. The quickest way to do this is to feel the pulses (Fig. 12.8). You should also observe colour, assess capillary filling time, feel for temperature and look for ankle oedema
- Skin: look for any obvious lesions (Fig. 12.9)
- Neurological assessment. Both motor and sensory systems are particularly important in patients with diabetes.

Skin manifestations of dyslipidaemias

Tendon xanthomata, which are observed usually on the Achilles tendon or extensor tendons on the back of the hand, are often diagnostic of dyslipidaemias.

Physical examination	Symptoms and signs	Possible diagnosis
Nails:	**Clubbing** 4 stages: **1** Increased fluctuancy of nail bed **2** Loss of angle between nail and nail bed **3** increased curvature in all directions **4** drumsticking **Stages of clubbing** 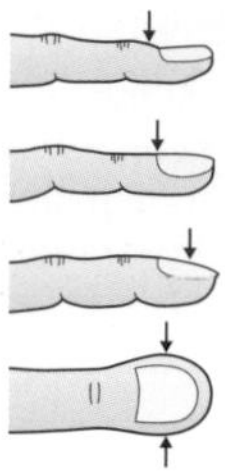 **Stage 1** Normal appearance and angle but increased fluctuancy of nail bed **Stage 2** Loss of angle between nail and nail bed **Stage 3** Increased curvature of nail **Stage 4** Expansion of terminal phalanx Drum stick appearance	**Respiratory causes** Cystic fibrosis and other lung diseases including bronchial carcinoma. Also note there are cardiovascular and other causes including thyroid disease, and even congenital causes. **Gastrointestinal causes (3 C's)** Coeliac disease, Crohn's disease, and Cirrhosis of the liver caused by: • haemochromatosis (↑ iron) • Wilson's disease (↑ copper) • glycogen storage disorders (very rare) • alcohol
	Koilonychia Spoon-shaped brittle nails, may be ridges	Iron-deficiency anaemia
Palms:	**Palmar erythema** Reddening of palms indicative of a hyperdynamic circulation	Liver cirrhosis caused by: • alcoholism or iron or copper deposition • thyrotoxicosis • pregnancy

Fig. 12.7 Main metabolic signs observed on examination of the hands.

Eruptive xanthomata are a consequence of severe hypertriglyceridaemia.

Gout
This can affect any joint in the body. In an acute attack, look for a red, inflamed, painful joint. In chronic gout, look for gouty tophi: deposits of urate crystals around joints, tendons and the cartilage of ear lobes, causing yellow discolouration of the overlying skin.

Head and neck

Face

A number of metabolic and nutritional disorders result in clinical signs evident on the face. For ease, the signs observed are divided into those affecting either the eyes (Fig. 12.10) or the lips and mouth (Fig. 12.11).

Neck

With the exception of iodine deficiency and thyroid disease, there are very few metabolic or nutritional disorders that manifest as signs in the neck.

Thyroid disease

Look at the patient's neck and ask the patient to swallow. You will often observe a prominent goitre (a diffuse enlargement of the thyroid gland). Goitre, can be due to iodine deficiency and can also be seen in thyroid diseases such as Graves' disease and Hashimoto's thyroiditis. All thyroid lumps ascend on swallowing because they are attached to the trachea.

Clinical Note

Structure to examine a lump (to help differentiate nature of the lump; benign or malignant).

Inspection: The 5 S's: **S**ite, **S**ize, **S**hape, **S**urface, **S**urroundings (state of adjacent tissues and overlying skin).

Palpation: The 4 T's: **T**emperature, **T**enderness, **T**ransillumability and **T**exture.

Extras: Colour, edge, composition, reducibility, pulsatility, and any findings on **percussion and auscultation.**

Always mention the need to assess neurovascular status in more detail.

Fig. 12.8 Peripheral pulses provide a quick assessment of vascular supply in the limbs.

Physical examination	Symptoms and signs	Possible diagnosis
Arm pulses: • Radial: assess rate, rhythm and volume • Brachial	↑ rate: tachycardia	• Anaemia, acute blood loss/shock • Thyrotoxicosis • Hypoglycaemia
	↓ rate: bradycardia	• Hypothermia • Hypothyroidism treatment with beta-blockers
	Irregular rhythm	Atrial fibrillation: hyperthyroidism
Leg pulses: • Femoral • Popliteal • Posterior tibial • Dorsalis pedis	↓ or absent peripheral pulses (may also hear bruit over the femoral artery, indicating turbulent blood flow caused by stenosis of arteries)	Peripheral vascular disease seen in diabetes or patients with dyslipidaemias
Blood pressure (BP)	High	May occur secondary to endocrine or renal disease or to obesity in 95% of cases, cause of high BP is unknown; 'essential' hypertension
	Low	• Severe anaemia • Hypovolmia; acute blood loss/shock • Diabetic ketoacidosis • Hypothyroidism

Thorax

The signs associated with thorax can be divided into those related to respiratory and cardiovascular systems.

Respiratory system

Few metabolic disorders result in obvious respiratory signs. Therefore, only a brief discussion is included here on acid base disorders.

Checklist for examination of the respiratory system (Figs 12.12 and 12.13)

Use the generic formula for examinations outlined at the start of this examination section. Specifically for a respiratory examination:

- Observe any respiratory distress, the level of consciousness, chest expansion (is it equal on both sides?), tachypnoea, and so on.

Remember for examination of any system follow the sequence: inspection, palpation, percussion and auscultation.

Cardiovascular system

As with the respiratory system, few metabolic disorders present with cardiovascular signs. However, anaemia of any cause can precipitate angina and eventually cause heart failure and, in extreme cases, shock.

Inspection and palpation

Metabolic signs that can be observed during a cardiovascular examination are listed in Fig. 12.14.

Percussion

Percussion may help to diagnose hepatomegaly in, e.g., cardiac failure.

Auscultation

Anaemia of any cause can lead to an innocent ejection systolic murmur. For heart failure, you may hear a third heart sound. Checklist for auscultation:

- Feel the pulse (carotid on one side) simultaneously to listening to identify systolic and diastolic sounds
- Are there two heart sounds present? The first heart sound is due to the closure of the mitral and tricuspid valves. The second heart sound is due to the closure of the aortic and pulmonary valves. Listen over all four areas (mitral, triscupid, aortic and pulmonary)

Fig. 12.9 Main metabolic signs observed on examination of the limbs: skin and joint problems associated with metabolic disorder.

Physical examination	Symptoms and signs	Possible diagnosis
Skin lesions: comment on: location, size, tenderness and discharge. With ulcers comment on: Base, Edge, Depth, Discharge (BEDD)		
Ischaemic/arterial skin ulcers	• Found at pressure areas: tips of toes/fingers • Painful • Deep and punched out • Discharge usually serum or pus, rarely blood-stained because of impaired blood supply • Surrounding tissues pale and cold	Ischaemic damage seen in: • Diabetes • Atherosclerosis
Venous ulcers	Found superior to the medial malleolus shallow depth painless	Venous damage venous insufficiency (Associated with obesity and varicose veins)
Neuropathic ulcers	• Usually found over pressure areas • Painless (lack of sensation) • Surrounding tissues are healthy because of good blood supply	Peripheral nerve lesions: chronic complication of diabetes
Gangrene (dead tissue)	• Brown/black tissue usually found on extremities and pressure points • Painless and senseless	Ischaemic damage
Tendon xanthomata	• Fatty deposits on the • Achilles tendon and finger extensors on back of hand leading to thickening • Fat deposits in palmar creases of hand called palmar xanthomata	Characteristic of dyslipidaemias (see Chapter 5)
Gouty tophi	• Deposits of urate crystals around joints, tendons and cartilage of ear lobes • Cause yellow discoloration of overlying skin	Gout
Joint problems	Signs of inflammation: Painful, red, hot, inflamed joint Acute onset	Acute gout Pseudogout

- Listen for extra third and fourth heart sounds
- Listen for murmurs. Murmurs are caused by turbulent blood flow. They are classified into systolic, diastolic or continuous, depending on their timing with the cardiac cycle
- Listen over the carotid, renal and femoral arteries for bruits. These indicate turbulent blood flow caused by stenosis of arteries; they are heard in patients with disseminated atherosclerosis.

Clinical Note

Identify murmurs with their timing (systolic or diastolic?), location – area where loudest, radiation, character, pitch, changes with respiration or position/movement or other accentuating manoeuvres.

Abdomen

Most metabolic disorders that produce abdominal signs do so as a result of excessive deposition of a metabolite or nutrient in organs such as the liver, or in arteries or the skin. This interferes with the correct functioning of the organ. For example:

- In glycogen storage diseases, the deposition of glycogen in the liver causes hepatomegaly
- Hepatomegaly may be caused by fat deposition (steatosis) in patient with dyslipidaemia
- In atherosclerotic disease, the deposition of fat in the walls of arteries leads to atherosclerotic plaque formation, resulting in turbulent blood flow which may be heard as bruits over carotid or renal arteries. Aortic aneurysm may cause a palpable pulsation in the abdomen (be very careful when examining

Fig. 12.10 Observation of the eyes for signs associated with metabolic disorder.

Physical examination	Symptoms and signs	Possible diagnosis
Jaundice: Observe colour of sclerae	Yellow discoloration of sclerae is a more sensitive indicator of jaundice than skin colour in mild-moderate disease (sclerae turn yellow first). With severe jaundice, skin is yellow-green	• liver disease • haemolytic anaemia (e.g. due to G6PDH or pyruate kinase deficiency)
Anaemia: observe colour of conjunctiva (pull down the lower eyelid) or buccal mucosa (most sensitive indicator: mucous membranes)	Pale/pink colour N.B. normal skin colour varies according to skin thickness, circulation and pigmentation So paleness may be normal for patient or indicative of anaemia N.B. it is a poor indicator of anaemia	• acute blood loss/infection • iron/B_{12}/folate deficiency • pernicious anaemia • haemolytic anaemia • hypothyroidism
Xanthelasma	Non-tender yellow fatty lumps in the skin particularly around the eyelids	• They may or may not indicate dyslipidaemia (see Chapter 5)
Corneal arcus (arcus senilis)	Observe white rim around outer edge of iris due to cholesterol deposition Sclerosis in cornea	• Common in elderly people • Significant in patients < 35 years old, as it may indicate hyperlipidaemia, such as FH or familial combined hyperlipidaemia (see Chapter 5)
Kayser-Fleischer rings: examine corneal-sclera junction for rings; N.B. they can only been seen with a slit lamp	Green-brown ring due to copper deposition in periphery of cornea	Wilson's disease: copper overload
Observe cornea and conjunctiva for dryness and ulceration	• Dryness and ulceration: xerophthalmia • White plaques on conjunctiva: Bitot's spots • Opaque scar tissue: keratomalacia and cataracts	All due to vitamin A deficiency
Progressive deterioration of vision	Loss of visual acuity	Diabetes mellitus

Fig. 12.11 Observation of the mouth and tongue for signs associated with metabolic disorder.

Physical examination	Symptoms and signs	Possible diagnosis
Colour of lips and tongue	Central cyanosis: purple-blue colour because of excess methaemoglobin in the tissues	• Inadequate perfusion of tissues, methaemoglobinaemia • Since methaemoglobin cannot carry oxygen, this leads to poor perfusion of tissues and cyanosis
Colour of tongue and tongue surface changes	Glossitis (red, smooth, sore tongue), loss of filiform papillae	• Iron/folate/B_{12} deficiency • Other B vitamin deficiencies: niacin, B_6 (pyridoxine)
Angular stomatitis: observe corners of mouth for cuts and infection	Angular stomatitis: inflamed, cracked corners of mouth; cracks may become infected with *Candida albicans*	Common in elderly due to iron deficiency or deficiency of B-group vitamins

Fig. 12.12 Examination of the respiratory system in metabolic disorder.

Physical examination	Symptoms and signs	Possible diagnosis
Signs of respiratory distress (rate, depth and rhythm of breathing are observed)	E.g. tachypnoea, use of accessory muscles of respiration, nasal flare and sternal recession	In starvation, severe muscle wasting can eventually cause wasting of the diaphragm, leading to respiratory distress and death
Shape of chest wall	• Pigeon chest, pectus carinatum: prominent sternum often accompanied by indrawing of softened ribs along attachment of diaphragm, Harrison's sulcus • Rickety rosary: expansion or swelling of ribs at costochondral junctions	Rickets in children
Cyanosis	• Central cyanosis: observe purple-blue colour of lips • Peripheral cyanosis: observe purple-blue colour of extremities (fingers and toes) caused by increased level of deoxygenated blood	Methaemoglobinaemia (see Fig. 12.11) Inadequate perfusion of tissues caused by peripheral vascular disease may be seen in diabetics patients
Respiratory rate: count for a minute; is it fast or laboured? normal is 15–20/min (for an adult)	• Hyperventilation • Deep Kussmaul respiration; deep, sighing breathing with rapid respiratory rate • Breath smells of acetone • Severe dehydration	Metabolic acidosis is a state that arises with a diabetic ketoacidosis or uraemia, and affects the respiratory system by causing a respiratory compensation – to correct the pH and acidosis → this is through increased respiratory rate and Kussmaul breathing

Fig. 12.13 Auscultation of the respiratory system: metabolic signs.

Physical examination	Symptoms and signs	Possible diagnosis
Breath sounds	↓ breath sounds	In obese people these may be difficult to hear
Crepitations/ crackles	Pulmonary oedema, often due to heart failure	Heart failure may be secondary to: • Anaemia from iron/folate/B_{12}/vitamin C deficiency wet beri-beri – B1 deficiency • Kwashiorkor

Fig. 12.14 Clinical signs that may be observed during cardiovascular examination.

Physical examination	Symptoms and signs	Possible diagnosis
Signs of shock and heart failure	Pallor, tachycardia, heart murmur, and cardiac enlargement. Untreated progresses to heart failure	Severe anaemia (haemoglobin < 8 g/dL) causes: • Blood loss • Iron/folate/B_{12} deficiency • Acute haemolytic crisis • Hypothyroidism
Apex beat	Visible on inspection	Thin, wasted individuals
Impalpable apex beat	Normally felt at the left fifth intercostal space, mid-clavicular line	Obesity
Displaced apex beat	Heart failure → cardiomegaly	Anaemia of any cause Kwashiorkor Hypercalcaemia

Fig. 12.15 Clinical signs that can be observed during an abdominal examination, and their underlying metabolic causes.

Physical examination	Symptoms and signs	Possible diagnosis
Abdominal distension: note shape, symmetry, size of any bulge or mass	General/localized swelling Asymmetrical enlargement	Obesity: pregnancy Ascites: kwashiorkor E.g. liver enlargement due to glycogen storage disorders, dyslipidaemias, kwashiorkor
Striae (stretch marks)	Purple abdominal striae	Cushing's syndrome Obesity
Spider naevi	Single, central arteriole feeding a number of small branches in a radial manner, with blanching (turning white) on pressure	Chronic liver failure and cirrhosis in: • Alcoholism • Haemochromatosis • Wilson's disease (copper overload) • Vitamin A toxicity (see Chapter 10)
Pigmentation	Slate-grey colour	Iron overload

this!). Think of an abdominal aortic aneurysm in elderlym male patients presenting with an abdominal or back pain. This is a medical emergency.

Useful points for the examination of the abdomen

When examining the abdomen:

- The patient should be lying as flat as possible, with arms by his or her sides
- The patient should be exposed from the nipples to the knees; however, in the interest of privacy, it is best to expose in stages, beginning with xiphisternum to pubis
- Kneel beside the bed so that you are at the same level as the patient
- As with any system of the body go through the sequence of inspection, palpation, percussion and auscultation.

Inspection

Observe the general symmetry and shape of the abdomen. The clinical signs that can be observed during an abdominal examination, and their underlying metabolic causes, are listed in Fig. 12.15. It is particularly relevant to comment on observing nutritional and hydration status in an abdominal examination.

Palpation

Points to remember when palpating the abdomen:

- Before you start, ask the patient 'Have you any pain anywhere in your abdomen?'. If the answer is 'yes', begin your palpation furthest from the pain
- The abdomen is divided either into nine areas (Fig. 12.16)

- Palpate all regions of the abdomen lightly then with greater pressure (deep palpation), then palpate the liver, spleen, while the patient takes deep breathes to feel the organs move with respiration. Ask the patient to breath normally again as you palpate in the midline for the abdominal aorta (to identify a pathological expansive mass indicating an aneursym; NB: a pulsative aorta can be normal in slim patients). Finally, ballot the kidneys
- The clinical signs with their underlying metabolic causes that can be detected on palpation of the abdomen are listed in Fig. 12.17.

Percussion

Abdominal percussion has two main roles:

- To outline the liver size. The liver is 'dull' to percussion and therefore, it is useful in determining the degree of hepatomegaly
- In the presence of abdominal distension, to determine whether it is due to solid, gas or free fluid (ascites) in the abdomen. The technique 'shifting dullness' can be used to distinguish the presence of ascites from solid or gas. Ascites is seen in congestive heart failure, liver cirrhosis and secondary to wet beriberi and kwashiorkor.

Also use percussion to demarcate the size of the spleen and bladder.

Auscultation

The clinical signs that can be detected on auscultation of the abdomen, with their underlying metabolic causes, are listed in Fig. 12.18.

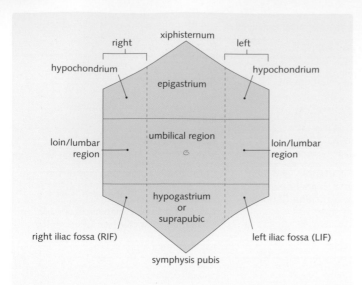

Fig. 12.16 Examination of the abdomen. A schematic representation of the abdomen showing nine areas

Fig. 12.17 Clinical signs that can be detected on palpation of the abdomen, with their underlying metabolic causes.

Physical examination	Symptoms and signs	Possible diagnosis
Abdominal pain: determine site (for clarity ask the patient to point to where the pain is) Onset (sudden/gradual) Character Radiation (to the back, groin) Associated symptoms (nausea) Timing (constant, colicky) Exacerbating or relieving factors Severity	Acute, severe upper abdominal pain ± guarding, rigidity and rebound tenderness (= cardinal signs of peritonism)	• Acute pancreatitis most commonly due to gallstones and alcohol, but also seen in type I familial lipoprotein lipase deficiency or apoC-II hyperlipidaemia (see Chapter 5) • Acute porphyria (see Chapter 7)
Liver enlargement (hepatomegaly)	• Liver edge is not normally palpable below costal margin • Gross hepatomegaly can fill whole abdomen	Causes: • Heart failure • Alcohol-induced liver disease • Haemolytic anaemia, e.g. G6PDH deficiency • Porphyria • Iron overload: haemochromatosis • Glycogen storage disorders (see Fig. 4.17) • Galactosaemia (see Chapter 4)
Spleen enlargement (splenomegaly)	Spleen supposedly has a palpable notch on its medial side but it is very difficult to feel	Causes: • Pernicious anaemia • Galactosaemia • Haemolytic anaemia
Kidneys	They are usually impalpable	• Lower pole of right kidney can be felt in very thin or wasted people • Renal disease and stones are associated with gout

Physical examination	Symptoms and signs	Possible diagnosis
Bowel sounds	Absent if there is mechanical obstruction	• Paralytic ileus • Gallstones
Bruits	Listen for bruits in the aorta (midline, above umbilicus), and for renal and femoral bruits 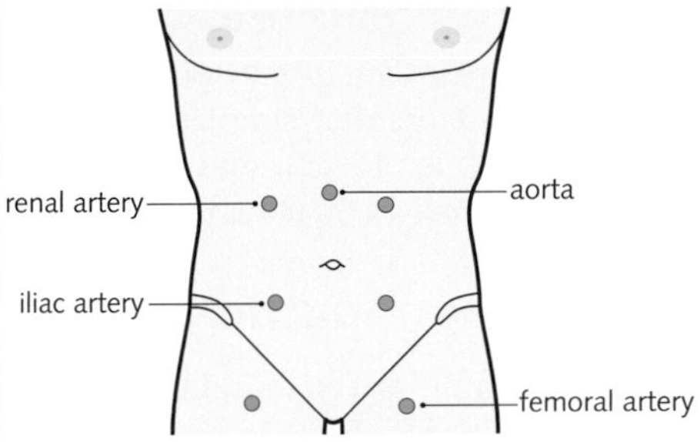 renal artery — aorta iliac artery — femoral artery	• Aortic aneurysm • Renal artery stenosis • Peripheral vascular disease, e.g. patients with diabetes or dyslipidaemias

Fig. 12.18 Clinical signs that can be detected on auscultation of the abdomen, and their underlying metabolic causes. (Figure taken from http://faculty.washington.edu/alexbert/MEDEX/Fall/ABDAscultation.jpg)

Figure 12.19 Physical clinical examination in disorders of nutrition.

Clinical signs can be a combination of any of the following:
- Wasting or cachexia
- Pallor; which indicates anaemia, possibly caused by an iron, vitamin B_{12} or folate deficiency
- Specific effects of vitamin deficiency; for example, deficiency of vitamin A causes Bitot's spots on the eyes, or deficiency of vitamin D and calcium causes rickets in children and osteomalacia in adults
- Oedema
- Bruising; for example, in vitamin K deficiency

Summary

The clinical signs of nutritional disorders are summarized in Fig. 12.19.

FURTHER INVESTIGATIONS

ROUTINE INVESTIGATIONS

This section describes selected aspects of clinical investigation relevant to metabolic disorder. It is not a comprehensive description of laboratory tests used in clinical practice. The main tests used every day to assess metabolic function can be divided into:

- 'First-line' tests, that is, the tests most frequently requested and often important for planning initial management
- 'Second-line' tests and specialist tests.

With all routine investigations, the results should not be interpreted separately; for example, in the diagnosis of anaemia, the haematology and clinical biochemistry tests are all part of the comprehensive patient assessment.

Haematology

The simplest, first-line haematology test is the full blood count (FBC). This measures red cell count and indices, total and differential white cell count and platelets. The 'second-line' tests include clotting studies and assessment of serum iron status and bone marrow iron stores (Fig. 12.20).

Clinical chemistry

First-line tests include urea and electrolytes (U&E), blood glucose, liver function tests (LFTs) and troponin (used in the diagnosis of myocardial infarction) (Fig. 12.21). Second-line tests include thyroid function tests, glycated haemoglobin, serum magnesium, ferritin, folate, lipid profile and C-reactive protein (important in the diagnosis and monitoring of infection). Other specialized tests include the measurements of vitamin and trace element concentrations performed in patients who receive total parenteral nutrition, and the specific diagnosis of genetic metabolic defects in paediatrics. The measurement of hormone levels in blood and tumour markers is a substantial part of specialized biochemistry testing.

HINTS AND TIPS

You do not need to learn normal range values for routine investigations as they will be given in exams. However, a familiarity with the common tests is helpful in appreciating the degree of abnormality when a result is abnormally high or low.

Urine

Urine is commonly tested for glucose, protein and ketones (dipstick tests). Although not as sensitive as blood tests, urinalysis provides a quick and easy method of investigation (Fig. 12.22). Note that urinary ketones are important in the diagnosis of diabetic ketoacidosis.

Histopathology

These tests are usually performed to confirm a diagnosis, usually after simpler biochemical tests have been done (Fig. 12.23), and are often performed together with medical imaging tests.

Immunopathology

An example of an immunopathological investigations is listed in Fig. 12.24.

Medical imaging

Medical imaging has an increasingly important role in medical investigations and diagnosis, with increased use of MRI, due to the advantageous safety profile.

Fig. 12.20 Haematological investigations.

Test	Normal range	Low/high
Full blood count (FBC)		
Haemoglobin g/dL	Men 13–18 Women 11.5–16	Low: anaemia High: polycythaemia
Red cell count ($\times 10^{12}$ /L)	Men 4.5–6.5 Women 3.9–5.6	Low: anaemia High: polycythaemia
Mean cell volume (MCV)	76–96 fL	Low: microcytic anaemia- iron deficiency Normal: normocytic anaemia- causes: chronic disease, mixed iron and B_{12}/folate deficiency High: macrocytic anaemia-B_{12}/folate deficiency
Mean cell haemoglobin (MCH)	27–32 pg	Low: iron deficiency High: B_{12}/folate deficiency
Reticulocyte count	0.8–2%	Low: iron/B_{12}/folate deficiency anaemia thalassaemia High: haemolytic anaemia
C-reactive protein		Increases with inflammation and infection
Bone marrow iron stores		Low: iron deficiency High: thalassaemia sideroblastic anaemia
Clotting studies: • prothrombin time • activated partial thrombo-plastin time (APTT)	10–14 s 35–45 s	Both high – vitamin K deficiency Prothrombin time is a good indicator of liver function (protein synthetic capacity)
Blood film	Normocytic, normochromic erythrocytes	Microcytic, hypochromic: iron deficiency, lead poisoning, thalassaemia
		Macrocytic, hypochromic: B_{12}/folate deficiency, alcohol abuse, liver disease Sickle cells: sickle cell anaemia Irregular 'blister' cells: G6PDH deficiency (very rare)

Fig. 12.21 First- and second-line biochemical investigations on blood or serum.

First-line biochemical investigations

Test	Normal range	Low/high
Liver function tests		
AST aspartate aminotransferase	< 35 U/L	High: hepatocellular damage, e.g. hepatitis cirrhosis fatty liver
ALT alanine aminotransferase	< 35 U/L	
Alkaline phosphatase (ALP)	<120 U/L (different isoenzymes present in liver, bone, placenta and intestine)	High: obstruction of biliary tract or intrahepatic cholestasis: cirrhosis
γ-glutamyl transferase (GGT)	<80 U/L	High: alcohol abuse obstructive liver disease carcinoma of head of the pancreas (fairly non-specific test of liver function)
Serum total bilirubin	<22 μmol/L	High: liver disease haemolytic anaemia anaemia
Urea and electrolytes (U&E)		
Sodium	135–145 mmol/L	High: dehydration Low: extracellular water excess
Potassium	3.5–5.0 mmol/L	High: diabetic ketoacidosis renal failure potassium-sparing diuretics Low: renal or intestinal loss surgical drainage of the bowel, vomiting insulin treatment of diabetic ketoacidosis hyperaldosteronism, diuretics
Bicarbonate	22–32 mmol/L	High: metabolic alkalosis Low: metabolic acidosis
Urea	2.5–6.7 mmol/L	High: renal disease catabolic state
Creatinine (U&E profile also includes chloride)	70–150 μmol/L	High: renal damage and failure Increased muscle bulk, e.g. athletes
Total protein	60–80 g/L	High: myeloma
Albumin	35–50 g/L	Low: chronic liver disease
Calcium	2.12–2.65 mmol/L	Low: vitamin D deficiency High: hyperparathyroidism, malignancy
Free T_4 (thyroxine)	9–22 pmol/L	High: hyperthyroidism
Free T_3 (triiodothyronine)	5–10.2 pmol/L	Low: hypothyroidism
Troponin	< 0.5 ng/mL	High: ↑ suspicion of myocardial infarction
Thyroid-stimulating hormone (TSH)	0.5–5.7 mU/L	Low: hyperthyroidism High: hypothyroidism

Second-line biochemical investigations

Test	Normal range	Low/high
Serum iron	13–32 μmol/L	Low: iron deficiency High: haemochromatosis thalassaemia
Total iron binding capacity (TIBC)	42–80 μmol/L	High: iron deficiency
Serum B_{12}	160–925 ng/L	Low: pernicious anaemia
Folate	4–18 μg/L	Low: pregnancy, cancer, drugs, e.g. methotrexate
Serum urate	< 0.48 mmol/L	High: hyperuricaemia and gout

Continued

Fig. 12.21 —cont'd

Test	Normal range	Low/high
Lipid profile: Total cholesterol Triacylglycerol (triglycerides) HDL-cholesterol	< 4.0 mmol/L < 1.7 mmol/L M: $\geq$ 1.0 mmol/L F: $\geq$ 1.2 mmol/L	High: dyslipidaemias chronic liver disease
Vitamin D: 25-hydroxyCC 1, 25-dihydroxyCC	37–200 nmol/L 60–108 pmol/L	Low: rickets or osteomalacia
Copper caeruloplasmin	12–25 µmol/L 0.20–0.45 g/L	High: Wilson's disease

Fig. 12.22 Examples of urine tests.

Test	Results
Glucose	High: diabetes, pregnancy, renal tubular damage, lowered renal treshold for glucose
Ketones	High: diabetic ketoacidosis and starvation
Protein	High: renal damage Urinary tract infections (leucocytes and nitrites may also be present)
Porphobilinogen (PBG) and δ-aminolevulinic acid (ALA)	High: acute porphyrias (see Chapter 7)
Bilirubin	High: hepatocellular or obstructive jaundice, haemolytic anaemia
Urobilinogen	High: haemolytic or hepatocellular jaundice Low: obstructive jaundice

There are many medical imaging tests used, from simple radiographs and ultrasound to magnetic resonance imaging and positron emission tomography scanning. Figure 12.25 illustrates some examples.

Clinical Note

Any patient presenting to casualty will require a combination of first-line tests. Including:
- Full blood count
- Urea and electrolytes
- Blood glucose. Bedside blood glucose can be life saving if a patient comes in unconscious or confused: he or she may be drunk or severely hypoglycaemic
- Liver function tests
- If there are signs of infection, blood, urine, sputum, wound swabs and CSF (if appropriate) samples must be taken for culture, and the measurement of C-reactive protein is useful
- Electrocardiogram and chest radiograph if necessary
- Troponin measurement if myocardial infarction is suspected.

Fig. 12.23 Examples of histopathology investigations.

Test	Results in metabolic disorder
Liver biopsy	Wilson's disease: increased copper deposition leading to liver cirrhosis Haemochromatosis: iron deposition may cause cirrhosis which may progress to hepatocellular carcinoma
Synovial joint fluid analysis	Gout: the presence of yellow, needle-shaped negatively birefringent monosodium urate crystals Pseudogout: blue positively birefringent calcium pyrophosphate crystals

Fig. 12.24 Example of immunopathology investigations.

Test	Normal result	Result
Direct Coombs' test (detection of antibodies to red blood cells)	Usually no antibodies are present and therefore there is no agglutination of erythrocytes	Positive test = agglutination of erythrocytes, e.g. in haemolytic disease of the newborn or in auto-immune haemolytic anaemia

Test	Examples of diagnostic utility
Chest X-ray (CXR)	Diagnosis of heart failure: anaemia of any cause, ischaemic heart disease, hypercalcaemia, or iron overload, can all result in heart failure; on a Chest X-ray this can show up as: (reference: oxford handbook of clinical medicine; 7th edition. permissions granted) A: **A**lveolar oedema/ perihilar shadowing ('bats wings') B: Kerley **B** lines (interstitial oedema) C: **C**ardiomegaly D: **D**ilated prominent upper lobe vessels E: pleural **E**ffusions
Bone X-ray, MRI	Defective bone mineralization: in rickets and osteomalacia: defective mineralization seen in pelvis, long bones and ribs in the early stages
Electrocardiogram (ECG)	Abnormalities of ECG pattern can be related to: • Ischaemic damage and myocardial infarction • Conduction defects (heart blocks) • Arrhythmias • Some electrolyte disturbances • Congenital heart defects
CT scan	Used to identify abnormalities and to exclude focal lesions due to tumours or infection; essential tool in the diagnosis of space-occupying lesions

Fig. 12.25 Examples of imaging investigations.

Investigation of glucose homeostasis

Measurement of blood glucose

Use
The measurement of blood glucose is used to confirm or reject a diagnosis of diabetes mellitus or impaired glucose tolerance and to monitor the control of blood glucose in diabetic patients.

Reference ranges for blood glucose levels are shown in Fig. 12.26.

Test
The estimation of blood glucose uses the glucose oxidase and peroxidase reaction.

Method
The test is based on the reaction catalysed by the enzymes glucose oxidase and peroxidase, and a peroxidase substrate (a dye). Glucose oxidase oxidizes glucose present in a deproteinized blood sample to gluconolactone and hydrogen peroxide. The hydrogen peroxide reacts with a dye to form a coloured complex, absorbance of which is read in a spectrophotometer. Under standard conditions, the amount of glucose in the unknown blood sample is equal to the amount of coloured product formed. Standardized solutions of glucose are processed at the same time in order to construct a calibration curve. Therefore, the amount of glucose in the unknown blood sample can be read off from the curve.

Advantages
The test is specific for glucose. A similar enzyme reaction is found in commercially available self-monitoring reagent strips: these are commonly used at home by patients with type 1 diabetes.

Fasting blood glucose

Use
The fasting blood glucose sample is usually used to diagnose diabetes mellitus in an asymptomatic patient or if the random blood glucose results are borderline.

Method
The patient should be fasted overnight (at least 10 hours) and have their blood glucose tested the following morning. Interpretation of fasting glucose results is shown in Fig 12.26.

Oral glucose tolerance test

Use
The oral glucose tolerance test (OGTT) is a reference method to diagnose disturbances in glucose homeostasis. However, fasting blood glucose provides very similar information and should be used first. The use of OGTT is restricted to the detection of borderline cases.

Fig. 12.26 Diagnostic intervals of fasting glucose for diabetes and impaired fasting glucose (IFG) and following this, diagnostic intervals for impaired glucose tolerance (IGT) from an oral glucose tolerance test (OGTT).

	Normal (mmol/L)	IFG (mmol/L)	Diabetes (mmol/L)
Fasting plasma glucose	< 6.0	6.0–6.9	≥7.0
Result	**Reference range**		
Impaired fasting glucose	Fasting plasma glucose 6–6.9 mmol/L		
Diabetic	Fasting blood glucose ≥ 7.0 mmol/L and/or 2 h value > 11.1 mmol/L in an OGTT		
	Normal (mmol/L)	**IGT (mmol/L)**	**Diabetes (mmol/L)**
2 h post-load blood glucose	< 7.8	7.8–11.1	≥11.1
Result	**Reference range**		
Normal	Returns to < 7.8 mmol/L		
Impaired glucose tolerance (IGT)	Fasting plasma glucose < 7.0 mmol/L and 2 h value between 7.8 and 11.1 mmol/L in an OGTT		

Method

Patients should make sure that they eat a normal diet, containing adequate carbohydrate, for the preceding 3 days. This ensures that the enzymes involved in glucose metabolism are present at normal levels. After an overnight fast, an initial basal blood sample is taken and the blood glucose concentration is determined; 75 g of glucose in 250–300 mL of water is drunk and the blood glucose is measured every 30 min for the next 2 h. The blood glucose concentration is determined by the glucose oxidase method. Patients must sit comfortably during the test because stress can lead to cortisol release, which antagonizes the action of insulin, therefore, increasing blood glucose concentration. Figs 12.26 and 12.27 illustrate the results of an OGTT.

Assessment of glycaemic control: glycated haemoglobin

Use

The concentration of glycated haemoglobin (HbA_{1c}) provides a measure of the average blood glucose concentration over the preceding 4–6 weeks, that is, the half-life of erythrocytes. This is useful for diabetic patients to show how well their blood glucose concentration has been controlled over a period of time and for the doctor to determine the true level of control – it is a good check on the validity of glucose values entered by patients in their glucose result log book. The higher the value of HbA_{1c} the less well-controlled the diabetes.

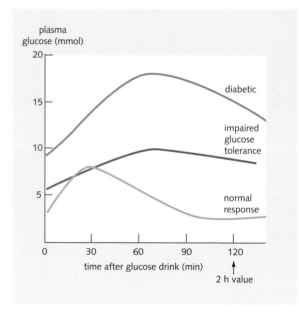

Fig. 12.27 Oral glucose tolerance test. Please note that persons with impaired glucose tolerance can have a normal fasting glucose concentration

Method

Glucose irreversibly attaches non-enzymatically to adult haemoglobin (HbA) over the lifetime of erythrocytes. The extent to which this occurs is proportional to the blood glucose concentration. The amount of glycated haemoglobin in the blood can be measured by a number of methods including high-pressure chromatography,

Fig. 12.28 Reference values for HbA$_{1c}$ expressed as a percentage of total haemoglobin.

Result	Reference values for HbA$_{1c}$
Desirable	< 6.5% (< 7.5% in patients at risk of severe hypoglycaemia)
Poorly controlled	> 10%

electrophoresis and immunoassay. It is usually expressed as a percentage of total haemoglobin (Fig. 12.28); reporting in mmol/mol units is now being introduced.

Investigation of lipid metabolism

Cholesterol and triacylglycerol (triglyceride) concentration

Uses

Coronary heart disease is a major cause of death in the UK. Plasma cholesterol levels are monitored routinely in 'at-risk' groups and when necessary in the rest of the population. 'At-risk' groups include:

- Patients with coronary heart disease (angina, post-myocardial infarction, post-angioplasty or coronary artery bypass graft), those with peripheral or cerebro-vascular disease, and patients with diabetes mellitus
- Patients with dyslipidaemias and their families, and patients with a family history of premature cardio-vascular disease
- Patients with multiple cardiovascular risk factors; for example, patients with high blood pressure, or high cholesterol (cardiovascular risk assessment charts can be found in the British National Formulary (BNF).

Investigations

Screening for cholesterol levels can be done on a non-fasting sample. If a raised cholesterol is found, a full lipid profile is performed, which measures the total cholesterol, high-density lipoprotein (HDL) cholesterol, and triacylglycerols (triglycerides). Blood taken for lipid studies is obtained after an overnight fast. Reference values for fasting plasma lipid concentrations are shown in Fig. 12.29.

Fig. 12.29 Desirable values for fasting plasma lipid concentrations in males ♂ and females♀.

Lipid	Plasma concentration (mmol/L)
Total cholesterol	< 4
LDL-cholesterol	< 2.0
HDL-cholesterol	Men: ≥ 1.0
Triacylglycerol (triglyceride)	Women: ≥ 1.2
	< 1.7

Low-density lipoprotein (LDL) cholesterol levels can also be obtained by calculation using the Friedewald equation. This is only valid if triacylglycerol levels are less than 4.5 mmol/L.

$$\text{LDL mmol/L} = \text{total cholesterol} - \text{HDL} - (\text{triacylglycerol}/2.2)$$

$$\text{LDL(mg/dL)} = \text{total cholesterol} - \text{HDL} - (\text{triacylglycerol}/5)$$

Triacylglycerol levels of greater than 10 mmol/L are associated with an increased risk of pancreatitis.

Enzymes as tissue markers

Glucose-6-phosphate dehydrogenase

Use

An enzyme assay is used for the diagnosis of glucose-6-phosphate dehydrogenase deficiency, the most common erythrocyte enzyme defect (see Chapter 4). It allows patients with glucose-6-phosphate dehydrogenase deficiency to be detected in between haemolytic attacks, such that diagnosis is not just dependent on the blood picture during an attack. An enzyme activity of < 2% of the normal level may be seen in very severe cases.

Pyruvate kinase assay

Use

Pyruvate kinase assay is used for the diagnosis of erythrocyte pyruvate kinase deficiency (see Chapter 4).

Test

The production of pyruvate is coupled to the reduction of a dye, with the colour change monitored spectrophotometrically. A decreased production of ATP can also be measured when radioactively labelled ^{32}P is added to erythrocytes and its incorporation into ATP is monitored.

Reference values

Patients typically need to have an enzyme level of 5–25% of the normal level to show clinical features.

Galactose and fructose

Both galactose and fructose are reducing sugars and are detected in the urine using alkaline copper (Cu^{2+}) reagents, such as Benedict's reagent.

Galactosaemia

Galactosaemia is caused by a deficiency of the enzyme galactose-1-phosphate uridyl transferase.

Tests

Screening tests are performed in infants with suspicious symptoms:

- Test for galactosuria: Clinitest tablets or reagent strips contain copper citrate, which is reduced by galactose. The colour change observed is clear blue to green to brown to a brick red precipitate if the reduction is complete. The presence of galactose in the urine along with positive symptoms should lead to the withdrawal of galactose and lactose from the diet until a diagnostic test can be performed
- Diagnostic test: assay erythrocytes for decreased galactose-1-phosphate uridyl transferase activity.

Fructokinase deficiency: essential fructosuria

The absence of fructokinase leads to a combination of a high fructose concentration in the blood and fructose accumulation in the urine. Both must be present to form a diagnosis. Fructose, like galactose, is a reducing sugar and its presence in urine can be detected with certain tablets. Bear in mind that this is a rare diagnosis, virtually always seen in paediatric practice.

Hormone assays

Thyroid-stimulating hormone

The measurement of thyroid-stimulating hormone (TSH) levels is used as a screening test for suspected hyperthyroidism and hypothyroidism. Both hyperthyroidism and hypothyroidism influence the basal metabolic rate by over-stimulating or under-stimulating lipid and carbohydrate metabolism respectively. Elevated TSH levels signify an inadequate thyroid hormone production, while suppressed levels signify excessive unregulated production of thyroid hormone. If TSH is abnormal, decreased levels of thyroid hormones, T3 and T4, may be present; these may be measured to confirm the diagnosis.

Other diagnostic endocrine tests you should be aware of include the dexamethasone suppression test, measuring ACTH in Cushing's syndrome (excess cortisol), and the Synacthen test in suspected Addison's disease (primary adrenal insufficiency), tests of levels of TSH, LH, FSH, cortisol, and use of the insulin tolerance test in the investigation of hypopituitarism.

Other investigations

Diagnosis of phenylketonuria

Every neonate is now screened for phenylketonuria as part of the neonatal screening (Guthrie test). Diagnosis is based on a high concentration of phenylalanine in the blood (see Chapter 6 for a full discussion).

Clinical Note

The most severe and devastating form of hypothyroidism is seen in young children with congenital thyroid hormone deficiency. If the condition is not corrected by supplemental therapy through oral administration of synthetic thyroid hormone soon after birth, the child will suffer from cretinism, a form of irreversible growth and mental retardation.

HINTS AND TIPS

It is worth knowing the different criteria for the diagnosis of diabetes and glucose intolerance as they are frequently asked in exams.

Screening test

A sample of capillary blood is taken from a heel-prick at 5–10 days after birth. The delay allows sufficient time for feeding, and therefore, for protein intake to be established and for the effect of the mother's metabolism to subside. This test used to be based on a microbiological technique, using a strain of *Bacillus subtilis* which only grows if excess phenylalanine is present. However, it is now based on chromatography. Increased plasma phenylalanine levels are indicative of phenylketonuria. The neonatal screening also includes the measurement of thyroid stimulating hormone (TSH), to screen babies for hypothyroidism.

ASSESSMENT OF NUTRITIONAL STATUS

For any individual, adequate nutrition is essential to maintain growth and development and recovery from illness. It is especially important in newborn babies, infants and during pregnancy, when nutritional deficiency can lead to wasting, severe mental retardation and even death. Malnutrition must be recognized and accurately assessed to enable decisions to be made about treatment and re-feeding methods. Assessment is divided into:

- Dietary history
- Anthropometry
- Physical examination
- Laboratory tests.

Medical, social and dietary history

The main aspect of this is the dietary history, but often weight loss and poor nutrition are related to medical, psychological or financial factors (see Fig. 12.2).

Medical history

Ask specifically about:

- Loss of appetite
- Weight loss or gain (quantified) and the time period
- Dysphagia, nausea, vomiting
- Symptoms of hyperthyroidism: weight loss, increased appetite, irritability, heat intolerance
- Relevant past medical history, periods of weight loss and gain in the past; use of laxatives
- Psychiatric history, especially if there is the possibility of depression or an eating disorder (e.g. anorexia nervosa).

Social history

In developed countries:

- Malnutrition may be related to the poor socio-economic status of a family
- Enquire about housing, social support and income support.

In the UK, nutritional deficiency is particularly seen in:

- Elderly people ('tea and biscuit brigade') living alone who are unable to cook or shop
- Young pregnant mothers who live off a staple diet of chips, pizzas and so on
- Chronic alcoholics.

In developing countries, nutritional deficiency may be related to war, poor crops and the poor socio-economic status of the entire country.

Dietary history

Dietary recall
Ask specifically:

- What do you eat in a typical day?
- What do you like and dislike eating ?
- Access to food or presence of financial problems?
- Do you watch what you eat; are you on any particular diet?
- Ask specifically about alcohol intake.

Patients are often asked to keep a food diary. This is usually more accurate than simply questioning the patient, although it relies on the patient's compliance to fill the diary in, and also their willingness to provide accurate information (patients with eating disorders are not usually willing to do so).

HINTS AND TIPS

The cause of weight loss or malnutrition is often not as simple as 'not eating enough'. You must eliminate serious underlying illnesses (such as cancer) before you consider psychiatric illnesses (depression or anorexia nervosa) or social/economic causes.

Anthropometric measurements

The basic anthropometric measurements are:

- Height
- Weight
- Calculation of the body mass index (BMI): weight $(kg)/height (m)^2$
- Mid-arm circumference: a measure of skeletal muscle mass (less frequently used)
- Skin-fold thickness. This helps to assess the amount of subcutaneous fat stores (needs to be done in a standardized way and is rarely used in routine practice).

For infants, it is difficult to measure skin-fold thickness accurately and it is therefore, of little value. The World Health Organization recommends that nutritional status is expressed as:

- % Weight/height: Measures wasting as an index of acute malnutrition
- % Height/age: Measures growth retardation/stunting as an index of chronic malnutrition.

In infants, regular growth measurements are very valuable in assessing their nutritional status. Therefore, all infants have their height and weight plotted on a growth chart (Fig. 12.30), which allows a decrease in the rate of growth to be easily recognized and monitored as an early sign of malnutrition.

Physical clinical examination in disorders of nutrition

Clinical signs

These can be a combination of any of the following:

- Wasting or cachexia
- Pallor, which indicates anaemia, possibly caused by an iron, vitamin B_{12} or folate deficiency
- Specific effects of vitamin deficiency; for example, deficiency of vitamin A causes Bitot's spots on the eyes, or deficiency of vitamin D and calcium causes rickets in children and osteomalacia in adults
- Oedema
- Bruising, for example in vitamin K deficiency.

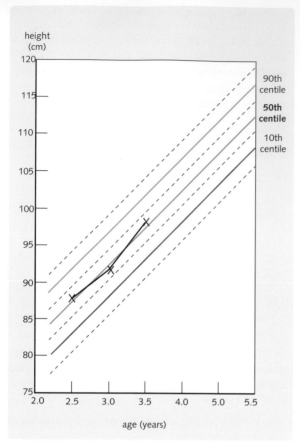

Fig. 12.30 Example of a growth chart often used to help in assessment of nutritional status in children. The line plotted here shows that the patient's height lies along the 50th centile, i.e. average height.

Biochemical tests

The tests for individual nutrients, vitamins and minerals are dealt with in Chapter 8. Here, the types of tests which can be employed are considered.

Types of biochemical tests

Direct measurement

These are the measurements of the concentration of a nutrient or a metabolite in body fluid, usually in the serum or urine.

Such measurements may exploit the activation of an enzyme by a vitamin. For example, thiamine is a cofactor for erythrocyte transketolase. In thiamine deficiency, the erythrocyte enzyme activity can be measured before and after the addition of thiamine pyrophosphate (the active form of thiamine). Addition of thiamine pyrophosphate to erythrocytes should lead to an increase in enzyme activity, proving thiamine deficiency.

Thiamine can also be measured directly using high-pressure liquid chromatography (HPLC).

Measurement of stores

We measure storage forms of nutrients because:

- A decrease in the dietary intake of a nutrient leads to the mobilization of that nutrient from its stores to maintain a normal plasma concentration
- Usually, only in severe deficiency does the plasma concentration drop significantly
- In some cases, by measuring a decrease in the body stores we can detect a deficiency earlier.

For example, the best way to assess iron deficiency is to measure a decrease in bone marrow iron stores (serum ferritin reflects iron stores and is low in iron deficiency), and the best way to assess vitamin C deficiency is to measure a decrease in white cell vitamin C content (Fig. 12.31).

A plasma albumin of less than 30 g/L is often used as an index of malnutrition. However, albumin level is very much affected by fluid and electrolyte disorders, and in these patients, albumin is not an accurate index of nutritional status. The diagnosis of severe malnutrition is usually made on the basis of clinical assessment.

Fig. 12.31 Some biochemical tests for nutrients (FBC, full blood count; MCV, mean cell volume).

Nutrient	Tests
Protein	Serum protein, albumin, prealbumin
Fat	Total cholesterol and triglycerides
Carbohydrate	Blood glucose
Vitamin A	Plasma vitamin A, retinol binding protein
Vitamin D	↓ calcium, ↓ phosphate, ↑ alkaline phosphatase. Measure vitamin D levels and parathyroid hormone
Vitamin K	↑ prothrombin time
Vitamin C	White cell vitamin C content (storage site)
B_1 (thiamine)	Erythrocyte thiamine
B_{12}	FBC, serum B_{12}, MCV
Folate	Serum and erythrocyte folate
Iron	FBC, ferritin, MCV etc., serum transferrin Best estimate is a fall in bone marrow iron stores

FBC, full blood count; MCV, mean cell volume.

Genetic testing

This is used in patients with high LDL cholesterol thought to be at risk of familial hypercholesterolaemia, in which many patients have mutations in the LDLR gene that encodes the LDL receptor protein. Genetic testing is relevant for risk estimation and management as patients who have one abnormal copy (heterozygotes) of the LDLR gene carry a risk of developing premature cardiovascular disease at the age of 30 to 40, and having two abnormal copies (homozygotes) may cause severe cardiovascular disease in childhood.

Best-of-five questions (BOFs)

Chapter 1

1. Which of the following statements is correct?
   a. Anabolic pathways degrade complex molecules into less complex components.
   b. Anabolic pathways release intrinsic chemical energy from biological molecules.
   c. Modulation of enzyme function is a major cellular regulation strategy.
   d. Cell membranes are freely permeable to most substrate molecules.
   e. Rate-limiting enzymes have the least influence on pathway activity.

2. Phosphorylation:
   a. Has little effect on an enzyme's activity.
   b. Typically occurs at phenylalanine residues within a protein.
   c. Always functions as a positive allosteric modulator.
   d. Is a covalent enzyme modification which alters enzyme activity.
   e. Is likely to have arisen via intelligent design.

3. Hormonal control of enzyme activity:
   a. Does not require a receptor to influence enzyme activity.
   b. Is of little importance in humans.
   c. Is exemplified by glucagon release following elevation of blood glucose.
   d. Affects only extracellular enzymes.
   e. Permits intracellular events to respond appropriately to organism energy status.

4. Regarding membrane transport:
   a. The Na^+/K^+ ATPase imports 2 K^+ ions for every 3 Na^+ ions exported.
   b. The Na^+/K^+ ATPase exemplifies secondary active transport.
   c. Sodium-glucose symports export glucose and sodium from cells.
   d. Secondary active transport is coupled directly to ATP hydrolysis.
   e. Steroid hormones require specialised transport mechanisms to cross cell membranes.

5. Concerning redox chemistry:
   a. Reduction is associated with a molecule losing a hydrogen atom.
   b. A molecule undergoing oxidation is termed the reaction "oxidant."
   c. Oxidation reactions do not necessarily require a simultaneous reduction.
   d. Oxidation is associated with a molecule losing electrons.
   e. NAD^+ and FAD are redox partners.

6. ATP:
   a. Is an important molecule cells use for storing energy.
   b. Has a long intracellular half-life.
   c. Plays no biological role in amphibians or marsupials.
   d. Is synthesised by substrate-level or oxidative phosphorylation.
   e. Contains six phospho anhydride bonds.

7. Acetyl CoA:
   a. Contains two acetyl groups.
   b. Is a product of lipogenesis.
   c. Can only generate ATP by substrate-level phosphorylation.
   d. Possesses a thiol group within the CoA component of the molecule.
   e. Is an important substrate in protein synthesis.

8. NAD^+ and FAD:
   a. Participate only occasionally in redox reactions.
   b. Act as cofactors for enzymes mediating redox reactions.
   c. Receive electron pairs from complexes in the electron transport chain.
   d. Are both derived from riboflavin.
   e. As long as one is present in sufficient quantity, the other is not necessary.

9. Exergonic reactions:
   a. Have positive δG values.
   b. Cannot occur spontaneously.
   c. Are energetically "favourable."
   d. Can also be called "exothermic."
   e. Can only occur if coupled to an endergonic reaction.

Chapter 2

10. The TCA cycle (I):
    a. Occurs in the mitochondrial matrix.
    b. Is solely a catabolic pathway.
    c. Contains 9 separate reactions.
    d. Generates ATP only by substrate-level phosphorylation.
    e. Contains four rate-limiting reactions.

11. TCA cycle (II):
  a. 12 ATP are generated (indirectly and directly) per 'turn' of the cycle.
  b. 1 $FADH_2$ and 3 $NADH + H^+$ are generated per 'turn'.
  c. Four highly endergonic reactions are present in the cycle.
  d. The TCA cycle's role is almost entirely anabolic.
  e. Occurs in mitochondrial intermembrane space.

12. Regulation of the TCA cycle:
  a. Rate-limiting enzymes of the TCA cycle exhibit reduced activity in the presence of Ca^{++} ions.
  b. Rate-limiting enzymes of the TCA cycle are allosterically inhibited by ATP.
  c. Low substrate availability does not influence TCA cycle activity.
  d. An increased rate of respiration imposes a reduced rate of TCA cycle activity.
  e. Malate dehydrogenase is a TCA cycle rate-limiting enzyme.

13. Which of the following does not require a TCA cycle intermediates for synthesis:

  a. Glucose.
  b. Porphyrins.
  c. Fatty acids.
  d. Cholesterol.
  e. Tryptophan

Chapter 3

14. ATP generation by substrate-level phosphorylation:
  a. Requires oxygen.
  b. Requires ADP as a substrate.
  c. Is less important than oxidative phosphorylation in anerobic scenarios.
  d. Occurs in the TCA cycle but not glycolysis.
  e. Is exergonic.

15. Oxidative phosphorylation:
  a. Requires oxygen and occurs at the OMM.
  b. Requires oxygen and occurs exclusively in the mitochondrial matrix.
  c. Electrons enter the electron transport chain within $NADH + H^+$ or $FADH_2$.
  d. The term is a misnomer as it does not require oxygen.
  e. Is less productive in terms of ATP generation than substrate-level phosphorylation.

16. Electron transfer during oxidative phosphorylation:
  a. Is in the direction oxygen $\rightarrow$ ETC complexes $\rightarrow$ NAD^+.
  b. Results in sequential reduction, then oxidation of each complex of the ETC.
  c. Terminates with transfer of electrons from oxygen to complex IV.

  d. Commences with arrival of $NADH + H^+$ at complex II.
  e. Is relevant only in prokaryotes.

17. Complexes I to V of the ETC:
  a. Contain no special structural features.
  b. Only complex I and II 'accept' electron pairs from $NADH + H^+$ and $FADH_2$.
  c. Are embedded in the OMM.
  d. Are all electron transfer/donor proteins.
  e. Are all sensitive to rotenone and cyanide.

18. The proton gradient:
  a. Is in the direction high$\rightarrow$low from the cytoplasm to the mitochondrial intermembrane space.
  b. "Discharges" via complex IV of the ETC.
  c. Is accumulated by complexes I, III and IV.
  d. Is not relevant to oxidative phosphorylation.
  e. Is only electrical in nature, not chemical.

19. ATP synthase:
  a. Consists of a single subunit.
  b. Is located at the OMM.
  c. Contains numerous pores through which protons may pass.
  d. Couples proton passage with electron transfer.
  e. Couples proton passage with ATP synthesis.

20. Transfer of $NADH + H^+$ from cytoplasm to mitochondria

  a. Is via direct transfer.
  b. Is only possible via the malate-aspartate shuttle.
  c. Is of no functional importance in terms of cell metabolism.
  d. Is necessary since $NADH + H+$ must locate in the mitochondria for participation in oxidative phosphorylation.
  e. Plays no role in sustaining a cytoplasmic pool of NAD^+.

Chapter 4

21. Carbohydrates:
  a. Sucrose is a triose sugar consisting of lactose and fructose.
  b. Fructose is a five-carbon carbohydrate.
  c. Carbohydrates contain only carbon, hydrogen and oxygen.
  d. Triose sugars comprise a pair of monosaccharides.
  e. Glycogen is a triose sugar.

22. Regarding glucose transfer:
  a. Glucose directly diffuses across phospholipid bilayers in the direction of the concentration gradient.
  b. When the concentration gradient is unfavourable for glucose entry into cells, ATP hydrolysis directly "powers" glucose import.

c. Glucose entry into cells occurs via facilitated diffusion.
d. Facilitated diffusion transporters are the main mechanism via which glucose enters gastrointestinal cells.
e. Glut-2 transporters are sensitive to insulin.

23. Glycolysis:
  a. Consists of 13 sequential reactions.
  b. Generates four ATP via substrate-level phosphorylation.
  c. Occurs in the mitochondrial matrix.
  d. Produces one pyruvate molecule for every glucose molecule entering the pathway.
  e. Can only occur in aerobic conditions.

24. Regarding the enzymes of glycolysis:
  a. There are three rate-limiting enzymes, catalysing reaction 1, 3, and 9.
  b. Phosphorylation is an important regulation mechanism used to modulate activity of the rate-limiting enzymes.
  c. ATP allosterically activates PFK-1, thus increasing pathway rate when ATP is abundant.
  d. Fru-2,6-BP, synthesised by PFK-2, allosterically activates hexokinase.
  e. PFK-2 is one of the rate-limiting enzymes of the glycolysis pathway.

25. Pyruvate dehydrogenase:
  a. Is a homodimer located in the mitochondrial matrix.
  b. Catalyses the conversion of pyruvate to acetyl CoA via a number of steps.
  c. Requires CoA, riboflavin and lipoic acid as cofactors to function.
  d. Is allosterically activated by $NADH + H^+$ and acetyl CoA.
  e. Is an unusual enzyme in that phosphorylation does not affect activity.

26. Gluconeogenesis:
  a. Is the production of glucose from non-carbohydrate molecules, and occurs in all cell types.
  b. Occurs in hepatocytes, partly in the cytoplasm and partly in the mitochondria.
  c. Is a net energy-generating pathway, although ATP is consumed.
  d. Is the first-line mechanism to activate to raise plasma glucose in response to falling plasma glucose.
  e. Fatty acids are the most common substrate for gluconeogenesis.

27. Regarding the differences between gluconeogenesis and glycolysis:
  a. The pyruvate → PEP conversion in gluconeogenesis is a two-step reaction, as opposed to PEP → pyruvate conversion in glycolysis which is a single reaction.

b. Both pathways occur exclusively in the cytoplasm.
c. Both pathways occur in all cells.
d. Conditions in which the glycolysis pathway is highly active also promote high activity in the gluconeogenesis pathway.
e. Both pathways have three rate-limiting enzymes.

28. Regarding glycogen:
  a. Glucose generated by glycogenolysis in muscle or hepatocytes is released into the bloodstream to maintain plasma glucose levels.
  b. The structure is composed exclusively of glucose monomers linked by (1–4) bonds.
  c. Synthesis occurs in the mitochondria, and requires UDP-glucose, ATP and a primer.
  d. Elongation and branch formation require different enzymes.
  e. Glycogen phosphorylase, which mediates glycogenolysis, is inactivated by phosphorylation by PKA.

29. The pentose phosphate pathway (PPP):
  a. Is an alternative rather than essential pathway.
  b. Consists of an initial, irreversible, oxidative phase and a reversible non-oxidative phase.
  c. The proportion of different intermediates generated by the pathway is relatively insensitive to cellular requirements.
  d. The PPP generates $NADP^+$, which is required for regeneration and reactivation of glutathione.
  e. Is unimportant in erythrocytes.

30. Regarding the section "fructose, galactose, sorbitol and ethanol":
  a. Fructose is absorbed into enterocytes via the GLUT-1 transporter, and then leaves via the same transporter.
  b. Fructokinase deficiency and fructose-1-phosphate aldolase deficiency are both X-linked genetic afflictions.
  c. Galactose enters enterocytes from the gut lumen via the sodium/glucose symport.
  d. Increased sorbitol production has no negative consequences for a cell.
  e. Ethanal is less toxic than ethanol.

Chapter 5

31. Fatty acids:
  a. Are synthesised de novo from pyruvate.
  b. Are catalysed by sequential oxidation of the α-carbon.
  c. Their catabolism generates $FADH_2$ and $NADH + H^+$ and acetyl CoA.
  d. Exist primarily in the non-ionised form at physiological pH, i.e. margaric acid rather than margarate.
  e. Polyunsaturated FA contain a single double bond.

32. The fatty acid (16:3cΔ4,5,14) has:
    a. no double bonds; it is fully saturated.
    b. 16 carbons and three double bonds at C4, C5 and C14.
    c. 15 carbons and double bonds at C4, C5 and C14.
    d. 14 carbons and double bonds at C3, C4 and C5.
    e. 16 carbons and one double bond at C2.

33. Fatty acid synthesis:
    a. Occurs in the mitochondria of all cell types.
    b. Requires $NADP^+$ and acetyl CoA.
    c. Is a simple reversal of the β-oxidation pathway.
    d. Consists of two completely disparate pathways, one for saturated FA and one for unsaturated FA.
    e. First requires acetyl CoA to export from mitochondria into cytoplasm via the citrate shuttle.

34. The following is a correct description of part of the sequence of fatty acid synthesis:
    a. Acetyl CoA transfer to cytoplasm, conversion to malonyl CoA, assembly of malonyl and acetyl groups on ACP, dehydration, condensation, reduction, dehydration.
    b. Acetyl CoA transfer to cytoplasm, conversion to malonyl CoA, assembly of malonyl and acetyl groups on ACP, condensation, dehydration, reduction, dehydration.
    c. Acetyl CoA transfer into mitochondria, conversion to malonyl CoA, assembly of malonyl and acetyl groups on ACP, condensation, reduction, dehydration, reduction.
    d. Acetyl CoA transfer to cytoplasm, conversion to malonyl CoA, assembly of malonyl and acetyl groups on ACP, condensation, reduction, dehydration, reduction.
    e. Acetyl CoA conversion to malonyl CoA, transfer of malonyl CoA to the cytoplasm, assembly of malonyl and acetyl groups on ACP, condensation, reduction, dehydration, reduction.

35. FA synthesis rate is not influenced by the following:
    a. Availability of acetyl CoA.
    b. TCA cycle activity.
    c. Citrate levels.
    d. $NADPH + H^+$ availability.
    e. $NADP^+$.

36. Triacylglycerols:
    a. Consist of three FA linked to maltitol.
    b. Can be synthesised from glycerol and FA in a three-stage process.
    c. Are synthesised in adipocyte mitochondria.
    d. Are split into FA and acetyl CoA by lipolysis.
    e. Catabolism (lipolysis) involves hydrolysis of the ester bond at C2.

37. Regarding fatty acid catabolism:
    a. Requires activated FA to access the cytoplasm from the mitochondrial matrix via the carnitine shuttle.
    b. Occurs in the mitochondrial matrix via a four-stage process.
    c. Commences with fatty acyl CoA being reduced by fatty acyl-CoA reductase.
    d. Involves conversion of a single bond between the C1 and C2 to a double bond.
    e. Includes thiolytic cleavage (releasing an acetyl CoA) prior to oxidation.

38. The following do *not* play an important role in regulation of lipolysis:
    a. Phosphorylation of hormone-sensitive lipase.
    b. Insulin.
    c. Availability of NAD^+.
    d. Availability of FAD.
    e. Vitamin K.

39. Cholesterol:
    a. Contains 30 carbon atoms.
    b. Is a vital structural component of cell membranes.
    c. Is only synthesised in the hepatocyte cytoplasm.
    d. Ingestion of cholesterol has a greater impact on blood cholesterol than ingestion of saturated fat.
    e. Cholesterol regulates its own synthesis via allosteric activation of HMG-CoA reductase.

40. Regarding lipid transport:
    a. Lipoprotein outer shells are hydrophobic on account of the phospholipid orientation.
    b. Apoproteins play a strictly structural role in lipoprotein particles.
    c. Chylomicrons transport dietary lipids from enterocytes to the liver via the hepatic portal vein.
    d. Chylomicron remnants lack E apoprotein.
    e. High [VLDL] in the bloodstream correlates to good cardiovascular health.

41. Regarding dyslipidaemias:
    a. Familial chylomicronaemia is a very common condition resulting for absence/deficiency of LPL.
    b. Acquired hypercholesterolaemia is very uncommon and is not detrimental to health.
    c. The mechanism by which statins lower blood cholesterol is inhibition of HMG-CoA reductase.
    d. High levels of plasma cholesterol are essential for effective neurotransmission in waterfowl.
    e. In placental mammals, atherosclerotic plaques are of no medical significance.

42. In relation to ketones:
    a. Acetoacetate, acetone and 3-epigallobutyrate are the three biologically significant ketones in humans.
    b. Hepatocytes, natural killer cells and enterocytes are all capable of ketogenesis.
    c. Ketone oxidation occurs in cell cytoplasm.
    d. Reduced TCA cycle activity increases ketogenesis by allowing more acetyl CoA to be diverted to ketogenesis.

e. Predominant catabolism (rather than synthesis) of lipids and high gluconeogenesis activity represses ketone synthesis.

Chapter 6

43. Amino acids:
a. Link via peptide bonds, forming polypeptides.
b. R-groups are the consistent feature between different amino acids.
c. Hydrogen bond interactions operate between C atoms of the $C=O$ component of one amino acid and the amino N atom of another amino acid.
d. Transamination and oxidative deamination both perform the same function; removal of the carboxyl group from an amino acid.
e. Oxidative deamination allows any amino acid to convert to alanine, glutamate or aspartate.

44. Regarding amino acid synthesis:
a. Only amino acids that cannot be synthesis endogenously are deemed essential.
b. Proline, glutamine and tryptophan are synthesised from glutamate.
c. Glycine biosynthesis occurs in the cytoplasm.
d. Phenylalanine is synthesised by hydroxylation of phenylalanine.
e. Absence of phenylalanine hydroxylase renders tyrosine an essential amino acid in individuals with phenylketonuria.

45. Regarding biological derivitives of amino acids:
a. Serotonin is synthesised from tryptophan by hydroxylation followed by decarboxylation.
b. Adrenaline, noradrenaline and dopamine are all synthesised from the amino acid methionine.
c. Tyrosine residues within thyroglobulin are fluorinated, ultimately allowing formation of T3 and T4.
d. Thyroid hormone generation is mediated by the enzyme thyroid transferase.
e. Amino acid decarboxylase requires TPP as a coenzyme.

46. Regarding amino acid catabolism:
a. "Transdeamination" describes transamination followed by oxidative deamination.
b. Transamination occurs in the mitochondria.
c. Oxidative deamination occurs in the cytoplasm.
d. Arginine generated by transamination (during transdeamination) enters the urea cycle.
e. Branched-chain amino acids can only be degraded in hepatocytes.

47. In the context of the urea cycle:
a. The urea cycle processes nitrogen (from amino acid catabolism and ammonia) for excretion as urea.
b. It occurs in cells of the renal cortex, across both the cytoplasm and the mitochondrial matrix.
c. Malate generated by cleavage of arginosuccinate is unable to participate in the TCA cycle.
d. Aspartate in the urea cycle must be generated in one of two ways: either by transamination of oxaloacetate or cleavage of arginosuccinate.
e. Urea can cause acidosis if the levels in the blood rise.

Chapter 7

48. 5,6,7,8-Tetrahydrofolate (THF): select the one false statement below
a. Is reduced from folate by the action of dihydrofolate reductase.
b. Is a carrier of one-carbon units in purine synthesis.
c. Certain anti-cancer drugs inhibit its synthesis.
d. The methionine salvage pathway is essential for maintaining a continual supply of THF
e. Folate deficiency can occur secondary to vitamin B_{12} deficiency.

49. Lesch-Nyhan syndrome: select the one false statement below
a. Is caused by a deficiency of the salvage enzyme, adenine phosphoribosyl transferase (APRT).
b. It is an X linked condition.
c. Causes patients to develop severe mental retardation and to self-mutilate.
d. The salvage pathway for guanine and hypoxanthine is virtually inactive.
e. Increased levels of guanine and hypoxanthine result in hyperuricaemia and gout.

50. Gout: select the one true statement below
a. Predominantly affects women.
b. May be caused by low levels of hypoxanthine-guanine-phosphoribosyl transferase (HGPRT).
c. Clinical features include chronic arthritis of the hips and knees.
d. Acute attacks are treated with xanthine oxidase inhibitors.
e. Is very effectively treated using aspirin.

51. Concerning gout: select the one false statement below
a. Gouty tophi are deposits of urate crystals in bone.
b. Initially, gout is characterized by swelling of a single joint.
c. Gouty tophi cause yellow discoloration of overlying skin.
d. Affected joints are tender.
e. Renal colic is a recognized complication.

52. Concerning porphyrias: select the one false statement below
a. Neurological symptoms are rare in chronic attacks.
b. Acute attacks commonly involve abdominal pain.
c. Mid-stream urine sample would be useful in diagnosis.

d. Are very rare.
e. Acute attacks often come in quick succession.

53. Haem: select the one false statement below
    a. Can reversibly bind O_2 for transport.
    b. Is produced mainly in erythrocytes.
    c. Synthesis is inhibited by lead.
    d. Breakdown occurs mainly in the reticuloendothelial system.
    e. Phenytoin leads to a decrease in haem concentration.

54. Gout: select the one false statement below

    a. May be caused by increased excretion of uric acid by the kidneys.
    b. May result from a partial deficiency of hypoxanthine-guanine phosphoribosyltransferase (HGPRT-).
    c. May result from overproduction of 5-phosphoribosyl 1-pyrophosphate (PRPP).
    d. Can be treated with allopurinol.
    e. May occur in myeloproliferative disorders.

Chapter 8

55. Type 1 diabetes: select the one true statement below
    a. Usually presents at old age.
    b. Is associated with HLA-DR7 antigens.
    c. Tends to occur in patients who are obese.
    d. Can be managed by changing the diet alone.
    e. Patients tend to develop ketoacidosis.

56. Glucagon: select the one true statement below
    a. Inhibits glucose uptake in the peripheral tissues.
    b. Decreases gluconeogenesis.
    c. Decreases ketone body synthesis.
    d. Increases lipogenesis.
    e. Stimulates protein breakdown.

57. The main metabolic changes found in diabetes mellitus are listed below: select the one false statement:
    a. Hyperglycaemia.
    b. An increase in the rate of gluconeogenesis.
    c. A decrease in ketone body synthesis.
    d. Hypertriglyceridaemia.
    e. An increase in lipolysis.

58. Concerning glucose homeostasis: select the one false statement below
    a. HBA_{1C} is a good marker of average blood glucose concentration.
    b. The oral glucose tolerance test involves drinking 75 g of glucose in 250–300 mL of water.
    c. 7.9 mmol/L is a normal fasting glucose level according to the WHO criteria.
    d. Serum fructosamine is a good marker of average blood glucose concentration.

e. Impaired glucose tolerance is normally diagnosed by an oral glucose tolerance test.

59. Secondary diabetes can occur in all of the following cases except:
    a. Chronic pancreatitis.
    b. Haemochromatosis.
    c. Cushing's syndrome.
    d. Long-term steroid use.
    e. Motor neuron disease.

60. Diabetic control: select the single best answer
    a. HbA1c provides a marker for the preceding 12 months of control.
    b. Impaired fasting glucose is defined as fasting plasma glucose 4–5 mmol/L.
    c. Impaired glucose tolerance is defined as fasting plasma glucose < 7.0 mmol/L and 2 h value between 7.8 and 11.1 mmol/L in an OGTT.
    d. Diagnosis of diabetes always requires the patient to be symptomatic.
    e. To be diagnosed with diabetes you always need to have both a fasting blood glucose ≥ 7.0 mmol/L and 2 h value > 11.1 mmol/L in an OGTT.

61. Gestational diabetes: select the single best answer
    a. Affects 50% pregnant women.
    b. Usually reverses after pregnancy.
    c. Eventually leads on to type 2 diabetes in 90% women.
    d. Is more likely to result in type 2 diabetes in patients with a low body mass index.
    e. Can occur in non pregnant individuals.

Chapter 9

62. Kwashiorkor: select the one false statement below
    a. Is an example of protein-energy malnutrition.
    b. Is always caused by a lack of protein and energy.
    c. Is rarely seen in the UK.
    d. Children are usually oedematous with scaly skin.
    e. Usually occurs when a child is weaned from breastfeeding because of the arrival of a second child.

63. Regarding the thyroid gland: select the single best answer
    a. Iodine deficiency is now rare due to fortification of bread.
    b. Triiodothyronine production has a negative feedback effect on the hypothalamus and anterior pituitary.
    c. High TSH levels cause hypoplasia of thyroid epithelium.
    d. The Guthrie test is only used on babies born to hypothyroid mothers.
    e. The anterior pituitary produces thyroid-releasing hormones.

64. Obesity: select the single best answer
    a. Can occur when energy intake is equal to energy expenditure.
    b. Is consistent with a body mass index of 20.
    c. Is more common in low socio-economic class in the West.
    d. Affects over 50% of women in the UK.
    e. Is commonly overcome in the long term by dieting.

65. Marasmus: select the one false statement below
    a. Is a protein and energy deficiency.
    b. Has a high mortality rate.
    c. Is characterized by a thin and emaciated appearance.
    d. Often occurs in children at the age below 18 months.
    e. Is treated first by correcting any infection, hypothermia or hypoglycaemia.

66. Obesity is associated with all of the following except:
    a. Osteoarthritis.
    b. Anxiety.
    c. Gallstones.
    d. Diabetes.
    e. The development of respiratory problems.

67. Coeliac disease: select the one false statement below
    a. Can result in calcium deficiency.
    b. May cause haematuria.
    c. Is always accompanied by normocytic anaemia.
    d. Is commonly associated with weight loss.
    e. May cause vitamin A deficiency.

68. Parenteral nutrition: select the one false statement below
    a. Is useful when enteral nutrition is not an option.
    b. Is indicated when a patient is eating less than 70% of their recommended daily intake.
    c. Can be complicated by infection.
    d. Can be complicated by hyperglycaemia.
    e. Is most often given through a central venous catheter into the superior vena cava.

69. Re-feeding syndrome: select the single best answer below
    a. Is result of high phosphate.
    b. Occurs several months after feeding commences.
    c. Can be prevented with thiamine before starting feeds.
    d. Never occurs in obese patients.
    e. Only arises when feeding patients with TPN (via parenteral route).

Chapter 10

70. Vitamin C: select the one true statement below
    a. Is a cofactor for proline and lysine hydroxylases involved in collagen synthesis.
    b. Is not an antioxidant.

c. Is a powerful oxidizing agent.
    d. Deficiency results in pellagra, characterized by swollen, sore gums and poor wound healing.
    e. Toxicity results in anaemia.

71. Vitamin A: select the one false statement below
    a. Is a fat-soluble vitamin.
    b. Increases epithelial cell turnover.
    c. Deficiency results in impaired dark adaptation and night blindness.
    d. Can be used in the treatment of severe acne.
    e. Is safe to use in pregnancy, even, in excess.

72. Regarding niacin: select the one false statement below
    a. It can be synthesized from the amino acid tryptophan.
    b. Deficiency results in beriberi.
    c. The nutritional requirement for niacin is decreased when the diet contains large amounts of protein.
    d. The clinical features of niacin deficiency include dermatitis, diarrhoea and dementia.
    e. Nicotinic acid can be used in the treatment of hyperlipidaemia.

73. Biotin: select the one false statement below
    a. Is synthesized by bacteria in the gut.
    b. Deficiency is rare in a normal diet.
    c. Deficiency can be induced by eating lots of raw egg whites.
    d. Deficiency results in night blindness.
    e. Deficiency may result in defective fatty acid synthesis.

74. Vitamin B_{12}: select the one false statement below
    a. Is only found in food of animal origin.
    b. Is the cofactor for methylmalonyl CoA mutase, involved in the breakdown of odd-numbered fatty acids.
    c. Intrinsic factor released by gastric parietal cells is required for its absorption.
    d. The stores of vitamin B_{12} are very small.
    e. Deficiency results in both neurological symptoms and megaloblastic anaemia.

75. Vitamin D: select the one true statement below
    a. Cannot be synthesized by the body in sufficient amounts.
    b. Active form is 25-hydroxycholecalciferol.
    c. Principal role is in calcium homeostasis.
    d. Is a recognized teratogen.
    e. Is an antioxidant.

76. Vitamins: select the one true statement below:
    a. A deficiency of vitamin A causes rickets in children.
    b. Vitamin B_{12}, C and E are all antioxidants.
    c. Vitamin A, D, E and C are all fat-soluble vitamins.
    d. A deficiency of vitamin B_{12} results in anaemia.

e. Both vitamin K and vitamin B$_{12}$ are synthesized by intestinal bacteria.

77. Osteomalacia: select the single best answer
   a. Bowed legs are a feature.
   b. Spontaneous fractures are a feature.
   c. Can be diagnosed by an increased alkaline phosphatase.
   d. Is common in childhood.
   e. Is commonly due to vitamin A deficiency.

78. Pernicious anaemia: select the single best answer
   a. Is the most common cause of vitamin B$_{12}$ deficiency.
   b. Is caused by a virus.
   c. Is diagnosed by an auto-antibody screen.
   d. Is treated by intramuscular injection of intrinsic factor.
   e. Is common in older men.

79. Vitamin K: select the single best answer
   a. Is a coenzyme for clotting factors III, V, IX and X.
   b. Needs to be taken in the diet regularly to avoid deficiency.
   c. Is given to children with intracranial haemorrhage.
   d. Deficiency will cause a decreased activated partial thromboplastin time (APTT).
   e. Is antagonized by oral anticoagulants such as warfarin.

80. Select the statement about vitamins which is true:
   a. Vitamin A, C and E are fat-soluble.
   b. They are required in relatively small amounts.
   c. Fat-soluble vitamins are stored in the kidney.
   d. The B-group vitamins are toxic in excess.
   e. Vitamin K deficiency is relatively common.

81. Rickets: select the one false statement below
   a. Is associated with mental retardation and seizures.
   b. Causes increased bone formation.
   c. Results in defective mineralization of the long bones visible on X-ray.
   d. Commonly develops in the children.
   e. Is characterized by delayed dentition.

82. Wernicke-Korsakoff syndrome: select the one false statement below
   a. Is due to dietary deficiency of folic acid.
   b. Causes ataxia.
   c. Can lead to short-term memory loss.
   d. Is seen in chronic alcoholics.
   e. Can be reversed.

Chapter 11

83. Zinc: Select the single best answer
   a. Is a not useful in wound healing.
   b. Absorption is increased in the presence of vitamin C.
   c. Deficiency causes acrodermatitis enteropathica.

d. Deficiency is not seen in patients on parenteral nutrition.
   e. Overload causes liver cirrhosis.

84. Iron: select the one false statement below
   a. Its absorption is favoured in the ferrous state (Fe^{2+}).
   b. Is stored in the body as ferritin.
   c. Deficiency results in microcytic anaemia.
   d. Overload can result in diabetes mellitus.
   e. Overload can be treated with penicillamine.

85. Calcium: select the one false statement below
   a. Is the most abundant mineral in the human body.
   b. Deficiency can occur secondary to vitamin D deficiency.
   c. Deficiency in children causes rickets.
   d. Is active in its ionized form, Ca^{2+}.
   e. In overload, it is deposited in the eyes producing Kayser–Fleischer rings on the cornea.

86. Regarding copper overload: select the one false statement below
   a. It is rare clinical problem in the UK.
   b. A 2-month course of chelation therapy normally resolves the problem.
   c. Any liver damage is irreversible.
   d. It is the result of a chromosome defect.
   e. The liver fails to excrete copper into the bile.

87. In the intestine: select the one false statement below
   a. Of neonates, there are no bacteria.
   b. Iron is absorbed in the ferrous (Fe^{2+}) form.
   c. Fat-soluble vitamins are absorbed along with glucose.
   d. Transferrin is involved in controlling iron absorption.
   e. Iron absorption is enhanced by ascorbic acid.

Chapter 12

History and examination

88. Common symptoms of anaemia include all of the following except:
   a. Fatigue.
   b. Headaches.
   c. Palpitations.
   d. Breathlessness.
   e. Tremor.

89. Tremor: select the one true statement below
   a. May be associated with hypothyroidism.
   b. is classed an essential tremor in Wernicke-Korsakoff syndrome .
   c. Can be caused by exercise.
   d. Of the flapping type is observed with outstretched arms and hands flat.
   e. Can be caused by hyperglycaemia.

90. Clubbing: select the one true statement below
    a. Is caused by iron-deficiency anaemia.
    b. Is defined as increased angle between the nail and nail bed.
    c. Can cause underlying nail fluctuance.
    d. Is a feature of cirrhosis.
    e. Is commonly seen as a result of glycogen storage disorder.

91. Regarding anaemia: select the one false statement below
    a. Iron deficiency will cause a decrease in haem and erythrocyte production.
    b. Macrocytic anaemia may be caused by a deficiency of erythrocyte enzymes.
    c. Pernicious anaemia is an auto-immune condition causing deficiency of B_{12} and folate.
    d. Lead poisoning inhibits three enzymes of haem synthesis, leading to anaemia.
    e. Sickle cell anaemia is a hereditary haemolytic anaemia.

92. Causes of clubbing include all of the following except:
    a. Chronic obstructive airway disease.
    b. Bronchial carcinoma.
    c. Cystic fibrosis.
    d. Coeliac disease.
    e. Liver cirrhosis.

93. Arterial ulcers are: select the single best answer below
    a. Painless.
    b. Shallow.
    c. Common at pressure areas.
    d. Common superior to the medial malleolus.
    e. Not know to discharge.

94. Classic signs and symptoms of peritonism in an abdomen examination include all of the following except:
    a. Guarding.
    b. Rebound tenderness.
    c. Rigidity.
    d. Pain.
    e. Distension.

Further investigations

95. Regarding urea and electrolytes: select the single best answer below
    a. Creatinine is low in renal disease.
    b. Low serum sodium concentration indicates dehydration.
    c. In renal failure, serum potassium is low.
    d. Creatinine can be raised in healthy athletes.
    e. Liver cirrhosis causes a high serum sodium.

96. Regarding haematological investigations: select the one false statement below
    a. A haemoglobin of 12 g/dL is normal in women.
    b. A red cell count of 8×10^{12}/L is consistent with polycythaemia.
    c. A prothrombin time of 12–16 seconds is normal.
    d. Mean cell haemoglobin is low in folate deficiency.
    e. Microcytic, hypochromic blood film is consistent with iron deficiency.

Extended-matching questions (EMQs)

1. Enzymes of glycolysis

A. Hexokinase.
B. Phosphoglucoisomerase.
C. Phosphofructokinase-1.
D. Phosphofructokinase-2.
E. Aldolase.
F. Triose phosphate isomerase.
G. Glyceraldehyde-3-phosphate dehydrogenase.
H. Phosphoglycerate kinase.
I. Phosphoglycerate mutase.
J. Enolase.
K. Pyruvate kinase.
L. Malate dehydrogenase.

For each of the following, select the SINGLE most appropriate response from the above list.

1. This enzyme catalyses the most exergonic reaction of glycolysis.
2. This enzyme the conversion of DHAP to GAP.
3. This enzyme has another isoform (glucokinase) in pancreatic islet cells and hepatocytes.
4. This enzyme catalyses a rate-limiting reaction which includes a phosphorylation, using ATP as the phosphoryl donor.
5. This catalyses the final substrate-level phosphorylation of glycolysis.

2. Enzymes of the TCA cycle

A. Citrate synthase.
B. Aconitase.
C. Isocitrate dehyrogenase.
D. α-ketoglutarate dehyrogenase.
E. Succinyl CoA synthetase.
F. Succinate dehydrogenase.
G. Fumarase.
H. Malate dehydrogenase.
I. Glycerol-3-phosphate dehydrogenase.
J. Phosphoglucoisomerase.
K. Pyruvate kinase.
L. Pyruvate dehydrogenase.

For each of the following, select the SINGLE most appropriate response from the above list.

1. This enzyme catalyses the reaction which generates GTP.
2. This enzyme catalyses the reaction which reduces FAD to $FADH_2$.
3. A rate-limiting enzyme that mediates a reaction that does not generate carbon dioxide as a product.
4. This enzyme catalyses the decarboxylation reaction that produces acetyl CoA from pyruvate.
5. An enzyme not associated with the TCA cycle.

3. Amino acids

A. Arginine.
B. Glutamate.
C. Glutamine.
D. Aspartate.
E. Tryptophan.
F. Isoleucine.
G. Alanine.
H. Tyrosine.
I. Cysteine.
J. Valine.
K. Serine.
L. Phenylalanine.

For each of the following, select the SINGLE most appropriate response from the above list.

1. Formed by cleavage of arginosuccinate.
2. Branched chain amino acid that is both ketogenic and glucogenic.
3. Pathological accumulation of this amino acid characterises phenylketonuria.
4. Amino acid that is a precursor of adrenaline.
5. This amino acid has a R-group containing sulphur.

For each scenario described below, choose the single most likely option from the list of options.
Each option may be used once, more than once or not at all.

4. Clinical aspects of diabetes

A. Antibiotics administration.
B. Autoimmune disease with peak age of onset at 15–20 years.
C. Diet and weight reduction.
D. Disease caused by a single gene defect.
E. Disease more common in Mediterranean than Caucasian populations.
F. Disease with typical age of onset from 60 years onwards.
G. Hypoglycaemia.
H. Hyperglycaemia.
I. Inhalation of insulin preparations.
J. Injection of insulin preparations.
K. Measurement of glycosylated haemoglobin.
L. Random blood glucose test.

For each of the following, select the SINGLE most appropriate option from the above list.

1. The onset of Type 1 diabetes.
2. The most common effective treatment of Type 1 diabetes.
3. The initial treatment of most patients with Type 2 diabetes.
4. Diabetic patient presenting with sweating, nausea, confusion and coma.
5. Method for measuring blood glucose control in the past month.

5. Inadequate or excessive micronutrient intake

A. Calcium.
B. Copper.
C. Folic acid.
D. Iron.
E. Pyridoxal phosphate (B_6).
F. Riboflavin.
G. Thiamine.
H. Vitamin A.
I. Vitamin C.
J. Vitamin D.
K. Vitamin E.
L. Vitamin K.

For each of the following, select the SINGLE most appropriate vitamin or mineral from the above list.

1. Lack of this substance may cause rickets.
2. Beri-beri may result from insufficient intake of this substance.
3. Deficiency in childhood causes xerophthalmia.
4. Lack of this substance causes macrocytic anaemia.
5. May contribute to osteoporosis in post-menopausal women.

6. Liver and alcohol abuse

A. Albumin.
B. Alcohol.
C. Bile salts.
D. Bilirubin.
E. Cholesterol.
F. Disulfiram.
G. γ-Glutamyl transferase.
H. Thiamine.
I. Urea.
J. Vitamin A.
K. Vitamin E.
L. Vitamin K.

For each of the following, select the SINGLE most appropriate response from the above list.

1. Jaundice arises from increased deposition of this in tissues.
2. Wernicke–Korsakoff syndrome can arise in alcoholics as a result of deficiency in this.
3. Increased risk of bruising and bleeding in alcoholics is due to deficiency in this.
4. Oedema can arise from severely depleted circulating levels of this.
5. This compound has been shown to have a beneficial effect on heart attacks and strokes when ingested in moderate amounts.

7. Causes of anaemia

A. Anaemia of chronic disease.
B. Autoimmune haemolytic anaemia.
C. Coeliac disease.
D. Glucose-6-phosphate dehydrogenase deficiency.
E. Hypothyroidism.
F. Iron deficiency.
G. Multiple myeloma.
H. Pernicious anaemia.
I. Sickle-cell anaemia.
J. Sideroblastic anaemia.
K. Thalassaemia.
L. Vitamin B_{12} deficiency.

For each of the following, choose ONE option from the list above.

1. A 10-year-old boy presents with painful joints in the hands and feet, jaundice and anaemia. He also has splenomegaly and his blood film shows target cells.
2. A 50-year-old man presents with macrocytic anaemia. He drinks alcohol regularly.
3. A 25-year-old Greek lady presents with anaemia and jaundice following anti-malarial treatment. She is noted to have Heinz bodies.
4. A 10-month-old baby presents with anaemia and failure to thrive. His blood film shows target cells, hypochromic and microcytic cells. HbF is still present.
5. A 40-year-old woman presents with lethargy and a sore red tongue. Her blood film shows hypersegmented polymorphs, an MCV > 110 fL and a low haemoglobin.

8. Nutritional deficiencies

A. Copper.
B. Folic acid.
C. Nicotinic acid.
D. Pyridoxine.
E. Selenium.
F. Thiamine.
G. Vitamin A.
H. Vitamin B_{12}.
I. Vitamin C.
J. Vitamin D.
K. Vitamin K.
L. Zinc.

For the following, select the MOST likely cause of nutritional deficiency from the above list.

1. A 15-year-old girl complains of not being able to see very well at night.
2. A 45-year-old man with poor diet complains that his gums are bleeding easily.
3. A 30-year-old man presents with nystagmus, opthalmoplegia and ataxia. He is known to drink at least 40 units of alcohol a week.
4. A 20-year-old woman with chronic diarrhoea complains of prolonged bleeding after a small cut to her index finger. The prothrombin time is increased.
5. A 25-year-old man was recently on anti-TB treatment and now presents with dermatitis, diarrhoea and depression.

9. Clinical Investigations

A. Chest X-ray.
B. CT scan.
C. Direct Coombs' test.
D. Fasting blood glucose.
E. Glycosylated haemoglobin.
F. Guthrie test.
G. Lipid profile.
H. Liver biopsy.
I. Oral glucose tolerance test.
J. Schilling test.
K. Serum iron.
L. Uric acid.

For the following statements, choose ONE clinical investigation from the above list.

1. The doctor suspects that the patient has been misleading him regarding the control of her blood glucose levels.
2. The patient, a teetotal, has macrocytic anaemia, despite eating a healthy and sensible diet.
3. The newborn baby had a blood sample taken from a heel-prick around 7 days after birth.
4. The patient is known to have a family history of coronary heart disease.
5. The patient complains of a painful and swollen big toe, following a heavy protein meal.

10. Disorders of metabolism

A. Albinism.
B. Alkaptonuria.
C. Glucose-6-phosphate dehydrogenase deficiency.
D. Histidinaemia.
E. Homocystinuria.
F. Lesch-Nyhan syndrome.
G. Maple syrup urine disease.
H. Menkes' kinky hair syndrome.
I. Phenylketonuria.
J. Porphyria.
K. Sickle cell anaemia.
L. Wilson's disease.

For the following statements, choose ONE disorder from the above list.

1. A 6-month-old baby presents with seizures and failure to thrive. His parents are advised to follow a food restriction diet.
2. The patient presents with painful joints and complains that his urine turns black on standing.
3. The patient presents with whitish hair, grey-blue eyes and pale skin. He is advised to use high sun protection when going out.
4. A 1-month-old baby presents with metabolic acidosis, hypoglycaemia and seizures. His parents complain that his urine smells sweet.
5. A 4-month-old baby presents with self-mutilation, spasticity and kidney stones. His parents complain of an 'orange' nappy.

BOF answers

Chapter 1

1. c. Modulation of enzyme function is a major cellular regulation strategy.
2. d. Is a covalent enzyme modification which alters enzyme activity.
3. e. Permits intracellular events to respond appropriately to organism energy status.
4. a. The Na^+/K^+ ATPase imports 2 K^+ ions for every 3 Na^+ ions exported.
5. d. Oxidation is associated with a molecule losing electrons.
6. d. Is synthesised by substrate-level or oxidative phosphorylation.
7. d. Possesses a thiol group within the CoA component of the molecule.
8. b. Act as cofactors for enzymes mediating redox reactions.
9. c. Are energetically "favourable."

Chapter 2

10. a. Occurs in the mitochondrial matrix.
11. b. 1 $FADH_2$ and 3 $NADH+H^+$ are generated per "turn."
12. b. Rate-limiting enzymes of the TCA cycle are allosterically inhibited by ATP.
13. e. Tryptophan

Chapter 3

14. b. Requires ADP as a substrate.
15. c. Electrons enter the electron transport chain within $NADH+H^+$ or $FADH_2$.
16. b. Results in sequential reduction, then oxidation of each complex of the ETC.
17. b. Only complex I and II "accept" electron pairs from $NADH+H^+$ and $FADH_2$.
18. c. Is accumulated by complexes I, III and IV.
19. e. Couples proton passage with ATP synthesis.
20. d. Is necessary since $NADH+H^+$ must locate in the mitochondria for participation in oxidative phosphorylation.

Chapter 4

21. c. Carbohydrates contain only carbon, hydrogen and oxygen.
22. c. Glucose entry into cells occurs via facilitated diffusion.
23. b. Generates four ATP via substrate-level phosphorylation.
24. b. Phosphorylation is an important regulation mechanism used to modulate activity of the rate-limiting enzymes.
25. b. Catalyses the conversion of pyruvate to acetyl CoA via a number of steps.
26. b. Occurs in hepatocytes, partly in the cytoplasm and partly in the mitochondria.
27. a. The pyruvate $\rightarrow$ PEP conversion in gluconeogenesis is a two-step reaction, as opposed to PEP $\rightarrow$ pyruvate conversion in glycolysis which is a single reaction.
28. d. Elongation and branch formation require different enzymes.
29. b. Consists of an initial, irreversible, oxidative phase and a reversible non-oxidative phase.
30. c. Galactose enters enterocytes from the gut lumen via the sodium/glucose symport.

Chapter 5

31. c. Their catabolism generates $FADH_2$ and $NADH+H^+$ and acetyl CoA.
32. b. 16 carbons and three double bonds at C4, C5 and C14.
33. e. First requires acetyl CoA to export from mitochondria into cytoplasm via the citrate shuttle.
34. d. Acetyl CoA transfer to cytoplasm, conversion to malonyl CoA, assembly of malonyl and acetyl groups on ACP, condensation, reduction, dehydration, reduction.
35. e. $NADP^+$.
36. b. Can be synthesised from glycerol and FA in a three-stage process.
37. b. Occurs in the mitochondrial matrix via a four-stage process.
38. e. Vitamin K.
39. b. Is a vital structural component of cell membranes.

40. c. Chylomicrons transport dietary lipids from enterocytes to the liver via the hepatic portal vein.

41. c. The mechanism by which statins lower blood cholesterol is inhibition of HMG-CoA reductase.

42. d. Reduced TCA cycle activity increases ketogenesis by allowing more acetyl CoA to be diverted to ketogenesis.

Chapter 6

43. a. Link via peptide bonds, forming polypeptides.

44. e. Absence of phenylalanine hydroxylase renders tyrosine an essential amino acid in individuals with phenylketonuria.

45. a. Serotonin is synthesised from tryptophan by hydroxylation followed by decarboxylation.

46. a. "Transdeamination" describes transamination followed by oxidative deamination.

47. a. The urea cycle processes nitrogen (from amino acid catabolism and ammonia) for excretion as urea.

Chapter 7

48. e. Folate deficiency can occur secondary to vitamin B_1 deficiency.

49. a. Is caused by a deficiency of the salvage enzyme, adenine phosphoribosyl transferase (APRT).

50. b. May be caused by low levels of hypoxanthine-guanine-phosphoribosyl transferase (HGPRT).

51. a. Gouty tophi are deposits of urate crystals in bone.

52. e. Acute attacks often come in quick succession.

53. b. Is produced mainly in erythrocytes.

54. a. May be caused by increased excretion of uric acid by the kidneys.

Chapter 8

55. e. Patients tend to develop ketoacidosis.

56. e. Stimulates protein breakdown.

57. c. A decrease in ketone body synthesis.

58. c. 7.9 mmol/L is a normal fasting glucose level according to the WHO criteria.

59. e. Motor neuron disease.

60. c. Impaired glucose tolerance is defined as fasting plasma glucose < 7.0 mmol/L and 2 h value between 7.8 and 11.1 mmol/L in an OGTT.

61. b. Usually reverses after pregnancy.

Chapter 9

62. b. Is always caused by a lack of protein and energy.

63. b. Triiodothyronine production has a negative feedback effect on the hypothalamus and anterior pituitary.

64. c. Is more common in low socio-economic class in the West.

65. e. Is treated first by correcting any infection, hypothermia or hypoglycaemia.

66. b. Anxiety.

67. c. Is always accompanied by normocytic anaemia.

68. b. Is indicated when a patient is eating less than 70% of their recommended daily intake.

69. c. Can be prevented with thiamine before starting feeds.

Chapter 10

70. a. Is a cofactor for proline and lysine hydroxylases involved in collagen synthesis.

71. e. Is safe to use in pregnancy, even in excess.

72. b. Deficiency results in beriberi.

73. d. Deficiency results in night blindness.

74. d. The stores of vitamin B_{12} are very small.

75. c. Principal role is in calcium homeostasis.

76. d. A deficiency of vitamin B_{12} results in anaemia.

77. b. Spontaneous fractures are a feature.

78. a. Is the most common cause of vitamin B_{12} deficiency.

79. e. Is antagonized by oral anticoagulants such as warfarin.

80. b. They are required in relatively small amounts.

81. a. Is associated with mental retardation and seizures.

82. a. Is due to dietary deficiency of folic acid.

Chapter 11

83. c. Deficiency causes acrodermatitis enteropathica.

84. e. Overload can be treated with penicillamine.

85. e. In overload, it is deposited in the eyes producing Kayser–Fleischer rings on the cornea.

86. b. A 2-month course of chelation therapy normally resolves the problem.
87. c. Fat-soluble vitamins are absorbed along with glucose.

Chapter 12

History and examination

88. e. Tremor.
89. c. Can be caused by exercise.
90. c. Can cause underlying nail fluctuance.

91. b. Macrocytic anaemia may be caused by a deficiency of erythrocyte enzymes.
92. a. Chronic obstructive airway disease.
93. c. Common at pressure areas.
94. e. Distension.

Further investigations

95. d. Creatinine can be raised in healthy athletes.
96. d. Mean cell haemoglobin is low in folate deficiency.

EMQ answers

1. Enzymes of Glycolysis

1. **K.** **Pyruvate kinase.** The most exergonic reaction of glycolysis is reaction 10; the conversion of phosphoenolpyruvate (PEP) to pyruvate. Transfer of the phosphoryl group from PEP to ADP results in pyruvate and ATP synthesis. This is catalysed by pyruvate kinase. The ΔG_O of this reaction is -31.4 kJ/mol.

2. **F.** **Triose phosphate isomerase.** This enzyme catalyses the isomerisation reaction converting dihydroxyacetone phosphate (DHAP) to glyceraldehyde-3-phosphate.

3. **A.** **Hexokinase.** This catalyses reaction 1 of glycolysis; the conversion of glucose to glucose-6-phosphate (Glc-6-P). The main functional difference is that hexokinase is allosterically inhibited by the reaction product Glc-6-P, whilst glucokinase is *in*sensitive to such inhibition. The isoforms also differ in affinity; low-affinity glucokinase requires higher [glucose] to perform equally as effectively as the high-affinity hexokinase dose at lower [glucose].

4. **H or A.** **Phosphofructokinase-1** or **Hexokinase.** Both these enzymes meet the question's criteria, i.e. catalysing rate-limiting glycolytic reactions where ATP is the phosphate donor in the reaction. Hexokinase catalyses reaction 1 of glycolysis, whilst phosphofructokinase-1 catalyses reaction 3 of glycolysis.

5. **K.** **Pyruvate kinase.** There are two substrate-level phosphorylation reactions in glycolysis. The first is catalysed by phosphoglycerate kinase (reaction 7) and the second is catalysed by pyruvate kinase (reaction 10).

2. Enzymes of the TCA cycle

1. **E.** **Succinyl CoA synthetase.** This enzyme catalyses the conversion of succinyl CoA to succinate in a substrate-level phosphorylation that directly generates GTP.

2. **F.** **Succinate dehydrogenase.** This enzyme catalyses the oxidation of succinate to fumarate. The coupled redox reaction is the reduction of FAD to $FADH_2$.

3. **A.** **Citrate synthase.** The three rate-limiting reactions of the TCA are reactions 1, 3 and 4; catalysed by citrate synthase, isocitrate dehydrogenase and α-ketoglutarate dehydrogenase respectively. However reaction 1 is the only reaction of these three that does not generate CO_2, making citrate synthase the answer.

4. **L.** **Pyruvate dehydrogenase.** This enzyme catalyses the conversion of pyruvate to acetyl CoA.

5. **I or J.** **Glycerol-3-phosphate dehydrogenase** or **Phosphoglucoisomerase.** These two enzymes are enzymes of glycolysis, therefore these two are the only members of the list not associated with the TCA cycle.

3. Amino acids

1. **A.** **Arginine.** One synthesis route for the basic amino acid arginine is a reaction within the urea cycle; arginosuccinate is cleaved by arginosuccinate lyase to form arginine and fumarate.

2. **F.** **Isoleucine.** Only three amino acids (of those discussed in this text) have branch-structure R-groups. These are Leucine, Isoleucine and Valine. However, of these three, only Isoleucine has a structure allowing catabolism to generate intermediates that can participate in both ketogenesis and gluconeogenesis.

3. **L.** **Phenylalanine.** Pathological accumulation of phenylalanine, resulting from deficiency or phenylalanine hydroxylase, characterises the autosomal recessive condition phenylketonuria.

4. **H.** **Tyrosine.** This amino acid is used as a substrate in the synthesis of dopamine, noradrenaline and adrenaline.

5. **I.** **Cysteine.** The only amino acids of physiological importance containing sulphur in their R-groups are methionine and cysteine. However, methionine is not present in the list.

4. Clinical aspects of diabetes

1. **B.** **Autoimmune disease with peak age of onset at 15–20 years.** Type 1 diabetes, also known as insulin-dependent diabetes or juvenile-onset diabetes, typically occurs in childhood or puberty.

2. **J.** **Injection of insulin preparations.** In type 1 diabetes, there is a complete deficiency of insulin that can only be corrected by life-long insulin treatment.

3. **C.** **Diet and weight reduction.** Type 2 diabetes is typically associated with obesity, and diet management is often the only treatment necessary when patients are first diagnosed. Weight loss can prevent or delay the development of type 2 diabetes.

4. **G.** **Hypoglycaemia.** Hypoglycaemia causes unpleasant autonomic symptoms, such as sweating, nausea and palpitations, and more severe neuroglycopenic symptoms as a result of a decrease in glucose supply to the brain: drowsiness, unsteadiness, confusion and coma.

5. **K.** **Measurement of glycated haemoglobin.** The concentration of glycated haemoglobin provides a measure of the average blood glucose concentration over the preceding 4–6 weeks, that is, the lifetime of an erythrocyte.

5. Inadequate or excessive micronutrient intake

1. **J.** **Vitamin D.** The main role of vitamin D is in calcium homeostasis, where a severe deficiency causes rickets in children and osteomalacia in adults.

2. **G.** **Thiamine.** Deficiency of thiamine causes two types of beri-beri: wet beri-beri which results in oedema and heart failure, and dry beri-beri which causes muscle wasting and peripheral neuropathy.

3. **H.** **Vitamin A.** Deficiency of vitamin A results in an increase in epithelial keratinization of the cornea leading to xeropthalmia.

4. **C.** **Folic acid.** A deficiency in folic acid results in decreased synthesis of purines and pyrimidines, leading to a decrease in nucleic acid synthesis and cell division. This shows up mostly in cells that rapidly divide such as red blood cells, presenting as large, immature red blood cells.

5. **A.** **Calcium.** There is a progressive reduction of total bone mass, due to the effects of oestrogen deficiency in post-menopausal women, and calcium deficiency increases the risk of osteoporosis.

6. Liver and alcohol abuse

1. **D.** **Bilirubin.** Jaundice refers to the yellow pigmentation of skin or sclerae of the eyes due to a raised plasma bilirubin level.

2. **H.** **Thiamine.** Alcohol inhibits the uptake of thiamine.

3. **L.** **Vitamin K.** Vitamin K is a coenzyme required for the γ-carboxylation of clotting factors II, VII, IX and X, activating them and thus, the clotting cascade.

4. **A.** **Albumin.** With reduced levels of serum albumin, fluid may escape into tissues to cause oedema or into body cavities to cause ascites or pleural effusions.

5. **B.** **Alcohol.** Regular consumption of moderate amounts of alcohol, i.e. one glass of red wine a day has been found to have a protective effect against heart attacks and strokes.

7. Causes of anaemia

1. **I.** **Sickle-cell anaemia.** A vaso-occlusive crisis occurs when the microcirculation is obstructed by sickled erythrocytes, causing ischaemic injury to joints, resulting in pain. The spleen can undergo a sudden very painful enlargement due to pooling of large numbers of sickled cells. This phenomenon is known as splenic sequestration crisis.

2. **L.** **Vitamin B_{12} deficiency.** B_{12} deficiency causes secondary folate deficiency, which leads to decreased production of DNA and defective cell division. As a result, the developing erythrocytes are megaloblastic, where the nuclei mature more slowly than the cytoplasm.

3. **D.** **Glucose-6-phosphate dehydrogenase deficiency.** Anti-malarial treatment is a precipitating factor here, resulting in oxidative stress and haemolysis of erythrocytes. Damage to the haemoglobin causes its oxidation to methaemoglobin, and the globin chains are precipitated as Heinz bodies.

4. **K.** **Thalassaemia.** The patient has β-thalassaemia, resulting in a deficiency of β-globin chains. As a result, fetal haemoglobin (HbF) persists in the circulation.

5. **H.** **Pernicious anaemia.** An auto-immune condition in which antibodies are made to intrinsic factor; preventing vitamin B_{12} absorption.

8. Nutritional deficiencies

1. **G.** **Vitamin A.** Vitamin A is required for proper function of 11-*cis* retinal, which binds to opsin to form rhodopsin, the visual pigment of rod cells in the retina involved in night vision.
2. **I.** **Vitamin C.** A deficiency in vitamin C results in scurvy which typically presents with swollen, sore, spongy gums with bleeding and loose teeth.
3. **F.** **Thiamine.** A deficiency of thiamine results in Wernicke's encephalopathy which typically presents with ataxia, nystagmus and opthalmoplegia.
4. **K.** **Vitamin K.** Vitamin K is a coenzyme required for the γ-carboxylation of clotting factors II, VII, IX and X, activating them and thus, the clotting cascade.
5. **C.** **Nicotinic acid.** Isoniazid treatment for tuberculosis inhibits nicotinic acid, which results in pellagra which presents with dermatitis, diarrhoea and depression.

9. Clinical investigations

1. **E.** **Glycated haemoglobin.** The concentration of glycated haemoglobin provides a measure of the average blood glucose concentration over the preceding 4–6 weeks, that is, the half-life of an erythrocyte.
2. **J.** **Schilling test.** The Schilling test measures the absorption of vitamin B_{12} and is usually used to diagnose pernicious anaemia.
3. **F.** **Guthrie test.** A sample of capillary blood is taken from a heel-prick at 5–10 days after birth and screened for phenylketonuria and hypothyroidism.

4. **G.** **Lipid profile.** Patients in 'at risk' groups have their cholesterol levels monitored routinely.
5. **L.** **Uric acid.** The patient has clinical symptoms of gout, which is usually due to a high level of uric acid in the blood which has precipitated out to form crystals.

10. Disorders of metabolism

1. **I.** **Phenylketonuria.** Phenylketonuria is an autosomal recessive disorder due to a deficiency of the enzyme phenylalanine hydroxylase, which results in accumulation of phenylalanine. Patients are advised to be on phenylalanine-restricted diet.
2. **B.** **Alkaptonuria.** Alkaptonuria is caused by a deficiency of the enzyme homogentisic acid oxidase. This results in the accumulation of homogentisate which is excreted in the urine, resulting in the urine turning black due to formation of alkapton.
3. **A.** **Albinism.** Albinism is a deficiency of the enzyme tyrosinase which converts tyrosine to melanin. People with pale skin which makes them more prone to sunburn and skin cancer, thus they are often advised to use high sun protection when going out.
4. **G.** **Maple syrup urine disease.** Patients with this disease excrete branched-chain amino acids in the urine, which gives it a maple syrup smell.
5. **F.** **Lesch-Nyhan.** A very rare X-linked disorder caused by absence of the enzyme hypoxanthine guanine phosphoribosyl transferase. It results in hyperuricaemia causing kidney stones, arthritis and gout as well as severe neurological disturbances such as spasticity and self-mutilation.

Acyl carrier protein A protein or a domain of a protein that contains thiol groups which provides attachment sites for malonyl CoA and growing fatty acid chains.

Adenosine diphosphate (ADP) A ribonucleotide diphosphate in which two phosphoryl groups are successively linked to the 5′ oxygen atom of adenosine.

Adenosine monophosphate (AMP) A ribonucleotide monophosphate in which a phosphoryl group is linked to the 5′ oxygen atom of adenosine.

Adenosine triphosphate (ATP) A nucleotide containing a purine base (adenine), a five-carbon sugar; ribose, and three phosphate groups.

Adipose tissue Also known as fat tissue. Animal tissue composed of specialized triacylgycerol-storage cells known as adipocytes. There is growing evidence that adipocytes are hormonally active secreting a range of so called adipokines (e.g. leptin is an adipokine).

Aerobic Occuring in the presence of oxygen.

Amino acid An organic acid consisting of an α-carbon atom to which an amino group, a carboxyl group, a hydrogen atom and a specific side chain (R group) are attached.

Anabolism The synthesis of complex molecules from simpler ones. Anabolism is associated with energy entrapment and storage.

Anaemia The blood haemoglobin below the normal range for the patient's age and sex. The normal range in males is 13.5–18.0 g/dL and in females is 11.5–16.0 g/dL.

Anaerobic Occuring in the absence of oxygen.

Atherogenic The ability to start or speed up the process of atherogenesis, which is the inflammation-driven formation of lipid deposits in the arteries leading to thickening and hardening of the arterial wall.

ATPase An enzyme that catalyses hydrolysis of ATP to ADP + Pi.

Autophosphorylation Phosphorylation of a protein kinase catalyzed by the same kinase.

Bioenergetics The study of the energy changes accompanying biochemical reactions.

Beta (β)-oxidation A cyclical sequence of reactions that degrades fatty acids to acetyl CoA. It consists of four steps: oxidation, hydration, further oxidation and thiolysis.

Carbohydrate A complex molecule in which the molar ratio of C:H:O is 1:2:1.

Carnitine shuttle A pathway that shuttles acetyl CoA from the cytosol to the mitochondria through the formation of acyl carnitine.

Catabolism The breakdown of energy-rich complex molecules (e.g. carbohydrate) to simpler ones (e.g. CO_2, H_2O). Catabolism is associated with energy release.

Chaperone A protein that forms complexes with newly synthesized polypeptide chains and assists in their correct folding into biologically functional conformations.

Chylomicron A plasma lipoprotein that transports dietary lipids absorbed from the intestine to the tissues.

Citrate shuttle A pathway that shuttles acetyl CoA from the mitochondria to the cytosol providing a substrate for fatty acid synthesis.

Condensation A reaction involving the joining of two or more molecules accompanied by the elimination of water.

Cori cycle An interorgan metabolic loop that distributes the metabolic burden between the muscle and the liver. Lactate, which builds up in muscle during intense activity, is taken to the liver to be converted back to glucose via gluconeogenesis. This replenishes fuel for the muscle and prevents lactic acidosis. The produced glucose returns to muscle as an energy source, completing the cycle.

C-terminus The amino acid residue bearing a free carboxyl group (–COOH) at one end of a peptide chain.

Cytochrome A haem-containing protein that is an electron carrier in processes such as respiration and photosynthesis.

De novo pathway A metabolic pathway in which a biomolecule is formed 'from scratch', from simple precursor molecules.

Deaminase An enzyme that catalyses the removal of an amino group from a substrate, releasing ammonia.

Dehydrogenase An enzyme catalysing oxidation–reduction reactions involving addition or extraction of hydrogen atoms.

Diabetes mellitus A syndrome caused by the lack, or diminished effectiveness, of insulin, resulting in a raised blood glucose (hyperglycaemia) and the presence of chronic vascular complications.

Dyslipidaemias A group of disorders caused by a defect in lipoprotein formation, transport or degradation.

Electron transport chain A series of enzyme complexes and associated cofactors that are electron carriers, passing electrons from reduced coenzymes or substrates to molecular oxygen (O_2), the terminal electron acceptor of aerobic metabolism.

Endergonic reaction A reaction during which there is a net gain of energy, $\Delta G > 0$. Such reactions do not occur spontaneously.

Endocytosis Process by which matter is engulfed by a plasma membrane and brought into the cell within a lipid vesicle derived from the membrane.

Endothermic reaction A reaction during which there is heat absorption; a positive enthalpy change ($+\Delta H$).

Enthalpy change (ΔH) A measure of the heat released or absorbed during a reaction.

Entropy change (ΔS) A measure of the change in disorder or randomness in a reaction.

Enzyme A biological catalyst, that is almost always a protein.

Essential amino acid An amino acid that cannot be synthesized by the body and must be obtained from the diet.

Essential fatty acid A fatty acid that cannot be synthesized by the body and must be obtained from the diet.

Exergonic reaction A reaction during which there is a net loss of energy, $\Delta G < 0$. Such reactions proceed spontaneously.

Exothermic reaction There is a release of heat during the reaction; a negative enthalpy change ($-\Delta H$).

Fatty acid breakdown The process in which a molecule of fatty acid is degraded by the sequential removal of two carbon units, producing acetyl CoA, which is then oxidized to CO_2 and H_2O by the TCA cycle.

Fatty acid synthesis A cyclical reaction in which a molecule of fatty acid is built up by the sequential addition of two carbons units derived from acetyl CoA.

Feedback inhibition Inhibition of an enzyme that catalyses an early step in a metabolic pathway by an end product of the same pathway.

Free energy change A thermodynamic state that defines the equilibrium in terms of the changes in enthalpy and entropy of a system at constant pressure, $\Delta G = \Delta H - T \times \Delta S$

Free radical A highly reactive atomic or molecular species with unpaired electron.

Gluconeogenesis Production of glucose from non-carbohydrate sources (e.g. amino acids, lactate, glycerol).

Glucose-alanine cycle An interorgan metabolic loop that transports nitrogen (as alanine) to the liver and transports energy (as glucose) from the liver to the peripheral tissues.

Glycation Non-enzymatic reaction resulting in binding of a sugar molecule to a protein.

Glycogen A large, highly branched polymer of glucose molecules joined by α-1,4 linkages with α-1,6 linkages at branch points.

Glycolysis Catabolic pathway consisting of ten enzyme-catalysed reactions by which one molecule of glucose is broken down into two molecules of pyruvate.

Glycoprotein A complex protein molecule containing carbohydrate residues: they are produced through the glycosylation of proteins in the endoplasmic reticulum or in the Golgi apparatus.

Glycosaminoglycan Long unbranched polysaccharides consisting of repeating disaccharide units. The disscharide unit consists of an N-acetyl-hexosamine and a hexose or hexuronic acid, either or both of which may be sulfated.

Glycosides A group of organic compounds, occurring abundantly in plants, that yield a sugar and one or more non-sugar substances on hydrolysis.

Glycosylation The addition of glycosyl groups to a protein to form a glycoprotein.

Haemoglobin A tetrameric, haem-containing globular protein in erythrocytes that carries oxygen to cells and tissues.

High-density lipoprotein (HDL) A type of plasma lipoprotein that is rich in protein and transports cholesterol and cholesteryl esters from tissues to the liver (this is known as the reverse cholesterol transport).

Hydrolase An enzyme that catalyses the hydrolytic cleavage of its substrate.

Hydrophilic 'Water loving'. A molecule that interacts with polar solvents, in particular with water, or with other polar groups.

Hydrophobie 'Water fearing'. Non-polar compounds that do not dissolve in water, such as oil.

Intermediate density lipoprotein (IDL) A type of plasma lipoprotein that is formed during the breakdown of VLDL. IDL are also called remnant lipoproteins and are atherogenic.

Isomerase An enzyme that catalyses a change in geometry or structure within one molecule.

Isozymes Different proteins from a single biological species that catalyse the same reaction.

Ketogenesis A five-step pathway that synthesizes ketone bodies from acetyl CoA in the mitochondrial matrix.

Ketone bodies Small molecules that are synthesized from acetyl CoA in the liver (acetoacetic acid, acetone, 3-hydroxybutyric acid).

Kinase An enzyme that catalyses the transfer of a phosphoryl group to an acceptor molecule.

Lipase An enzyme that catalyses the hydrolysis of triacylglycerols.

Lipid A water-insoluble organic compound found in biological systems.

Lipolysis The hydrolysis of triacylglycerols by lipase. (Note that lipolysis is different from fatty acid breakdown.)

Lipoprotein A macromolecular assembly of lipid and protein molecules with a hydrophobic core and a hydrophilic surface, present in plasma. Lipoproteins transport triglycerides and cholesterol between tissues.

Low density lipoprotein (LDL) A type of plasma lipoprotein that is formed during the breakdown of IDL and is enriched in cholesterol and cholesteryl esters. LDL are atherogenic. The measurement of plasma cholesterol reflects mainly the concentration of LDL.

Lysosome A specialized digestive organelle in eukaryotic cells.

Metabolism An integrated set of chemical reactions occurring in the body. The sum of chemical reactions in the body.

Micelle An aggregation of amphipathic (both water-repellent and water-friendly) molecules in which the hydrophilic portions of the molecules project into the aqueous environment and the hydrophobic portions point into the interior of the structure.

Mitochondrion An organelle that is the main site of oxidative energy metabolism in eurkaryotic cells.

Non-essential amino acid An amino acid that can be produced in sufficient quantity to meet metabolic needs.

N-terminus The amino acid residue bearing a free α-amino group ($-NH_2$) at one end of a peptide chain.

Nucleophilic A chemical compound or group that is attracted to nuclei and tends to donate or share electrons.

Nucleoside A compound containing a purine or pyrimidine and a sugar: purine or pyrimidine N-glycoside of ribose or deoxyribose.

Nucleotide The phosphate ester of a nucleoside, consisting of a nitrogenous base linked to a pentose phosphate.

Oxidase An enzyme that catalyses an oxidation-reduction reaction in which O_2 is the electron acceptor.

Oxidation The loss of electrons by a molecule, atom or ion. Gain of oxygen or loss of hydrogen by a molecule.

Oxidative deamination The removal of an amino group from an amino acid, which leaves behind the carbon skeleton.

Oxidative phosphorylation A process in which ATP is formed as electrons are transferred from NADH and $FADH_2$ to molecular oxygen, via a series of electron carriers that make up the electron transport chain.

Pentose phosphate pathway A pathway by which glucose-6-phosphate is metabolized to generate NADPH and ribose-5-phosphate.

Peptide Two or more amino acids covalently joined in a linear sequence by peptide bonds.

Peptide bond The covalent secondary amide linkage that joins the carbonyl oxygen atom, the amide hydrogen atom, and the two adjacent α-carbon atoms.

Peroxidase An enzyme that catalyses a reaction in which hydrogen peroxide is the oxidizing agent.

Phosphatase An enzyme that catalyses the hydrolytic removal of a phosphoryl group.

Phosphorylase An enzyme that catalyses the cleavage of its substrate via nucleophilic attack by inorganic phosphate.

Phosphorylation A reaction involving the addition of a phosphoryl group to a molecule.

P:O ratio The ratio of molecules of ADP phosphorylated to atoms of oxygen reduced during oxidative phosphorylation.

Polypeptide A polymer of many amino acid residues linked by peptide bonds.

Polysaccharide A polymer of many monosaccharide residues linked by glycosidic bonds.

Protease An enzyme that catalyses hydrolysis of peptide bonds.

Protein A biopolymer consisting of one or more polypeptide chains.

Protein glycosylation The covalent addition of carbohydrate to proteins.

Proteoglycans A special class of glycoproteins that are heavily glycosylated. They consist of a core protein with one or more covalently attached glycosaminoglycan chains.

Purine A nitrogenous base with a two-ring structure in which a pyrimidine is fused to imidazole (e.g. adenine, guanine).

Pyrimidine A nitrogenous base having a heterocyclic ring that consists of four carbon atoms and two nitrogen atoms (e.g. thymine, cytosine).

Reducing agent A substance that provides (as it itself loses) electrons in an oxidation-reduction reaction thereby becoming oxidized.

Reduction The gain of electrons by a molecule, atom or ion. Loss of oxygen or gain of hydrogen by a molecule.

Ribonucleic acid (RNA) A polymer consisting of ribonucleotide residues joined by 3'-5' phosphodiester bonds. The sugar moiety is ribose.

Ribose A five-carbon monosaccharide that is the carbohydrate component of RNA.

Salvage pathway A pathway in which a major metabolite, such as purine or pyrimidine nucleotide, can be synthesized from a preformed molecular entity, such as a purine or pyrimidine, rather than synthesized *de novo*.

Saturated fatty acid A fatty acid that does not contain a carbon-carbon double bond.

Standard redox potential (E_o) A measure of the tendency of a particular redox pair (e.g. NAD^+ and NADH) to lose electrons.

Steroid A lipid characterized by a carbon skeleton with four fused rings. All steroids are derived from the acetyl CoA.

Sterol A steroid containing a hydroxyl group.

Substrate-level phosphorylation Formation of ATP by direct phosphorylation of ADP, without requiring mitochondrial respiratory chain.

Transaminase An enzyme that catalyses the transfer of an α-amino group (NH_3^+) from an amino acid to an α-keto acid.

Triacylglycerol A lipid containing three fatty acyl residues esterified to a glycerol backbone.

Tricarboxylic acid cycle (TCA) A cyclical sequence of eight reactions that completely oxidize one molecule of acetyl CoA to two molecules of CO_2, generating energy either directly as ATP or in the form of reducing equivalents (NADH or $FADH_2$).

Ubiquitin A small basic protein that binds to a protein and targets it for degradation.

Unsaturated fatty acid A fatty acid with at least one carbon-carbon double bond.

Urea cycle A metabolic cycle consisting of five reactions that synthesize the organic compound urea from two inorganic compounds; CO_2 and NH_4^+.

Very low density lipoprotein (VLDL) A type of plasma lipoprotein that transports mostly endogenous triacylglycerols, and also cholesterol and cholesteryl esters from the liver to the tissues.

Vitamin An organic micronutrient that cannot be synthesized by the body and must be obtained from the diet.

Water-soluble vitamin An organic micronutrient that is soluble in water.

References

CHAPTER 8

American Diabetes Association. http://www.diabetes.org/
diabetes-basics/prevention/pre-diabetes/pre-diabetes-faqs.
html Accessed (accessed July 2011).

Department of Health. http://www.dh.gov.uk/en/
Publicationsandstatistics/Publications/
PublicationsPolicyAndGuidance/Browsable/DH_4902982
(accessed July 2011).

Diabetes UK. http://www.diabetes.org.uk/Guide-to-diabetes/
Complications/Hyperosmolar_Hyperglycaemic_State_
HHS/ (accessed July 2011).

Marrero DG. The prevention of type 2 diabetes: an overview.
Journal of Diabetes Science and Technology 2009;3:
756–60.

Mokdad AH, Bowman BA, Ford ES, Vinicor F, Marks JS,
Koplan JP. The continuing epidemics of obesity and diabetes
in the United States. The Journal of the American Medical
Association 2001;286: 1195–200.

National Diabetes Fact Sheet. American Diabetes Association
Available from: http://www.diabetes.org/diabetes-basics/
(accessed July 2011).

National Institute for Health and Clinical Excellence (NICE).
Type 2 diabetes: the management of type 2 diabetes. http://
www.nice.org.uk/CG066 (accessed July 2011).

National Institute for Health and Clinical Excellence (NICE).
Type 2 Diabetes: National clinical guideline for management
in primary and secondary care. http://www.nice.org.uk/
nicemedia/live/11983/40803/40803.pdf (accessed July
2011).

CHAPTER 9

Baynes J, Dominiczak MH 2009 Medical Biochemistry, 3rd edn.
Mosby, Chapter 21, Pages 305 and 205.

http://en.wikipedia.org/wiki/Refeeding_syndrome.

http://www.burgerman.info/www-nursing/macro-micro-
nutrients.htm.

http://www.nature.com/nature/journal/v404/n6778/images/
404652aa.2.jpg (accessed July 2011).

Mehanna HM, Moledina J, Travis J. Refeeding syndrome: what
it is, and how to prevent and treat it, British Medical Journal
2008;336(7659): 1495–8. http://www.bmj.com/content/
336/7659/1495.long.

National Institute for Health and Clinical Excellence (NICE)
2002 NICE issues guidance on surgery for morbid obesity.
NICE. http://www.nice.org.uk/guidance/index.jsp?action=
article&o=32423 last updated 2010.

National Institute for Health and Clinical Excellence (NICE).
http://www.nice.org.uk/nicemedia/pdf/
CG43quickrefguide2.pdf.

Obesity resources

Colquitt JL, Picot J, Loveman E, Clegg AJ 2009 Surgery for
obesity. Cochrane Database of Systematic Reviews Art.
No.: CD003641. DOI: 10.1002/14651858.CD003641.
pub3.

National Institute for Health and Clinical Excellence (NICE).
NICE issues guidance on surgery for morbid obesity. http://
www.nice.org.uk/guidance/index.jsp?action=article&o=
32423 (accessed July 2011).

National Institute for Health and Clinical Excellence (NICE).
Quick reference guide 2: obesity. http://www.nice.org.uk/
nicemedia/pdf/CG43quickrefguide2.pdf (accessed July
2011).

World Health Organisation. Obesity. http://www.who.int/
topics/obesity/en/ (accessed July 2011).

Refeeding syndrome resources

Hearing SD 2004 Refeeding syndrome. British Medical Journal.
2004. 908–9.

Mehanna HM, Moledina J, Travis J 2008 Refeeding syndrome:
what it is, and how to prevent and treat it. British Medical
Journal 336(7659): 1495–1498. http://www.bmj.com/
content/336/7659/1495.long.

National Institute for Health and Clinical Excellence 2006
Nutrition support in adults. Clinical guideline CG32, NICE.

CHAPTER 12

Drinkaware.co.uk. http://www.drinkaware.co.uk/tips-and-
tools/drink-diary/ (accessed July 2011).

http://faculty.washington.edu/alexbert/MEDEX/Fall/
ABDAscultation.jpg (accessed July 2011).

http://en.wikipedia.org/wiki/Refeeding_syndrome (accessed
July 2011).

http://en.wikipedia.org/wiki/Familial_hypercholesterolemia
(accessed July 2011).

http://www.askdoctorclarke.com/content/c95.pdf (accessed
July 2011).

Rader DJ, Cohen J, Hobbs HH 2003 Monogenic
hypercholesterolemia: new insights in pathogenesis and
treatment. The Journal of Clinical Investigation 2003.
1795–803. http://www.ncbi.nlm.nih.gov/pmc/articles/

PMC161432/ doi:10.1172/JCI18925. PMID 12813012. Full text at PMC: 161432.

Wilkinson IB, Longmore M, Turmezei T, Cheung CK 2008 Oxford Handbook Clinical Medicine, 7th edn. Oxford University Press.

Mehanna HM, Moledina J, Travis J 2008 Refeeding syndrome: what it is, and how to prevent and treat it. British Medical Journal 336(7659): 1495–1498. http://www.bmj.com/content/336/7659/1495.long.

Index

Note: Page numbers followed by *b* indicate boxes, *f* indicate figures and *ge* indicate glossary terms.